PREDICTABILITY IN PSYCHOPHARMACOLOGY
Preclinical and Clinical Correlations

Predictability in Psychopharmacology
Preclinical and Clinical Correlations

Edited by

Abraham Sudilovsky, M.D.
Assistant Clinical Research Director
The Squibb Institute for Medical Research
Princeton, New Jersey, and
Research Assistant Professor of Psychiatry
Department of Psychiatry
N.Y.U. Medical Center
New York, New York

Samuel Gershon, M.D.
Professor of Psychiatry
Director, Neuropsychopharmacology
* Research Unit*
Department of Psychiatry
N.Y.U. Medical Center
New York, New York

Bernard Beer, Ph.D.
Assistant Director
Department of Pharmacology
The Squibb Institute for
* Medical Research*
Princeton, New Jersey

Raven Press ■ New York

Made in the United States of America

International Standard Book Number 0-89004-017-6
Library of Congress Catalog Card Number 74-14483

Foreword

The subject of this book — predictability in psychopharmacology — clearly identifies an important problem that exists in psychiatric medicine and one that must be pursued with vigor by those involved in the discovery and development of new drug substances for the treatment of mental disease. Although we believe we are able to communicate objectively and articulately with the patient, there can be no doubt about the many subtleties involved in attempting to interpret human behavioral patterns, not only in the clearly ill patient but also, particularly, in those who represent cases bordering between health and disease. A new magnitude of difficulty is encountered in the attempt to interpret behavioral effects in animals, since the animal cannot communicate. Indeed, a given set of animal behavioral data presented to several psychopharmacologists or psychiatrists may well be interpreted in several different ways.

Herewith the dilemma: How do we pick the best compounds for study in specific disease states in man? At a time when regulatory requirements and costs of drug development are increasing around the world, it is imperative that the pharmaceutical industry, regulatory authorities, and academic centers interested in new developments in the areas of diseases of the central nervous system cooperate in their efforts to bridge the gaps of predicting drug effects across species lines.

To this end, the present volume is most welcome. It delineates experimental procedures already under investigation as well as others that may soon come under scrutiny. It is obviously essential that experimental approaches be actively pursued if we are to improve the reliability with which results obtained in animals predict a drug's ultimate effectiveness in treating man. I am hopeful that this effort will be only the first in a series of continuing dialogues among industry, regulatory authorities, and academic institutions for the ultimate benefit of the individual patient and society at large.

C. G. Smith, Ph.D.
Vice-President, Research and Development
Director, The Squibb Institute
for Medical Research

Acknowledgment

We are indebted to the CNS Area Team of the Squibb Institute for Medical Research for support of the Symposium on which this volume is based. We wish to express our appreciation to all those persons who participated in the symposium, particularly to Dr. Frank Ayd, Jr. and Dr. William W. K. Zung for helpful pointers during its planning stage.

We also thank Dr. David Frost, Science Editor of the Squibb Institute, and Virginia B. Martin, Managing Editor of Raven Press, for editorial advice. The philosophically constructive attitude of the publisher, Dr. Alan Edelson, contributed greatly to making our task more enjoyable. Finally, we are most appreciative of Miss Jo Embessi's secretatial skill and diligence.

The Editors

Preface

The search for an understanding of the mechanisms involved in the production of diseases and their appropriate therapy has never been undertaken from such a multiplicity of avenues as at present. However, advance in some fields, and particularly in that of behavioral derangements, has been held back by the use of diverse clinical criteria for diagnosis and by the lack of animal models that are identical with, or at least parallel to, disease entities. The ability to diagnose, determine etiology, and prescribe appropriate treatment is an integral requirement of medical practice. We can often travel this route through diagnosis, isolation, and identification of the pathogen in infectious diseases, and the final and important therapeutic step, determination of the sensitivity of the organism to appropriate medication. For infectious diseases, therapeutic predictability is usually quite precise. In psychiatry, we have not reached this level of precision. Traditionally, new drugs for use in psychiatric disorders are first tested in various animal models, then pharmacologic properties of these drugs are investigated in man, and their therapeutic effects are correlated with those of other agents used in the disease state. Awareness of the pitfalls and needs in the latter stages of investigation might provide fresh insights into the development of human and animal models with more accurate predictability than was previously available.

This volume deals with some of the problems in this area, both at the clinical and preclinical levels. Insight into the difficulties with which we are confronted is essential if we are to make progress; the work goes beyond this by proposing interim measures as well as by exploring new, unique, and stimulating procedures and hypotheses. Most of the chapters included were presented at the First CNS Symposium of The Squibb Institute for Medical Research (June 28–29, 1974); each is followed by an edited transcription of the discussions recorded during the sessions. Other (invited) chapters cover areas of interest that were not explored during the meeting because of limitations on time and material.

The two chapters on clinical nosology and typology spell out the current *modi operandi* in psychiatric diagnosis and present clear data on the limitations of this approach, especially with regard to functional psychoses. When we have diagnostic concordance rates as low as those described, it is deafeningly clear that prediction from results in animals to effects in human psychopharmacology is impaired at this first level of operations by the problems of diagnostic heterogeneity. A proposal elaborated in the first chapter suggests that, even under these conditions, significant progress can be made. In the second chapter, the convergence of diagnostic processes for depression serves to illustrate the effort to disentangle semantic confusion. That the approach to the issue under scrutiny in this volume is still debatable is made clear in a recent editorial [Fink, M. (1974): Psychiatric diagnosis: Phenotypic or pathophysiologic? *Biol. Psychiatry,* 9:3:227–229], stimulated by the Symposium discussions, that analyzes the relevance of biologic features for the classification of populations.

Other issues of interest are taken up in subsequent chapters in which use is made of normal human subjects to examine the effects of psychoactive compounds. Included are the predictability of computerized EEG measures for determining specific psychiatric indications of potential psychotropic drugs and the utilization of this method to study drug bioavailability in the central nervous system, the utility and viability of small sample sizes for early assessment of clinical activity, and some specific suggestions for new approaches to the evaluation of antianxiety properties of new chemical agents.

The remainder of the book deals with animal models as predictors of potential psychotropic drug therapeutic activity and provides some tantalizing possibilities for the solution of some of the problems that are faced at the preclinical stage of drug development.

The present volume attempts in a critical and imaginative way to permit us to further our search for the effective pharmacologic treatment of psychopathologic conditions. The primary aim is to eliminate the difficulties inherent in the clinical phase of assessment, for which suggestions are offered. A number of possible new methods and concepts are presented in the specific area of predicting drug activity. It is hoped that the promise of these approaches will be fulfilled, and that new benchmarks will be achieved in predicting clinical results from preclinical experimentation.

Abraham Sudilovsky
Samuel Gershon
Bernard Beer
(May 1975)

Contents

Contributors

G. K. Aghajanian, M.D.
Department of Psychiatry
Yale University School of Medicine
and
Connecticut Mental Health Center
34 Park Street
New Haven, Connecticut 06508

B. Beer, Ph.D.
The Squibb Institute for Medical Re-
  search
P. O. Box 4000
Princeton, New Jersey 08540

B. Blackwell, M.D.
Department of Psychiatry
University of Cincinnati Medical Center
234 Goodman Street
Cincinnati, Ohio 45229

B. S. Bunney, M.D.
Department of Psychiatry
Yale University School of Medicine
and
Connecticut Mental Health Center
34 Park Street
New Haven, Connecticut 06508

D. E. Clody, Ph.D.
The Squibb Institute for Medical Re-
  search
P. O. Box 4000
Princeton, New Jersey 08540

E. F. Domino, M.D.
Department of Mental Health
Lafayette Clinic
951 East Lafayette
Detroit, Michigan 48207

D. Domizi, M.D.
Department of Psychiatry
University of Chicago
950 East 59 Street
Chicago, Illinois 60637

F. Dorsey, Ph.D.
Department of Community Health Sci-
  ences
Duke University Medical Center
Durham, North Carolina 27710

E. Ellinwood, M.D.
Department of Psychiatry
Duke University Medical Center
Durham, North Carolina 27710

J. Endicott, Ph.D.
Biometrics Research
New York State Psychiatric Institute
722 West 168 Street
New York, New York 10032

M. Fink, M.D.
Departments of Psychiatry and Behav-
  ioral Science
Health Sciences Center—School of
  Medicine
State University of New York at Stony
  Brook
Stony Brook, New York 11790

B. Gurland, M.D.
Biometrics Research
New York State Psychiatric Institute
722 West 168 Street
New York, New York 10032

Z. P. Horovitz, Ph.D.
The Squibb Institute for Medical Re-
  search
P. O. Box 4000
Princeton, New Jersey 08540

P. Irwin, B.A.
Departments of Psychiatry and Behav-
  ioral Science
Health Sciences Center—School of
  Medicine
State University of New York at Stony
  Brook
Stony Brook, New York 11790

G. L. Klerman, M.D.
Department of Psychiatry
Harvard Medical School
Massachusetts General Hospital
2 Fruit Street
Boston, Massachusetts 02114

J. Kuriansky, Ed.M.
Biometrics Research
New York State Psychiatric Institute
722 West 168 Street
New York, New York 10032

B. Migler, Ph.D.
The Squibb Institute for Medical Research
P. O. Box 4000
Princeton, New Jersey 08540

L. A. Nelson, B.A.
Department of Psychiatry
Duke University Medical Center
Durham, North Carolina 27710

E. Robins, M.D.
Department of Psychiatry
Washington University School of Medicine
St. Louis, Missouri 63110

C. R. Schuster, Ph.D.
Department of Psychiatry
University of Chicago
950 East 59 Street
Chicago, Illinois 60637

P. Sibony, B.A.
Department of Psychiatry
New York Medical College
New York, New York 10029

S. H. Snyder, M.D.
Departments of Pharmacology and Experimental Therapeutics
Johns Hopkins University School of Medicine
725 North Wolfe Street
Baltimore, Maryland 21205

R. L. Spitzer, M.D.
Biometrics Research
New York State Psychiatric Institute
722 West 168 Street
New York, New York 10032

M. Stern, M.A.
Department of Psychiatry
University of Chicago
950 East 59 Street
Chicago, Illinois 60637

A. Sudilovsky, M.D.
The Squibb Institute for Medical Research
P. O. Box 4000
Princeton, New Jersey 08540

E. H. Uhlenhuth, M.D.
Department of Psychiatry
University of Chicago
950 East 59 Street
Chicago, Illinois 60637

W. Whitehead, M.D.
Department of Psychiatry
University of Cincinnati Medical Center
234 Goodman Street
Cincinnati, Ohio 45229

W. W. K. Zung, M.D.
Department of Psychiatry
Duke University Medical Center
Durham, North Carolina 27705

Predictability in Psychopharmacology: Preclinical and Clinical Correlations, edited by A. Sudilovsky, S. Gershon and B. Beer. Raven Press, New York, © 1975.

Preliminary Report of the Reliability of Research Diagnostic Criteria Applied to Psychiatric Case Records

Robert L. Spitzer, Jean Endicott, Eli Robins,* Judith Kuriansky, and Barry Gurland

*Biometrics Research, New York State Department of Mental Hygiene, New York State Psychiatric Institute, New York, New York 10032 and *Washington University School of Medicine, St. Louis, Missouri 63110*

A crucial problem in psychiatry that effects both clinical work as well as the research study of methods to improve psychiatric treatment is the generally low reliability of current psychiatric diagnostic procedures. This sad state of affairs is well recognized in our field, has been amply demonstrated in numerous studies, and is responsible in part for the low regard with which psychiatric diagnosis is often held both within psychiatry and the general field of medicine. Furthermore, inability to agree on the names of the conditions we treat and study hinders any attempt to study the etiology, course, and treatment of these conditions.

The sources of diagnostic unreliability have been studied and can be divided into problems in eliciting data from the patient and problems in synthesizing these data according to the diagnostic criteria (Beck, 1962; Beck, Ward, and Mendelson, 1962). Most studies have shown that the primary source of unreliability is the variability among clinicians in the diagnostic criteria that they use. Although the Diagnostic and Statistical Manual of the American Psychiatric Association (DSM-II) provides some general guidelines for differential diagnosis by describing the major features of each of the conditions, the paucity of specific criteria in this manual forces the clinician to rely heavily on his own concepts of the diagnostic categories that he has formed, based on his particular training, experience, and interests.

An alternative approach toward the diagnostic procedure is the development of specific inclusion and exclusion criteria for each diagnosis that the clinician is required to use, regardless of his own personal concept of the disorder. With this approach, the clinician's task is twofold: to determine the presence or absence of specific clinical phenomena, and then to apply the comprehensive rules provided for making the diagnoses. A consequence of this approach is the need for an "undiagnosed psychiatric disorder" category for those patients who do not fulfill the criteria of any of the conditions. This approach, unlike the standard approach to diagnosis, seeks to identify relatively homogeneous subgroups of patients by minimizing false positives and tolerating a small number of false negatives.

This chapter is a preliminary report of the reliability of a set of specific diagnostic criteria for a selected group of functional psychiatric disorders, called the Research Diagnostic Criteria (RDC), wherein we present the reliability of these criteria as applied to psychiatric case records. A future chapter will present a more extensive exposition of the rationale and development of the RDC.

THE RDC

The RDC were developed by Spitzer, Endicott, and Robins with the assistance of the other participants in a collaborative project on the psychology of depressive disorders. This project is sponsored and coordinated by the Clinical Research Branch of the NIMH. The latest version of the RDC appears as an appendix following this chapter. The RDC is an elaboration and expansion of the specified criteria developed by a group of psychiatrists at Washington University School of Medicine in St. Louis for a smaller number of diagnoses (Feighner, Robins, and Guze, 1972). They have offered considerable evidence for the validity of these conditions as separate diagnostic entities. In developing the RDC, additional diagnoses were added, such as schizo-affective disorders, some personality disorders, and a category called borderline or atypical psychosis. In addition, many different nonmutually exclusive ways of categorizing major depressive illness were provided for studies focusing on depressive illness.

Often the criteria in the RDC take the form of listing specific symptoms, and/or clinical characteristics, a number of which are necessary for the criteria to be fulfilled. Many conditions have exclusion as well as inclusion criteria. A consequence of this approach is the recognition of the need for an "undiagnosed psychiatric disorder" category for the patients who do not meet the criteria for any of the specific disorders, yet exhibit significant psychopathology.

Each diagnosis is judged either as absent, probable, or definitely present. When two or more diagnoses are mutually exclusive (for example, depressive personality and minor depressive illness) they are so noted in the criteria. Otherwise, more than one diagnosis may be given to the same patient for the same period of illness, or for different periods of illness (for example, schizophrenia and alcoholism).

Some of the diagnostic terms in the RDC are different from those used in traditional nomenclatures. This is done to help avoid confusion when the category is defined in such a way that it has only partial correspondence with a traditional category. For example, the traditional category of neurotic depression includes patients who would be categorized in the RDC as either major or minor depressive illness. For several of the diagnostic categories, the criteria differ little, if at all, from those generally used (for example, the diagnosis of obsessive-compulsive neurosis or phobic neurosis). For other categories where a consensus as to the diagnostic criteria does not exist in the field, it was necessary to adopt what seemed to us as reasonable, although admittedly arbitrary, criteria. For example, the RDC schizo-affective schizophrenia includes the symptom picture of both schizophrenia and affective illness but none of the criteria relate to acuteness of onset, although many clinicians include this variable in their use of the term. Of course, it will be possible to examine the data for all schizoaffectives and compare them with those whose onset of illness is acute, to determine if use of this additional criterion increases diagnostic validity.

STUDY

An initial version of the RDC was used in a study of 120 case records of patients from the New York State Psychiatric Institute. The purpose of this study was to determine the reliability of the RDC as applied by research assistants to a large sample of heterogeneous patients, and to compare the reliability of these diagnoses using the RDC with the reliability of diagnoses made by experienced psychiatrists using the official nomenclature of the DSM-II, under conditions approximating those usually present in most research studies in which clinical diagnoses are made using the DSM-II categories.

This case record study was possible because Ms. Judith Kuriansky and Dr. Barry Gurland of the Psychopathology and Diagnosis Section of Biometrics Research had a set of case records used in a previous study of diagnostic practice conducted at the New York State Psychiatric Institute (Kuriansky, Deming, and Gurland, 1974). That study involved an examination of the case records from two decades in which the hospital diagnosis of schizophrenia had more than doubled (from 28% during the decade 1932–1941 to 77% during the decade 1947–1956).

The study used 128 records of patients aged 20 to 59; 64 cases were selected from each decade to reproduce the original proportions of the hospital diagnoses. The case records were xeroxed and all references to diagnosis and year of admission were obliterated. Since the RDC used in this study are only for functional conditions, we excluded eight cases in which the diagnosis of an organic brain syndrome was noted as possibly present in the case record. This left a total of 120 cases.

Three independent diagnoses on each case were available: those made by the hospital psychiatrist, by Gurland, a British trained psychiatrist, and by one of a group of 16 experienced North American psychiatrists, who acted as re-diagnosticians of the cases. Both Gurland and the re-diagnosticians used the DSM-II when making their diagnoses.

Because the earlier study focused on diagnostic practice, no attempt was made to alter the diagnostic practices of the re-diagnosticians in an effort to achieve high interrater reliability. Therefore, they did not meet together or participate in any special training sessions and the degree to which they referred to the DSM-II manual is unknown. The design of the earlier study was such that any lack of reliability among the re-diagnosticians would have no systematic biasing effect on their comparison of the patients from the two decades.

All of the cases were read and diagnosed independently by Spitzer and six of his research assistants who were paired in varying combinations for each case. Each research assistant read from 30 to 60 cases. Only one of the research assistants had professional training in psychopathology (psychiatric social work). However, all of the research assistants had considerable on-the-job training in making psychiatric ratings and in the use of the RDC and most had attended a 10-session seminar on descriptive psychiatry given by Spitzer to the first-year psychiatric residents at the Psychiatric Institute.

RESULTS

Reliability was determined using the statistic kappa (Spitzer, Cohen, Fleiss, and Endicott, 1967). Kappa is the proportion of agreement corrected for chance agreement as a function of the base rates. It varies from negative values for less than chance-expected agreement through 0 for exactly chance-expected agreement to +1 for perfect agreement.

The reliability of the RDC for the entire set of 120 cases is shown in the first three columns of Table 1. The first column gives the agreement between Spitzer (RLS) and the first Biometrics research assistant who read the case. The second column gives the agreement between RLS and the second Biometrics research assistant who read the case. The third column gives the agreement between the two Biometrics research assistants. The results indicate very good agreement for all of the major categories. To our knowledge, reliabilities for schizophrenia and affective illness are higher than have been reported in diagnostic studies of this kind. [In a review of such studies (Spitzer and Fleiss, 1974) the range of kappa values for schizophrenia over six studies where the data were available for such calculations was .32 to .77, and for affective illness over five studies it was .19 to .59.]

The reliabilities for the specific diagnostic categories are generally very high with the exception of schizo-affective schizophrenia and borderline or atypical psychosis, two categories that are by their very nature difficult to define with precision. We believe that an additional reason for the low reliabilities obtained here is that the criteria in these two categories were modified to a greater degree than were other categories while the study was in progress. In the case of schizo-affective schizophrenia, one of the first Biometric raters seemed to overdiagnose the condition and, by chance, was

TABLE 1. *Kappa coefficients of agreement for major diagnosis by various pairs of raters on 120 case records*

| | Diagnostic system used | | | | |
| | Both RDC | | | RDC and DSM-II | Both DSM-II |
Illness	RLS vs biom. 1	RLS vs biom. 2	biom. 1 vs biom. 2	RLS vs BG	BG vs re-diag.
Schizophrenia	.78	.84	.84	.67	.48
Other schizophrenia	.68	.82	.70	.70	.49
Schizo-affective	.22	.54	.24	.19	.37
Affective Illness	.70	.74	.70	.65	.48
Manic illness	.82	.92	.76	.42	.37
Major depressive illness[a]	.67	.74	.66	.55	.25
Minor depressive illness[b]	.56	.66	.56	—[c]	.07
Other	.69	.70	.74	.63	.61
Briquet's syndrome	—	—	1.00	—	—
Antisocial personality	—	—	.66	—	—
Alcoholism	1.00	.66	.66	1.00	—
Drug dependence	1.00	1.00	1.00	—	—
Obsessive-compulsive neurosis	.64	.52	.65	.59	.42
Anxiety neurosis	.65	.59	.52	.53	.06
Phobic neurosis	.66	.39	.66	—	.32
Borderline or atypical Psychosis	.24	.06	.20	—	—
Undiagnosed illness	.45	.30	.59	—	—

[a] Equivalent to any psychotic depressive illness in DSM-II.
[b] Equivalent to neurotic depression in DSM-II.
[c] A dash indicates that either the diagnostic category was not available to one or both raters, or that none or only one of the raters ever used it.

given many more cases than the other raters when this was the major differential diagnostic problem. We believe that the kappa of .54 between RLS and the second Biometrics rater is a better estimate of what can be achieved with the criteria in their present form. In the case of borderline or atypical psychosis, this category is more often given as a subsidiary diagnosis than as the major diagnosis. The average agreement for this category among the three pairs of raters as either major or subsidiary diagnosis is .39 which, although low, is higher than when the category is used as the major diagnosis.

Interrater agreement using the RDC with specially trained research assistants was considerably higher than that between Barry Gurland (BG) and the 16 re-diagnosticians using the DSM-II categories for the major categories of schizophrenia and affective illness. This was also the case for all of the specific diagnoses with the exception of schizo-affective schizophrenia.

How does the reliability obtained by BG and the re-diagnosticians using the DSM-II categories compare with other studies of diagnostic reliability? The kappa values between BG and the re-diagnosticians for schizophrenia and affective illness (.48 for both) is approximately in the middle of the range of values previously noted in this chapter as having been obtained in studies of the reliability of psychiatric diagnoses. Thus the reliability of diagnostic judgment obtained by BG and the re-diagnosticians is approximately that obtained in the usual research study employing psychiatric diagnoses.

Examination of the agreement between RLS and BG (Table 1, fourth column) yields kappa values that are generally intermediate between those obtained when both raters use the RDC and when both raters use the DSM-II categories. The most likely explanation for these results is that BG, although using DSM-II categories, was trained in England, has a special interest in diagnosis, and has a diagnostic orientation that is more similar to the orientation made explicit in RDC than the more direct approach characteristic of the 16 North American psychiatrists. The good agreement between RLS using the RDC system and BG using the DSM-II categories was also reflected in very similar distributions across all diagnoses for the total sample of cases. This indicates that the RDC is a refinement of the standard nomenclature rather than a different system yielding high reliability at the expense of being at variance with expert diagnostic practice.

Several issues must be considered in appraising these results. First, this study dealt with case records rather than actual patient interviews. Is it possible that the high values obtained here are inflated because case records present stereotypes which are easier to categorize than live patient evaluations? This is unlikely for several reasons. The case records usually contained voluminous progress notes that often presented conflicting diagnostic cues which actually increased the difficulty in arriving at a diagnosis. In addition, the actual agreement values for the case records are in the same range as were obtained in a previous study using diagnoses based on interviews of newly admitted inpatients. Since the agreement between the re-diagnosticians and BG was not particularly good, this indicates that the use of case records did not guarantee a high reliability.

Could the higher agreement values obtained with the RDC primarily be a function of the time spent by the Biometrics raters in training and working together and developing a shared concept of the various categories, as contrasted with the absence of such shared experiences on the part of the psychiatrists using the DSM-II categories? If BG and the re-diagnosticians had worked together, they would have improved their reliability. However, previous studies of diagnostic reliability using the standard nomenclature have employed psychiatrists who worked together in an attempt to improve agreement, yet the reliabilities obtained in these studies are well below those obtained here with the RDC. Furthermore, it is likely that a large part of "working together" actually consists of supplementing the general criteria which are provided in DSM-II with specific criteria to aid the differential diagnostic process. Unfortunately, such working rules are of no value to the profession as a whole unless they are made available for general use. This is precisely what the RDC attempts to do.

The results of this study indicate that the RDC may be a technique for greatly increasing the reliability of psychiatric diagnosis. We recognize that several of the categories need further work before they, too, can be reliably diagnosed. In addition, it is recognized that the demonstration of reliability is only a partial requirement of a diagnostic system. The fundamental requirement, of course, is validity. It is possible for a classification system to be reliable but not valid. Therefore, validity studies will be required before this approach can be shown to be generally useful. However, we believe that these initial results are promising and justify further work on the RDC.

ACKNOWLEDGMENTS

This work was supported by NIMH grant 23864, "NIMH Clinical Research Branch Collaborative Depression Studies, II: SADS" and Biometrics Research, New York State Department of Mental Hygiene.

REFERENCES

Beck, A. T. (1962): Reliability of psychiatric diagnosis: 1. A critique of systematic studies. *Am. J. Psychiatry,* 119:210.
Beck, A. T., Ward, C. H., and Mendelson, M. (1962): Reliability of psychiatric diagnosis: 2. A study of consistency of clinical judgments and ratings. *Am. J. Psychiatry,* 119:351.
Feighner, J. P., Robins, E., and Guze, S. B. (1972): Diagnostic criteria for use in psychiatric research. *Arch. Gen. Psychiatry,* 26:57–63.
Kuriansky, J. P., Deming, E. W., and Gurland, B. J. (1974): On trends in the diagnosis of schizophrenia. *Am. J. Psychiatry,* 131:402–408.
Spitzer, R. L., Cohen, J., Fleiss, J. L., and Endicott, J. (1967): Quantification of agreement in psychiatric diagnosis. *Arch. Gen. Psychiatry,* 17:83–87.
Spitzer, R. L., and Fleiss, J. L. (1974): A reanalysis of the reliability of psychiatric diagnosis. *Br. J. Psychiatry,* 124 (*in press*).

APPENDIX

RESEARCH DIAGNOSTIC CRITERIA (RDC)* FOR A SELECTED GROUP OF FUNCTIONAL DISORDERS

* Developed by Robert L. Spitzer, Jean Endicott, and Eli Robins, with the assistance of the other participants in the NIMH Clinical Research Branch Collaborative Program on the Psychobiology of Depression. These diagnostic criteria are an expansion and elaboration of some of the criteria developed by the Renard Hospital group in St. Louis. Investigators wishing to use these criteria should contact Drs. Spitzer and Endicott at Biometrics Research, New York State Psychiatric Institute, 722 West 168th Street, New York, New York 10032.

I. Introduction and Instructions

The Research Diagnostic Criteria (RDC) were developed to enable research investigators to apply a consistent set of criteria for the description or selection of samples of subjects with functional psychiatric illnesses. This work is part of a collaborative project on the psychobiology of the depressive disorders sponsored by the Clinical Research Branch of the NIMH. Although this project focuses on the depressive disorders, the ubiquity of depressive symptoms in other psychiatric disorders required the development of criteria for nonaffective illnesses as well. The affective disorders are subclassified into a number of nonmutually exclusive subcategories to permit testing of a number of hypotheses relevant to affective illness. Investigators who use these criteria where the focus is on other conditions, may wish to further subdivide them into subtypes appropriate to their own research. They may also choose to ignore some or all of the subtypes of depressive illness noted here.

The purpose of this approach to psychiatric diagnosis is to obtain relatively homogeneous groups of patients who meet specified diagnostic criteria. For this reason patients who do not meet any of the specified diagnostic criteria but have evidence of psychiatric disturbance, are classified as Other Psychiatric Disorder. We are assuming that for research purposes it is better to avoid false positives (cases incorrectly diagnosed as a particular condition), than false negatives (cases incorrectly diagnosed as Other Psychiatric Disorder).

Some of the diagnostic terms used here are different from those used in the traditional nomenclature. This is done hopefully to avoid confusion when the category is defined here in such a way that it has no corresponding traditional category. For example, the traditional category of Neurotic Depression includes patients who would be categorized here as either Major Depressive Disorder or Minor Depressive Disorder. Many of the new terms and criteria used in the RDC are likely to be part of the revised nomenclature of the American Psychiatric Association, DSM-III.

The source of data for making the diagnostic judgments will usually be a direct examination of the patient. The examination can be based on a focused clinical interview or a structured interview guide and rating scale designed specifically for eliciting information relevant to these categories—the Schedule for Affective Disorders, and Schizophrenia (SADS). The RDC can also be used with detailed case record material. Another version of the RDC, the Family History–Research Diagnostic Criteria, is appropriate for making diagnostic judgments about subjects when the source of information is limited to a relative's or other informant's account of the illness.

Consider each of the diagnoses relevant to your study and the criteria noted here and indicate whether, in your judgment, it applies or not, even if it is not a label that you personally use. All diagnoses are judged as either No, Probable, or Definite (and coded for statistical purposes as 1, 2, and 3, respectively). In most instances, explicit criteria will indicate the criteria for Probable or Definite. For example, in diagnosing Major Depressive Disorder, 5 criteria (A through E) must be met for the episode of illness being considered. Criterion B contains a list of depressive symptoms. For criterion B to be met at least 4 symptoms must be present. The diagnosis is Probable if A through E are met and if only 4 of the symptoms in B are present. The diagnosis is Definite if 5 or more symptoms in criterion B are met. The Probable diagnosis can also be used when the patient appears to meet the criteria for Definite but the rater is not certain about 1 of the criteria. An example with Major Depressive Disorder would be 5 symptoms present for criterion B, but the rater was unsure about some feature of criterion C.

The specific criteria refer to either symptoms, duration or course of the illness, or level of severity of impairment. For some of the diagnoses, certain symptoms or symptom patterns are of diagnostic significance only if they persist beyond a certain stated duration. When no duration is noted in the criteria, a symptom is considered of diagnostic significance regardless of its duration, if it is definitely present.

Since Probable implies more than 50% certainty, it should not be used for 2 mutually exclusive conditions for the same episode of illness (e.g., Schizophrenia and Manic Disorder). Otherwise, more than 1 diagnosis may be given to the same patient for the same episode of illness, or for different episodes of illness (e.g., Schizophrenia and Alcoholism).

Most diagnoses are noted for the present illness and/or for a previous episode of illness followed by remission of at least 2 months (for those illnesses which can be episodic). Some diagnoses are not noted for either present illness or previous episode of illness but just as occurring during the patient's life-time (such as Antisocial Personality and Bipolar Disorder). In some cases 2 diagnoses which are mutually exclusive for the same episode of illness (e.g., Schizo-affective Disorder and Manic Disorder) are appropriate for different episodes. This approach makes it possible to look at cases which are consistent over time, as well as those rarer cases in which the clinical picture for 2 episodes of illness suggests 2 different conditions.

Whenever a diagnosis is made of a present illness, its duration in weeks should be noted. Do not include a previous period of the same condition in calculating duration of present illness if it was followed by a period of remission (more or less return to premorbid level) that lasted more than 2 months.

Many known organic conditions can produce psychiatric disturbances which are difficult to distinguish from many of the conditions described in the RDC. All of the conditions in the RDC (with the exception of Alcoholism, Drug Abuse, and Other Psychiatric Disorder) are to be diagnosed only when there is no likely known organic etiology for the symptoms. Therefore, before the RDC can be properly used, patients should be screened to exclude those in whom known organic factors, such as recent childbirth (1 week), hyperthyroidism, amphetamine intoxication, ingestion of a hallucinogen, fever, or arteriosclerosis may play a significant role in the development of the psychiatric disturbance. Patients who have symptoms which strongly suggest organicity, such as memory impairment or disorientation, should also be excluded even if a known organic etiology cannot be established. When a psychosis has developed some time after the ingestion of a hallucinogen, the rater will have to use his judgment in assessing the relative importance of this known organic factor.

II. Definitions of Critical Terms

1. Formal Thought Disorder

There is no generally accepted definition of formal thought disorder. In this manual, the term is used to describe four readily identifiable, nonmutually exclusive forms of disturbance in speech which, in certain contexts, strongly suggest Schizophrenia. These forms of speech should not be counted as evidence of formal thought disorder if they are explainable by acute or chronic brain syndrome (including due to alcohol or drugs), elevated mood, a transient overwhelming affect (e.g., anger, fear), sarcasm, humor, limited intelligence or education, or language or cultural differences. Neologisms and blocking, which are often thought of as indicative of formal thought disorder, are not included here because of the general unreliability of clinical judgments of these phenomena, and because it is unlikely that either of these would be the only manifestation of formal thought disorder.

There is a tendency to overrate thought disorder. Therefore, the rater should never rate any of these 4 types of formal thought disorder unless he can give a specific example from the patient's speech.

A. Incoherence. Understandability of speech is impaired by distorted grammar, incomplete sentences, lack of logical connection between phrases or sentences, or sudden irrelevancies.

> Example: "I don't quite gather. I know one right and one left use both hands, but I can't follow the system that's working. The idea is meant in a kind way, but it's not the way I understand life." (Mayer-Gross, W., Slater, E., Roth, M.: *Clinical Psychiatry,* Baltimore, Williams & Wilkins, 1969)

B. Loosening of associations. Repeatedly saying things in juxtaposition which lack a logical or inherent relationship, or shifting idiosyncratically from one frame of reference to another.

> Examples: "I'm tired. All people have eyes." In response to questions about concern that he will be deserted by his friends, patient replies: "I wonder what's for dessert today?" (Bemporad, Jules and Pinsker, Henry: *American Handbook of Psychiatry,* Basic Books, 1974)

C. Illogical thinking (other than as evidenced by delusions, hallucinations, incoherence, loosening of associations, phobias, or compulsions). Thinking in which facts are obscured, distorted, or excluded. This is a complex and subtle judgment which usually requires a knowledge of the patient's reasoning for some behavior or belief.

Examples: Patient refuses to sit on the chair because it is yellow. Patient explains that she gave her family IBM cards she punched in an effort to overcome communication difficulties with them. In answering questions about his first hospitalization patient says, "It could have been a few years before or after I was born."

D. Poverty of content of speech. Speech is adequate in amount but conveys little information because of vagueness, talking past the point, empty repetitions or use of stereotyped or obscure phrases. Does not include poverty in the amount of speech. As Wing has noted, "This symptom may appear to be readily recognizable in some of one's colleagues, therefore only rate it when it is really pathological."

Example: When asked how he liked it in the hospital the patient answered: "Well, er . . . not quite the same as, er . . . don't know quite how to say it. It isn't the same being in the hospital as, er . . . working, er . . . the job isn't quite the same, er . . . very much the same but, of course, it isn't exactly the same." (John Wing, *Present State Examination,* 9th edition, Institute of Psychiatry, 1971)

2. Thought Broadcasting

The belief or experience that his thoughts, as they occur, are broadcast from his head into the external world so that others can hear them. This phenomena may occur as a delusion and/or a hallucination. When a hallucination, the patient hears his own thoughts from the outside, not just within his head.

Example: A man believed that his thoughts were being picked up by a hidden microphone and broadcast on T. V.

3. Thought Insertion

The belief or experience that thoughts, which are not his own, are inserted into his mind. This symptom, which is often falsely rated as present, should not be confused with the belief that he has been caused to have unusual thoughts (for example, evil thoughts caused by the Devil), which are, nevertheless, his own thoughts. Do not include elated subjects who may speak as if their thoughts are coming from God. In such cases the subject knows they are his thoughts.

Example: A man believed that thoughts were being put into his mind by radar.

4. Thought Withdrawal

The belief that thoughts have been removed from his head resulting in a diminished number of thoughts remaining. This is extremely rare and should only be rated when the examiner is convinced that it is present.

5. Delusions of Control (or Influence)

The belief or experience that his feelings, impulses, thoughts, or actions are not his own and are imposed on him by some external force. It does not include the mere conviction that he is acting as an agent of God, or has had a curse placed on him, or that he is the victim of fate, or is not sufficiently assertive, or that someone is attempting to control him. This symptom is frequently rated present when in fact the essential requirement, that the patient experiences his will, thoughts, or feelings as replaced by some other force, is absent.

Examples: A man claimed that his words were not his own but those of his father. A student believed that his actions were under the control of a yoga. A housewife believed that sexual feelings were being put into her body.

6. Other Bizarre Delusions

Bizarre delusions other than those noted above, in the absence of the manic or depressive syndrome, suggest Schizophrenia even if the delusions are of short duration. In judging whether a delusion is bizarre, consider the extent to which the belief is patently absurd, fantastic, or implausible. Do not include as bizarre delusions which are the elaboration of common implausible ideas or subcultural beliefs, such as communicating with God, the Devil, ghosts, or ancestors, or being under the influence of curses, spells, voodoo, or hypnosis.

Examples of bizarre delusions: A man believed that when his adenoids had been removed as a child, a box had been inserted in his head, and that wires had been placed in his head so that the voice he heard was that of Governor Rockefeller. A woman believed that an underground radio station was broadcasting through noise that emanated from her washing machine.

Examples of nonbizarre delusions: A man believed that his appearance had changed and that people therefore no longer respected him. A woman believed that her dead child was still alive but had been kidnapped by some neighbors.

7. Multiple Delusions

Multiple delusions in the absence of the manic or depressive syndrome suggest Schizophrenia, even if the delusions are of short duration. Multiple delusions are counted as present when there are at least 2 separate delusional beliefs which are not the elaboration of a single central theme. The multiple delusions may be all of the same type (e.g., paranoid).

Example of multiple delusions: A woman patient felt that the nurses approached her with homosexual intentions, that the patients were really nurses and doctors in disguise planted there to assist her, and that people could read her mind by looking at her hands.

Example of a non-multiple delusion that is merely an elaboration of a single theme: A man believed that some unknown force had enlisted his family, friends and associates in a scheme to kill him, and that they poisoned his food and tapped his phone.

8. Flight of Ideas

Accelerated speech with abrupt changes from topic to topic usually based on understandable associations, distracting stimuli, or play on words.

An extreme example of this disorder is "You have to be quiet to be sad. Everything having to do with 's' is quiet—on the q.t.—sit, sob, sigh, sin, sorrow, surcease, sought, sand, sweet mother's love and salvation. This is my first case—I am a kind of a bum lawyer or liar—too damned honest to be a lawyer, so had to be a liar." (Kolb, Lawrence, *Noyes' Modern Clinical Psychiatry,* Philadelphia, Saunders, 1968)

9. Catatonic Motor Behavior

These symptoms are very rare nowadays and should only be considered present when they are obvious.

Catatonic stupor. Marked decrease in reactivity to environment and reduction of spontaneous movements and activity. The patient may appear to be unaware of the nature of his surroundings.

Catatonic rigidity. Maintaining a rigid posture against efforts to move him.

Waxy flexibility. Maintaining postures into which he is placed for at least 15 seconds.

Catatonic excitement. Apparently purposeless and stereotyped excited motor activity not influenced by external stimuli.

10. Nonaffective Verbal Hallucinations Spoken to the Subject

A voice or voices are heard by the subject speaking directly to him, the content of which is unrelated to depressive or elated mood. Do not rate as present if limited to voices saying only one or two words.

Example: A woman heard voices telling her that she was having a nervous breakdown and should go to the hospital.

III. Diagnostic Criteria

1. Schizophrenia

Present episode:[1]	1. No 2. Probable 3. Definite	Duration of present episode[1]: _____ (weeks)	Age at first episode: ____	Previous episode followed by significant improvement:[1]	1. No 2. Probable 3. Definite

---

[1] Since episodes of Schizophrenia are often followed by considerable residual impairment, the term "remission" is not used here as it is in most of the other episodic disorders. Patients who show only minimal signs of Schizophrenia during the present episode of illness and who only met the criteria during a previous episode of illness should be coded as No for Present Illness and Probable or Definite for Previous Episode Followed by Significant Improvement. If the patient has met the criteria during both the Present Illness and a Previous Episode, and has probably met the criteria more or less continuously between episodes (e.g., formal thought

There are many different approaches to the diagnosis of Schizophrenia. The approach taken here avoids limiting the diagnosis to cases with a chronic deteriorating course. However, the criteria are designed to screen out borderline conditions, brief hysterical or situational psychoses, and paranoid states. Patients with a full depressive or manic syndrome who would otherwise meet the Schizophrenia criteria are excluded and are diagnosed as either Schizo-affective Disorder, Major Depressive Disorder, or Manic Disorder.

A through C are required for the episode of illness being considered.

A. At least 2 of the following are required for definite, and 1 for probable.

    (1) Thought broadcasting, insertion, or withdrawal (as defined in this manual).

    (2) Delusions of control, other bizarre delusions, or multiple delusions (as defined in this manual).

    (3) Delusions other than persecutory or jealousy, lasting at least 1 week.

    (4) Delusions of any type if accompanied by hallucinations of any type for at least 1 week.

    (5) Auditory hallucinations in which either a voice keeps up a running commentary on the patient's behaviors or thoughts as they occur, or 2 or more voices converse with each other.

    (6) Nonaffective verbal hallucinations spoken to the subject (as defined in this manual).

    (7) Hallucinations of any type throughout the day for several days or intermittently for at least 1 month.

    (8) Definite instances of formal thought disorder (as defined in this manual).

    (9) Obvious catatonic motor behavior (as defined in this manual).

B. A period of illness lasting at least 2 weeks.

C. At no time during the active period of illness being considered did the patient meet the criteria for either probable or definite manic or depressive syndrome (criteria A and B under Major Depressive or Manic Disorders) to such a degree that it was a prominent part of the illness.

Subtypes of Schizophrenia.

This section is for studies in which there is interest in subtypes of Schizophrenia.

1a. Subtypes based on the course of Schizophrenia up to the present.

        1. Acute   2. Subacute   3. Subchronic   4. Chronic

The following 4 mutually exclusive categories should be considered for each patient who has met the criteria for Probable or Definite Schizophrenia. Note: Some patients diagnosed initially as Acute will later show a Subacute, Subchronic, or even Chronic course.

---

disorder), then the duration of the Present Illness should include the total time that the patient has probably met the criteria. On the other hand, if between the episodes, the patient probably did not meet the criteria and either recovered or only had minimal symptoms, then the Duration of the Present Episode should be limited to the duration of the present condition.

(1) Acute Schizophrenia: A through C are required.

    A. Sudden onset—less than 3 months from first signs of increasing psychopathology to any of the core symptoms (criterion A).

    B. Short course—continuously ill with significant signs of Schizophrenia[2] for less than 3 months.

    C. Full recovery from any previous episode.

(2) Subacute Schizophrenia: Course is closer to that of Acute Schizophrenia than that of Chronic Schizophrenia.

    Example: First episode with fairly rapid onset and duration of 5 months.

    Example: Second episode with onset for this episode over a period of 6 months and full recovery from first episode.

(3) Subchronic Schizophrenia: Course is closer to that of Chronic Schizophrenia than that of Acute Schizophrenia.

    Example: Significant signs of Schizophrenia[2] more or less continuously present for at least the last 1 year.

    Example: Second episode following a previous episode from which he did not fully recover.

(4) Chronic Schizophrenia: Significant signs of Schizophrenia[2] more or less continuously present for at least the last 2 years.

1b. Subtypes based on the phenomenology of the present episode of schizophrenic illness.

1. Paranoid   2. Disorganized   3. Confusional turmoil   4. Catatonic   5. Undifferentiated

The following mutually exclusive categories should be considered for each patient who has met the criteria for Probable or Definite Schizophrenia to describe the phenomenology of the present episode of schizophrenic illness.

(1) Paranoid. Throughout the active period of the episode of illness the clinical picture is dominated by the relative persistence of, or preoccupation with, 1 or more of the following:

    1. Persecutory delusions.

    2. Grandiose delusions.

    3. Delusions of jealousy.

    4. Hallucinations with a persecutory or grandiose content.

(2) Disorganized (Hebephrenic). A through C are required.

    A. Marked formal thought disorder (as defined in this manual).

    B. Either 1 or 2:

        1. Fluctuating affect which is shallow, incongruous, or silly.

---

[2] Significant signs of Schizophrenia include any of the core symptoms listed in criterion A for Schizophrenia or extreme social withdrawal, eccentric behavior, or unusual thoughts or perceptual experiences.

    2. Fragmentary delusions or hallucinations with content not organized into a coherent theme.

  C. Not associated with marked emotional turmoil.

(3) Confusional Turmoil. A through C are required.

  A. Emotional turmoil.
  B. Perplexity.
  C. Either 1, 2, or 3.
    1. Dream-like dissociation.
    2. Disorientation to time, place, or person.
    3. Ideas of reference.

(4) Catatonic. Throughout the active period of the episode of illness the clinical picture is dominated by any of the following catatonic symptoms:

  1. Catatonic stupor (marked decrease in reactivity to environment and reduction of spontaneous movements and activity).
  2. Catatonic rigidity (maintaining a rigid posture against efforts to move him).
  3. Catatonic excitement (apparently purposeless and stereotyped excited motor activity not influenced by external stimuli).
  4. Catatonic posturing (voluntary assumption of inappropriate or bizarre posture).

(5) Undifferentiated. Present episode of illness meets the criteria for more than one of the previous categories, or for none of them.

2. Schizo-affective Disorder, Manic Type

Present episode:[1]	1. No 2. Probable 3. Definite	Duration of present episode[1]: _____ (weeks)		Age at first episode: ___	Previous episode followed by significant improvement[1]:	1. No 2. Probable 3. Definite

This category is for patients with an episode of illness that fulfills the criteria for manic syndrome (A and B) but who also have at least 1 of the symptoms suggesting Schizophrenia listed here in C. It includes chronic forms even though the term is sometimes limited to acute or episodic psychoses. It also includes forms in which the schizophrenic symptoms are of brief duration compared to the affective symptoms or the converse. The term Schizo-affective Disorder rather than Schizophrenia is used to reflect the current uncertainty as to whether this condition is a subgroup of Schizophrenia or more closely related to affective illness.

A through E are required for the episode of illness being considered.

  A. One or more distinct periods with a predominantly elevated or irritable mood. The elevated or irritable mood must be relatively persistent and prominent during some part of the illness or occur frequently. It may alternate with depressive mood. If the disturbance in mood only occurs during periods of alcohol or drug intake or withdrawal from them, it should not be considered here.

B. If mood is elevated at least 3 of the following symptoms must be definitely present to a significant degree (4 if mood is only irritable):

(1) More active than usual—either socially, at work, sexually, or physically restless.

(2) More talkative than usual or felt a pressure to keep on talking.

(3) Flight of ideas (as defined in this manual) or subjective experience that thoughts are racing.

(4) Inflated self-esteem (grandiosity, which may be delusional).

(5) Decreased need for sleep.

(6) Distractability, i.e., attention is too easily drawn to unimportant or irrelevant external stimuli.

(7) Excessive involvement in activities without recognizing the high potential for painful consequences, e.g., buying sprees, sexual indiscretions, foolish business investments, reckless driving.

C. At least 1 of the following symptoms suggestive of Schizophrenia is present:

(1) Delusions of control or of thought broadcasting, insertion or withdrawal (as defined in this manual).

(2) Hallucinations of any type throughout the day for several days or intermittently throughout a 1 week period unless all of the content is clearly related to depression or elation.

(3) Auditory hallucinations in which, either a voice keeps up a running commentary on the patient's behaviors or thoughts as they occur, or 2 or more voices converse with each other.

(4) At some time during the period of illness had delusions or hallucinations for more than 1 week in the absence of prominent affective (depressed or manic) symptoms.

(5) At some time during the period of illness had more than 1 week when he exhibited no prominent manic symptoms but had several instances of formal thought disorder (as defined in this manual).

D. Duration of episode at least 1 week (or any duration if hospitalized).

E. Affective symptoms overlap temporally to some degree with the active period of schizophrenic-like symptoms (delusions, hallucinations, thought disorder, bizarre behavior).

The following qualifying categories should be considered for each patient who has met the criteria for Probable or Definite Schizo-affective Disorder, Manic Type.

2a. Subtypes based on the course of symptoms suggestive of Schizophrenia up to the present.

1. Acute 2. Subacute 3. Subchronic 4. Chronic

The following 4 mutually exclusive categories should be considered for each patient who has met the criteria for Probable or Definite Schizo-affective Disorder. Note: Some patients diagnosed initially as Acute will later show a Subacute, Subchronic, or even Chronic course.

(1) Acute Schizo-affective Disorder: A through C are required.

    A. Sudden onset—less than 3 months from first signs of increasing psychopathology to any of the core schizophrenic symptoms (criterion C).

    B. Short course—continuously ill with significant signs of Schizophrenia[3] for less than 3 months.

    C. Full recovery from any previous episode.

(2) Subacute Schizo-affective Disorder: Course is closer to that of Acute Schizo-affective Disorder than that of Chronic Schizo-affective Disorder.

    Example: First episode with fairly rapid onset and duration of 5 months.

    Example: Second episode with onset over a period of 6 months for this episode and full recovery from first episode.

(3) Subchronic Schizo-affective Disorder: Course is closer to that of Chronic Schizo-affective Disorder than that of Acute Schizo-affective Disorder.

    Example: Significant signs of Schizophrenia[3] more or less continuously present for at least the last 1 year.

    Example: Second episode following a previous episode from which he did not fully recover.

(4) Chronic Schizo-affective Disorder: Significant signs of Schizophrenia[3] more or less continuously present for at least the last 2 years.

2b. Temporal relationship of affective and schizophrenic-like features for current episode.

        1. Mainly schizophrenic   2. Mainly affective   3. Other

(1) Mainly schizophrenic: Either A or B.

    A. Core schizophrenic symptoms listed under C in the Schizo-affective criteria are present for at least 1 week in the absence of affective features.

    B. Prior to the onset of the affective features, patient exhibited the following features which are often associated with Schizophrenia: social withdrawal, impairment on occupational functioning, eccentric behavior, or unusual thoughts or perceptual experiences.

(2) Mainly affective: A and B are required.

    A. Affective symptoms began prior to the onset of any of the schizophrenic symptoms listed under C in the Schizo-affective criteria.

    B. Good premorbid social and occupational adjustment.

(3) Other: Does not clearly fit either (1) or (2).

2c. Length of time from first signs of increasing psychopathology to any of the core schizophrenic symptoms noted in C.

---

[3] Significant signs of Schizophrenia include any of the symptoms suggestive of Schizophrenia listed in criterion C for Schizo-affective Disorder or extreme social withdrawal, eccentric behavior, or unusual thoughts or perceptual experiences.

1. Less than 2 days   2. Less than 1 week   3. Less than 1 month   4. Less than 2 months
5. More than 2 months

3. Schizo-affective Disorder, Depressed Type

Present episode:[1]	1. No 2. Probable 3. Definite	Duration of present episode[1]: _____ (weeks)	Age at first episode: ____	Previous episode followed by significant improvement[1]:	1. No 2. Probable 3. Definite

This category is for patients with an episode of illness that fulfills the criteria for depressive syndrome (A and B) but who also have at least 1 of the symptoms suggesting Schizophrenia listed here in C. It includes chronic forms even though the term is sometimes limited to acute or episodic psychoses. It also includes forms in which the schizophrenic symptoms are of brief duration compared to the affective symptoms or the converse. The term Schizo-affective Disorder rather then Schizophrenia is used to reflect the current uncertainty as to whether this condition is a subgroup of Schizophrenia or more closely related to affective illness.

A through E are required for the episode of illness being considered.

A. One or more distinct periods with dysphoric mood characterized by symptoms such as the following: depressed, sad, blue, hopeless, low, down in the dumps, empty, "don't care anymore," irritable, worried. The dysphoric mood must be a major part of the clinical picture during some part of the illness and relatively persistent or occur frequently. It may not necessarily be the most dominant symptom. It does not include momentary shifts from one dysphoric mood to another dysphoric mood, e.g., anxiety to depression to anger such as are seen in states of acute psychotic turmoil.

B. At least 5 of the following symptoms are required for definite and 4 for probable (for past episodes because of memory difficulty, the criteria are 4 and 3 symptoms).

(1) Poor appetite or weight loss or increased appetite or weight gain (change of 1 lb a week over several weeks or 10 lbs a year when not dieting).
(2) Sleep difficulty or sleeping too much.
(3) Loss of energy, fatigability, or tiredness.
(4) Psychomotor retardation or agitation (but not mere subjective feeling of restlessness or being slowed down).
(5) Loss of interest or pleasure in usual activities, including social contact or sex (do not include if limited to a period when delusional or hallucinating).
(6) Feelings of self-reproach or excessive inappropriate guilt (either may be delusional).
(7) Complaints or evidence of diminished ability to think or concentrate such as slowed thinking or mixed-up thoughts (do not include if associated with obvious formal thought disorder).

(8) Recurrent thoughts of death or suicide, including thoughts of wishing to be dead.

C. At least 1 of the following is present:

   (1) Delusions of control or of thought broadcasting, insertion, or withdrawal (as defined in this manual).

   (2) Hallucinations of any type throughout the day for several days, or intermittently throughout a 1 week period, unless all of the content is clearly related to depression or elation.

   (3) Auditory hallucinations in which, either a voice keeps up a running commentary on the patient's behaviors or thoughts as they occur, or 2 or more voices converse with each other.

   (4) At some time during the period of illness had delusions or hallucinations for more than 1 month in the absence of prominent depressive symptoms (although typical depressive delusions, such as delusions of guilt, sin, poverty, nihilism, or self-deprecation, or hallucinations with similar content are not included).

   (5) Preoccupation with a delusion or hallucination to the relative exclusion of other symptoms or concerns (other than delusions of guilt, sin, poverty, nihilism, or self-deprecation or hallucinations with similar content).

   (6) Definite instances of formal thought disorder (as defined in this manual).

D. Duration at least 1 week (or any duration if hospitalized).

E. Affective symptoms overlap temporally to some degree with the active period of schizophrenic-like symptoms (delusions, hallucinations, thought disorder, bizarre behavior).

The following qualifying categories should be considered for each patient who has met the criteria for Probable or Definite Schizo-affective Disorder, Depressed Type.

3a. Subtypes based on the course of symptoms suggestive of Schizophrenia up to the present.

1. Acute   2. Subacute   3. Subchronic   4. Chronic

The following 4 mutually exclusive categories should be considered for each patient who has met the criteria for Probable or Definite Schizo-affective Disorder. Note: Some patients diagnosed initially as Acute will later show a Subacute, Subchronic, or even Chronic course.

(1) Acute Schizo-affective Disorder: A through C are required.

   A. Sudden onset—less than 3 months from first signs of increasing psychopathology to any of the core schizophrenic symptoms (criterion C).

   B. Short course—continuously ill with significant signs of Schizophrenia[3] for less than 3 months.

   C. Full recovery from any previous episode.

(2) Subacute Schizo-affective Disorder: Course is closer to that of Acute Schizo-affective Disorder than that of Chronic Schizo-affective Disorder.

   Example: First episode with fairly rapid onset and duration of 5 months.

Example: Second episode with onset over a period of 6 months for this episode and full recovery from first episode.

(3) Subchronic Schizo-affective Disorder: Course is closer to that of Chronic Schizo-affective Disorder than that of Acute Schizo-affective Disorder.

Example: Significant signs of Schizophrenia[3] more or less continuously present for at least the last 1 year.

Example: Second episode following a previous episode from which he did not fully recover.

(4) Chronic Schizo-affective Disorder: Significant signs of Schizophrenia[4] more or less continuously present for at least the last 2 years.

3b. Temporal relationship of affective and schizophrenic-like features for current episode.

1. Mainly schizophrenic   2. Mainly affective   3. Other

(1) Mainly schizophrenic: Either A or B.

A. Core schizophrenic symptoms listed under C in the Schizo-affective criteria are present for at least 1 week in the absence of affective features.
B. Prior to the onset of the affective features, patient exhibited the following features which are often associated with Schizophrenia: social withdrawal, impairment in occupational functioning, eccentric behavior, or unusual thoughts or perceptual experiences.

(2) Mainly affective: A and B are required.

A. Affective symptoms began prior to the onset of any of the schizophrenic symptoms listed under C in the Schizo-affective criteria.
B. Good premorbid social and occupational adjustment.

(3) Other: Does not clearly fit either (1) or (2).

3c. Length of time from first signs of increasing psychopathology to any of the core schizophrenic symptoms noted in C.

1. Less than 2 days   2. Less than 1 week   3. Less than 1 month   4. Less than 2 months
5. More than 2 months

4. Manic Disorder (may immediately precede or follow Major Depressive Disorder)

Present illness:	1. No 2. Probable 3. Definite	Duration of present illness: ____ (weeks)		Age at first episode: ____	Previous episode followed by remission:	1. No 2. Probable 3. Definite

---

[4] Significant signs of Schizophrenia include any of the symptoms suggestive of Schizophrenia listed in criteria C for Schizo-affective Disorder or extreme social withdrawal, eccentric behavior, or unusual thoughts or perceptual experiences.

This category is for an episode of illness characterized by predominantly elevated or irritable mood accompanied by the manic syndrome. It should also be used for mixed states in which manic and depressive features occur together, or when a patient cycles from a period of depression to a period of mania, or the reverse.

A through E are required for the episode of illness being considered.

A. One or more distinct periods with a predominantly elevated or irritable mood. The elevated or irritable mood must be a prominent part of the illness and relatively persistent although it may alternate with depressive mood. If the disturbance in mood only occurs during periods of alcohol or drug intake or withdrawal from them, it should not be considered here.

B. If mood is elevated at least 3 of the following symptom categories must be definitely present to a significant degree (4 symptoms if mood is only irritable):

   (1) More active than usual – either socially, at work, sexually, or physically restless.
   (2) More talkative than usual or felt a pressure to keep talking.
   (3) Flight of ideas (as defined in this manual) or subjective experience that thoughts are racing.
   (4) Inflated self-esteem (grandiosity, which may be delusional).
   (5) Decreased need for sleep.
   (6) Distractability, i.e., attention is too easily drawn to unimportant or irrelevant external stimuli.
   (7) Excessive involvement in activities without recognizing the high potential for painful consequences, e.g., buying sprees, sexual indiscretions, foolish business investments, reckless driving.

C. Overall disturbance is so severe that at least 1 of the following is present:

   (1) Meaningful conversation is impossible.
   (2) Serious impairment socially, with family, at home, or at work.
   (3) In the absence of (1) or (2), hospitalization.

D. Duration of manic features at least 1 week (or any duration if hospitalized).

E. None of the following which suggests Schizophrenia is present:

   (1) Delusions of control or thought broadcasting, insertion, or withdrawal (as defined in this manual).
   (2) Hallucinations of any type throughout the day for several days or intermittently throughout a 1 week period unless all of the content is clearly related to depression or elation.
   (3) Auditory hallucinations in which either a voice keeps up a running commentary on the patient's behavior as it occurs, or 2 or more voices converse with each other.
   (4) At some time during the period of illness had delusions or hallucinations for more than 1 week in the absence of prominent affective (depressed or manic) symptoms.
   (5) At some time during the period of illness had more than 1 week when he exhibited no prominent manic symptoms but had several instances of formal thought disorder (as defined in this manual).

5. Hypomanic Disorder (may immediately precede or follow Major Depressive Disorder)

Present illness:	1. No 2. Probable 3. Definite	Duration of present illness: _____ (weeks)		Age at first episode: ____	Previous episode followed by remission:	1. No 2. Probable 3. Definite

This category is for describing manic-like episodes that are not of sufficient intensity to meet either criterion B or C for Manic Disorder.
A through D are required.

A. Has had a distinct period with a predominantly elevated or irritable mood. The elevated or irritable mood must be relatively persistent or occur frequently. It may alternate with depressive mood. If the disturbance in mood occurs only during periods of alcohol or drug intake or withdrawal from them, it should not be considered here.

B. If the mood is elevated, at least 2 of the symptoms noted in Manic Disorder B must be present (3 symptoms if mood is only irritable).

C. Duration of mood disturbance at least 2 days. Definite if elevated or irritable mood lasted for 1 week, probable if 2–6 days.

D. The episode being considered does not meet the criteria for Schizophrenia, Schizo-affective Disorder, or Manic Disorder.

6. Bipolar Depression with Mania (Bipolar 1)

1. No   2. Probable   3. Definite

Has met the criteria for Manic Disorder and Major or Minor Depressive Disorder. Probable if the Manic Disorder is only probable.

7. Bipolar Depression with Hypomania (Bipolar 2)

1. No   2. Probable   3. Definite

Has met the criteria for both Hypomanic Disorder and Major or Minor Depressive Disorder and has never met the criteria for Manic Disorder. Probable if the Hypomanic Disorder is only probable.

8. Major Depressive Disorder (may immediately precede or follow Manic Disorder)

Present illness:	1. No 2. Probable 3. Definite	Duration of present illness: _____ (weeks)		Age at first episode: ____	Previous episode followed by remission:	1. No 2. Probable 3. Definite

This category is for episodes of illness in which a major feature of the clinical picture is dysphoric mood accompanied by the depressive syndrome. This category is distinguished from less severe disturbances of mood which are not accompanied by the full syndrome and which in this classification are called Minor Depressive Disorder. This category should also be used for mixed states, in which manic and depressive features occur together, or when a patient cycles from a period of mania to a period of depression, or the reverse. Note: This category should also be considered for patients with a pre-existing psychiatric condition, including Schizophrenia.
A through E required for the episode of illness being considered.

A. Dysphoric mood characterized by symptoms such as the following: depressed, sad, blue, hopeless, low, down in the dumps, "don't care anymore," irritable, worried. The mood disturbance must be prominent and relatively persistent but not necessarily the most dominant symptom. It does not include momentary shifts from 1 dysphoric mood to another dysphoric mood, e.g., anxiety to depression to anger, such as are seen in states of acute psychotic turmoil.

B. At least 5 of the following symptoms are required for definite and 4 for probable (for past episodes, because of memory difficulty, the criteria are 4 and 3 symptoms).
   (1) Poor appetite or weight loss or increased appetite or weight gain (change of 1 lb. a week over several weeks or 10 lbs. a year when not dieting).
   (2) Sleep difficulty or sleeping too much.
   (3) Loss of energy, fatigability, or tiredness.
   (4) Psychomotor agitation or retardation (but not mere subjective feeling of restlessness or being slowed down).
   (5) Loss of interest or pleasure in usual activities, or decrease in sexual drive (do not include if limited to a period when delusional or hallucinating).
   (6) Feelings of self-reproach or excessive or inappropriate guilt (either may be delusional).
   (7) Complaints or evidence of diminished ability to think or concentrate, such as slow thinking, or mixed-up thoughts (do not include if associated with obvious formal thought disorder).
   (8) Recurrent thoughts of death or suicide, including thoughts of wishing to be dead.

C. Dysphoric features of illness lasting at least 1 week. Definite if lasted more than 2 weeks, probable if 1 to 2 weeks.

D. Sought help from someone during the dysphoric period or had impaired functioning socially, with family, at home, or at work.

E. None of the following, which suggests Schizophrenia is present.
   (1) Delusions of control or thought broadcasting, insertion, or withdrawal (as defined in this manual).
   (2) Hallucinations of any type throughout the day for several days or intermittently throughout a 1 week period unless all of the content is clearly related to depression or elation.
   (3) Auditory hallucinations in which either a voice keeps up a running com-

mentary on the patient's behaviors or thoughts as they occur, or 2 or more voices converse with each other.

(4) At some time during the period of illness had delusions or hallucinations for more than 1 month in the absence of prominent affective (manic or depressive) symptoms (although typical depressive delusions, such as delusions of guilt, sin, poverty, nihilism, or self-deprecation or hallucinations of similar content are permitted).

(5) Preoccupation with a delusion or hallucination to the relative exclusion of other symptoms or concerns (other than delusions of guilt, sin, poverty, nihilism, or self-deprecation or hallucinations with similar content).

(6) Definite instances of formal thought disorder (as defined in this manual).

☐ If has not met criteria for probable or definite Major Depressive Disorder, check here and skip to Minor Depressive Disorder.

Subtypes of major depressive disorder.

This section is primarily for studies in which there is interest in one or more subtypes of Major Depressive Disorder. The diagnoses in this section describe different ways of categorizing such patients who meet the criteria of Probable or Definite Major Depressive Disorder and therefore many patients will meet the criteria for several categories. Probable in this section refers to the subtype, not the certainty that the condition meets the criteria for Major Depressive Disorder.

8a. Primary Major Depressive Disorder

	No	Probable	Definite		No	Probable	Definite
Present illness:	1	2	3	Previous episode followed by remission:	1	2	3

The first appearance of probable or definite Major Depressive Disorder was not preceded by any of the following (either probable or definite) although these conditions may have occurred afterwards: Schizophrenia, Panic Disorder, Phobic Disorder, Obsessive Compulsive Disorder, Briquet's Disorder, Antisocial Personality, Alcoholism, Drug Abuse, Preferential Homosexuality, a serious physical illness which led to major changes in living conditions, or a physical illness which often is associated with psychological symptoms (e.g., thyrotoxicosis).

Episodes of Manic Disorder or Hypomanic Disorder may or may not have been present.

8b. Secondary Major Depressive Disorder

	No	Probable	Definite		No	Probable	Definite
Present illness:	1	2	3	Previous episode followed by remission:	1	2	3

A period of Major Depressive Disorder (either probable or definite) was preceded by any of the conditions listed below (either probable or definite). (Note that it is possible for a patient to have had both Primary and Secondary Depressive Disorders, for example, depression at age 20 and 40 and alcoholism beginning at age 30.) Check the condition which existed prior to the development of the Secondary Major Depressive Disorder.

_____ Schizophrenia
_____ Schizo-affective Disorder
_____ Obsessive Compulsive Disorder
_____ Panic Disorder
_____ Phobic Disorder
_____ Briquet's Disorder
_____ Antisocial Personality
_____ Alcoholism
_____ Drug Abuse

_____ Preferential Homosexuality (not limited to discrete periods of life)
_____ a serious physical illness which led to major changes in living conditions
Specify illness _____
_____ a physical illness which often is associated with psychological symptoms (e.g., thyrotoxicosis)
Specify illness _____

8c. Recurrent Major Depressive Disorder

1. No   2. Probable   3. Definite

This is for individuals who have had 2 or more episodes that met criteria for probable or definite Major Depressive Disorder separated by at least 2 months of return to more or less usual functioning in the absence of Manic Disorder or Hypomanic Disorder.

8d. Psychotic Major Depressive Disorder

	No	Probable	Definite		No	Probable	Definite
Present illness:	1	2	3	Previous episode followed by remission:	1	2	3

This category is applied to patients with a Major Depressive Disorder (either probable or definite) who have had any of the symptoms in either A, B, or C. Note that the term Psychotic Depressive Reaction in the standard nomenclature often involves the additional concepts of severity of functional impairment and endogenous phenomena which are not included in this category and are covered separately in other subtypes. The category here is not used in the sense of a psychotic-neurotic dichotomy and thus there is no implication that patients not so classified thereby have a neurotic depression.

Either A, B, or C is required.

A. Delusions.

B. Hallucinations.

C. Depressive stupor (mute and unresponsive).

8e. Incapacitating Major Depressive Disorder

	No	Probable	Definite		No	Probable	Definite
Present illness:	1	2	3	Previous episode followed by remission:	1	2	3

This category is considered for all patients who have had a probable or definite Major Depressive Disorder. It is applied to patients who might be classified as Psychotic Depressive Reaction in the standard nomenclature on the basis of severity of functional impairment.

Either A or B is required.

A. Unable to function at work or at school, or to take care of the house for at least 1 week (or if hospitalized was so impaired that obviously could not work).

B. Unable to feed or clothe himself or maintain minimal personal hygiene without assistance.

8f. Endogenous Major Depressive Disorder

Present Illness: 1. No   2. Probable   3. Definite

This category is considered for all patients with a current episode that meets the criteria for probable or definite Major Depressive Disorder. It is applied to those patients who show a particular symptom picture that many research studies indicate is associated with good response to somatic therapy. Ignore the presence or absence of precipitating events even though this feature is often associated with the term "endogenous."

At least 4 symptoms are required for probable and 6 for definite, with at least 1 symptom from group A.

A. (1) Distinct quality to depressed mood, i.e., depressed mood is perceived as distinctly different from the kind of feeling he would have or has had following the death of a loved one.
   (2) Lack of reactivity to environmental changes (once depressed doesn't feel better, even temporarily, when something good happens).
   (3) Mood is regularly worse in the morning.

B. (1) Feelings of self-reproach or excessive or inappropriate guilt.
   (2) Early morning awakening or middle insomnia.
   (3) Psychomotor retardation or agitation (more than mere subjective feeling of being slowed down or restless).
   (4) Poor appetite.
   (5) **Weight loss (2 lbs a week over several weeks or 20 lbs in a year when not dieting).**
   (6) Loss of interest or pleasure in usual activities or decreased sexual drive.

8g. Agitated Major Depressive Disorder

Present Illness: 1. No   2. Probable   3. Definite

This category is considered for all patients with a current episode that meets the criteria for probable or definite Major Depressive Disorder. At least 2 of the following manifestations of psychomotor agitation (not mere subjective anxiety) are required for several days during the current episode.

(1) Pacing

(2) Handwringing.

(3) Unable to sit still.

(4) Pulling or rubbing on hair, skin, or clothing.

(5) Outburst of complaining or shouting.

(6) Talks on and on or can't seem to stop talking.

8h. Retarded Major Depressive Disorder

Present Illness: 1. No   2. Probable   3. Definite

This category is considered for all patients with a current episode that meets the criteria for probable or definite Major Depressive Disorder.
At least 2 of the following manifestations are required for at least 1 week during the current episode.

(1) Slowed speech.

(2) Increased pauses before answering.

(3) Low or monotonous speech.

(4) Mute or markedly decreased amount of speech.

(5) Slowed body movements.

8i. Situational Major Depressive Disorder

Present Illness: 1. No   2. Probable   3. Definite

This category is considered for all patients with a current episode that meets the criteria for a probable or definite Major Depressive Disorder. It is applied to those patients in whom the depressive illness has developed after an event or in a situation that seems likely to have contributed to the appearance of the episode at that time. In making this judgment consider the amount of stress inherent in the event or situation, the cumulative effect of such stresses, and the closeness of the events to the onset or exacerbation of the depressive episode.

Definite is for situations in which, in the absence of the external events, the episode almost certainly would not have developed at that time.

Example: depressive episode immediately following sudden death of a loved one.

Probable is for situations in which, in the absence of the external events, the episode probably would not have developed at that time.

Example: depressive episode several months after increasing business difficulties.

8j. Simple Major Depressive Disorder

Present Illness: 1. No   2. Probable   3. Definite

This category is considered for all patients with a current episode that meets the criteria for probable or definite Major Depressive Disorder. It is applied to depressive episodes that develop in a person who has shown no significant signs of psychiatric disturbance in the year prior to the development of the current episode, with the exception of symptomatology associated with either Major or Minor Depressive Disorder, Manic or Hypomanic Disorder.

Often depressive episodes begin with symptoms other than those in the classic depressive syndrome, such as phobias, panic attacks or excessive somatic concerns. In such instances, these symptoms should be regarded as part of the depressive episode unless the duration of the other symptoms is sufficient to warrant a separate diagnosis.

Note that the concept of Simple Major Depressive Disorder is not identical with the concept of Primary Major Depressive Disorder. An individual who had had Alcoholism followed by more than 1 year of abstinence who then developed a depression would be categorized as having a Simple and a Secondary Major Depressive Disorder.

8k. Predominant mood of current episode of Major Depressive Disorder

(Check 1 only.)

(1) _____ Mainly depressed (sad, blue, hopeless)

(2) _____ Mainly depressed interspersed with periods of euphoric mood

(3) _____ Mainly anxious (fearful, tense, nervous, jittery)

(4) _____ Anxious and depressed without either predominating

(5) _____ Mainly hostile (angry, irritable, resentful)

(6) _____ Mainly apathetic (empty, don't care)

(7) _____ Other

9. Minor Depressive Disorder

Present illness:	1. No 2. Probable 3. Definite	Duration of present illness: _____ (weeks)	Age at first episode: ____	Previous episode followed by remission:	1. No 2. Probable 3. Definite

This category is for nonpsychotic episodes of illness in which the most prominent disturbance is a mood of depression without the full depressive syndrome that characterizes Major Depressive Disorder. This category is distinguished from Generalized Anxiety Disorder in which there is a clear predominance of anxious mood.

A through F are required for the episode of illness being considered.

A. An episode of illness in which relatively persistent depressed mood dominates the clinical picture (or is coequal with anxiety). The depressed mood may be described as depressed, sad, blue, hopeless, low, down in the dumps, or "don't care anymore."

B. Two or more of the symptoms listed below:
   (1) Poor appetite or weight loss or increased appetite or weight gain (change of 1 lb. a week over several weeks or 10 lbs. a year when not dieting).
   (2) Sleep difficulty or sleeping too much.
   (3) Loss of energy, fatigability, or tiredness.
   (4) Psychomotor agitation or retardation (but not mere subjective feeling of restlessness or being slowed down).
   (5) Loss of interest or pleasure in usual activities, or decrease in sexual drive (do not include if limited to a period when delusional or hallucinating).
   (6) Feelings of self-reproach or excessive or inappropriate guilt (either may be delusional).
   (7) Complaints or evidence of diminished ability to think or concentrate, such as slow thinking, or mixed-up thoughts (do not include if associated with obvious formal thought disorder).
   (8) Recurrent thoughts of death or suicide, including thoughts of wishing to be dead.
   (9) Crying.
   (10) Pessimistic attitude.
   (11) Brooding about past or current unpleasant events.
   (12) Preoccupation with feelings of inadequacy.

C. Duration at least 2 weeks.

D. The episode of illness being considered does not meet the criteria for Major Depressive Disorder, Schizophrenia, Briquet's Disorder, Unspecified Psychosis, or Manic Disorder.

E. The episode of illness may be superimposed on another pre-existing psychiatric disorder, for example, Alcoholism, Phobic or Obsessive Compulsive Disorders. This category should be given as an additional diagnosis only if the depressed mood, by virtue of its intensity or effect on functioning, can be clearly distinguished from the patient's usual condition.

F. When the episode of illness is not superimposed on another pre-existing psychiatric disorder, it must result in either impairment in social functioning with family, at home, or at work, taking medication, or seeking help from someone.

9a. With Significant Anxiety

1. No   2. Probable   3. Definite

Current episode associated with significant anxiety.

10. Panic Disorder

Present illness:	1. No 2. Probable 3. Definite	Duration of present illness: _____ (weeks)	Age at first episode: ____	Previous episode followed by remission:	1. No 2. Probable 3. Definite

This category is for nonpsychotic episodes of illness in which the most prominent disturbance is panic attacks. This category is distinguished from Generalized Anxiety Disorder in which there is anxiety but without frequent panic attacks.

A through E are required for the episode of illness being considered.

A. At least 6 panic attacks, distributed over a 6 week period and occurring at times other than during marked physical exertion or a life-threatening situation, and in the absence of a medical illness that could account for symptoms of anxiety.

B. The panic attacks are manifested by discrete periods of apprehension or fearfulness with at least 3 of the following symptoms present during the majority of attacks required for definite and 2 for probable (for past episodes, because of memory difficulty, the criteria are 2 and 1 symptoms).

   (1) dyspnea, (2) palpitations, (3) chest pain or discomfort, (4) choking or smothering sensations, (5) dizziness, vertigo or feelings of unreality, (6) paresthesias (tingling), (7) sweating, (8) faintness, (9) trembling or shaking, (10) fear of dying during attack.

C. Nervousness apart from the anxiety attacks over the 6 week period.

D. The anxiety symptoms, or reactions to them are a major part of the clinical picture during some phase of the period of illness being considered.

E. The condition has resulted in either impairment in social functioning, seeking help from someone, or taking medication, or abusing alcohol or drugs.

Patients with probable or definite Major Depressive Disorder, Schizophrenia or Schizo-affective Disorder who manifest recurrent anxiety attacks do not receive the additional diagnosis of Panic Disorder for the same period of illness if the anxiety attacks largely overlap temporally with those of the other disorder. However, some patients may have a period of illness that meets the criteria for more than 1 of the following conditions: Panic Disorder, Phobic Disorder, or Obsessive Compulsive Disorder. In such instances, more than 1 diagnosis should be given.

Recent work suggests that panic attacks occurring spontaneously should be distinguished from panic attacks that occur under stereotyped, if irrational circumstances.

11. Generalized Anxiety Disorder

Present 1. No   Duration   Age at   Previous episode 1. No
illness: 2. Probable of present   first   followed by   2. Probable
      3. Definite   illness: _____ episode: ___ remission: 3. Definite
                      (weeks)

This category is for the nonpsychotic episodes of illness in which the most prominent disturbance is a generalized anxiety without the frequent panic attacks that characterize Panic Disorder or the full depressive syndrome that characterizes Major Depressive Disorder. This category is distinguished from Minor Depressive Disorder by the clear predominance of the depressed mood in the latter.

A through F are required for the episode of illness being considered.

A. An episode of illness in which relatively persistent generalized anxious mood dominates the clinical picture. The anxious mood may be described as anxious, nervous, jittery, tense, restless, or "up tight."

B. At least 1 of the following:

    (1) Difficulty falling asleep.
    (2) Sweating, blushing, dizziness, palpitations, or shortness of breath.
    (3) Muscular tension or tremors.
    (4) Persistent worrying about future events.
    (5) Fidgeting or inability to sit still.

C. Duration at least 2 weeks.

D. The episode of illness being considered does not meet the criteria for Major Depressive Disorder, Schizophrenia, Briquet's Disorder, Unspecified Psychosis, or Manic Disorder.

E. The episode of illness may be superimposed on another pre-existing psychiatric disorder, for example, Alcoholism, Phobic or Obsessive Compulsive Disorders. This category should be given as an additional diagnosis only if the anxious mood, by virtue of its intensity or effect on functioning, can be clearly distinguished from the patient's usual condition.

F. When the episode of illness is not superimposed on another pre-existing psychiatric disorder, it must result in either impairment in social functioning with family, at home, or at work, taking medication, or seeking help from someone.

11a. With Significant Depression

1. No   2. Probable   3. Definite

Current episode associated with significant depression. Note if the anxiety is coequal with depression, the diagnosis should be Minor Depressive Disorder with significant anxiety.

12. Cyclothymic Personality

1. No   2. Probable   3. Definite

Since early adulthood the following traits have been present to a noticeably greater degree than in most people and were not limited to discrete affective episodes: A through C are required.

A. Recurrent periods of depression lasting at least a few days alternating with similar periods of clearly better than normal mood, with or without normal interval period.

B. Usually not in normal mood.

C. Changes in mood often unrelated to external events or circumstances.

13. Depressive Personality

1. No   2. Probable   3. Definite

This category is for individuals who characteristically are bothered by depressive moods not attributable to any other psychiatric condition described in these criteria. Patients with this condition may also have other episodic conditions superimposed on them, including Major Depressive Disorder or an episode of a psychotic illness. A through D are required.

A. Since early adulthood has been bothered by depressive mood (e.g., sad, blue, hopeless, low, "don't care anymore") to a noticeably greater degree than most people, for at least several days of almost every month of almost every year. The depressive mood or the symptoms in B dominate the clinical picture. (Includes a person in his 20s who has been this way for at least 5 years.)

B. Since early adulthood at least 3 of the following traits have been present to a noticeably greater degree than in most people and were not limited to discrete affective episodes of illness:

(1) Easily disappointed, self-pity, or feelings of being short-changed.
(2) Over-reactive to stressful situations.
(3) Pessimistic.
(4) Feelings of inadequacy.
(5) Bothered by low energy or fatigue.
(6) Preoccupation with negative aspects or events or situations.
(7) Demanding or complaining behavior.
(8) Dramatic attention-seeking behavior.

C. The chronic condition (other than a superimposed episode of another condition) has resulted in 1 of the following:

(1) Impairment in functioning socially, with family, at work, or at home.
(2) Taking medication.
(3) Seeking help from someone.
(4) A suicidal gesture or attempt.
(5) Someone has complained about some manifestation of the condition.

D. Depressive mood can not be attributed to any other psychiatric condition noted in this manual, such as Cyclothymic Personality, Briquet's Disorder, or to premenstrual tension.

14. Briquet's Disorder

1. No   2. Probable   3. Definite

This condition is a chronic or recurrent polysymptomatic disorder that begins early in life, and is characterized by multiple somatic complaints not explained by known medical illness. While most people have various aches and pains and other physical complaints not explained by known medical illness, they will rarely mention them in a psychiatric interview. An essential feature of Briquet's Disorder is the readiness with which patients with this condition will mention such symptoms.

The results of many research studies justify the separation of this condition from simple conversion reaction and hysterical personality.

A and B are required.

A. In the judgment of the rater, the patient has had a dramatic, vague or complicated medical history, with onset prior to age 25.

B. For women a minimum of at least 1 reported manifestation in each of at least 5 of the following 6 groups is required for a definite diagnosis. For a probable diagnosis at least 1 manifestation in each of at least 4 groups is required. Since 1 of the groups of symptoms can only apply to women, 1 group less is required for diagnosing men.

The rater need not obtain confirmatory evidence that the symptom was actually present, e.g., vomiting spells. The mere report of such by the patient is sufficient. However, only physical symptoms that in the judgment of the rater are not explained by some physical illness are considered significant. This judgment often will require asking additional questions about the presence of other symptoms, what treatment was given, what the doctor said was wrong, etc. In addition, physical symptoms that only occurred during periods of other psychiatric illness (e.g., Schizophrenia or Major Depressive Disorder) or that developed for the first time after the age of 40 are not considered significant.

Group 1. Patient believes that he has been sickly for most or a good part of his life.

Group 2. Loss of sensation, loss of voice and unable to whisper, trouble walking, any other pseudoneurological conversion reaction (e.g., paralysis, blindness) or dissociative reaction (e.g., amnesia, loss of consciousness).

Group 3. Abdominal pain or vomiting spells.

Group 4. (Judged by the patient as occurring more frequently or severely than with most women): Dysmenorrhea, menstrual irregularity, or excessive menstrual bleeding.

Group 5. (For major portion of life after opportunities for a sex life) Sexual indifference (uninterested in having sex), lack of pleasure during intercourse, or pain during intercourse.

Group 6. Back pain, joint pain, pain in extremities, or more headaches than most people.

15. Antisocial Personality

1. No   2. Probable   3. Definite

This category is for patients who have a chronic or recurrent disorder with the appearance of at least 1 of its manifestations before age 15 and some of the manifestations have occurred after age 15. A minimum of at least 1 manifestation in each of at least 4 of the following 8 categories is required for a definite diagnosis. For a probable diagnosis at least 1 manifestation in each of at least 3 categories is required.

If the patient has had a serious alcohol or drug problem count only those manifestations of Antisocial Personality which occurred during periods in which there was no problem with alcohol or drugs. Do not count symptoms limited to a period of Manic Disorder.

Because of the difficulty in distinguishing between behaviors due to Schizophrenia from similarly appearing behaviors due to Antisocial Personality, the latter diagnosis should not be made when a diagnosis of Schizophrenia or Schizo-affective Disorder has been made.

(1) School problems as manifested by any of the following: truancy (positive if more than once per year for at least 2 years, not including the last year of school), suspension, expulsion, or fighting that leads to trouble with teachers or principals.

(2) Running away from home overnight at least twice while living in parental or parental surrogate home.

(3) Trouble with the police as manifested by any of the following: 2 or more arrests for non-traffic offenses, 4 or more arrests (including tickets only) for moving traffic offenses, or at least 1 felony conviction.

(4) Poor work history as manifested by being fired, quitting 3 or more jobs without another job to go to, or frequent job changes not accounted for by normal seasonal economic fluctuations. Include never worked if due to antisocial behavior.

(5) Marital difficulties manifested by any of the following: 2 or more divorces, deserting family, frequent separations due to marital discord, recurrent physical attacks upon spouse.

(6) Repeated outbursts of rage or fighting not on the school premises: if prior to age 18 must occur at least twice and lead to difficulty with adults; after age 18 this must occur at least twice, or if a weapon (e.g., club, knife, or gun) is used, only once is enough to rate this category positive.

(7) Vagrancy or wanderlust, e.g., at least several months of wandering from place to place with no prearranged plans (other than vacations).

(8) Persistent and repeated lying.

The criteria for this category are based on the results of a number of research studies. The criteria of callousness, exploitativeness, and lack of loyalty to individuals, groups or social values, which are part of the traditional concept of Antisocial Personality are not noted here because they are difficult to define behaviorally. However, the disorder defined here is highly predictive of these and other antisocial traits.

16. Alcoholism

Present illness:	1. No 2. Probable 3. Definite	Duration of present illness: _____ (weeks)	Age at first episode: ___	Previous episode followed by remission:	1. No 2. Probable 3. Definite

A and B are required for the episode of illness being considered.

A. Duration at least 1 month.

B. At least 3 manifestations for definite, and 2 for probable.
  (1) Patient thinks he drinks too much.
  (2) Others complain of his drinking.
  (3) Admits he often can't stop drinking when he wants to.
  (4) Frequent drinking before breakfast.
  (5) Frequently missed work, had impaired performance on the job, or unable to take care of household responsibilities because of drinking.
  (6) Job loss where drinking was the primary reason according to the patient.
  (7) Frequently has difficulties with family members, friends, or associates because of his drinking.
  (8) Divorce or separation, where drinking was the primary reason according to the patient.
  (9) Alcoholic benders — on 3 or more occasions drank steadily for 3 or more days more than a fifth of whiskey daily (or 24 bottles of beer, or 3 bottles of wine).
  (10) Physical violence associated with drinking on at least 2 occasions.
  (11) Traffic difficulties due to drinking, e.g., reckless driving, accidents, speeding.
  (12) Picked up by police due to behavior associated with drinking (other than traffic difficulties) e.g., disturbance of the peace, fighting, public intoxication.
  (13) Frequent blackouts (memory loss for events that occurred during a drinking episode while conscious).
  (14) Frequent tremors most likely due to drinking.
  (15) Delirium tremens with disorientation after stopping drinking.
  (16) Hallucinations after stopping drinking on at least 2 occasions.
  (17) Withdrawal seizures in a non-epileptic, limited to periods when he stopped drinking.
  (18) Cirrhosis of the liver attributed to alcohol by an M.D.

(19) Polyneuropathy most likely due to drinking.
(20) A diagnosis of Korsakoff's syndrome (chronic brain syndrome with anterograde amnesia as the predominant feature).

17. Drug Abuse

Present illness:	1. No 2. Probable 3. Definite	Duration of present illness: _____ (weeks)	Age at first episode: ___	Previous episode followed by remission:	1. No 2. Probable 3. Definite

This category is for patients who are addicted to, dependent on, or abuse drugs other than alcohol, tobacco, and ordinary caffeine-containing beverages. Dependence on medically prescribed drugs is also excluded so long as the drug is medically indicated and the intake is proportional to the medical need.

Narcotics (natural or synthetic)

A. Probable — used 2+ days per week for more than a month, or drug free but taking a narcotic substitute or blocking agent.

B. Definite — withdrawal as shown by 4 or more of the following symptoms: insomnia, sweating or flushing, runny nose, chills, cramps, diarrhea, muscle pain, nausea, gooseflesh, twitching.

Amphetamines or cocaine

A. Probable — used more than 25 times during a 3 month period, and at least once used it more than 3 days in a row.

B. Definite — probable plus needed to increase the amount to get the same high (tolerance) or had ideas of reference, or felt paranoid, or heard voices, or had visions, when taking them.

Sedatives, hypnotics (including barbiturates and non-barbiturates), or tranquilizers. Excludes up to 3 times usual prescribed dose for night-time hypnotics or day-time tranquilizers.

A. Probable — 4 or more times greater than the usual prescribed dosage for more than 1 month.

B. Definite — probable plus needed to increase the amount to get the same effect (tolerance) or stopping led to weakness, insomnia, delirium, or having a convulsion, or 6 or more times greater than the usual prescribed dosage for more than 2 weeks, or several instances of serious side effects, "very stoned" or attempts to get high.

Marijuana or hashish

A. Probable — used almost daily or more during a 1 month period and uncomfortable without it.

B. Definite — probable plus felt apathetic and uninterested in things previously involved with.

LSD or other hallucinogens

A. Probable — used 10 times or more.

B. Definite — used 50 times or more.

Glue, gasoline, chloroform, ether, other volatile solvents

A. Probable — used 10 times or more.

B. Definite — probable plus needed to increase the amount to get the same effect.

18. Obsessive Compulsive Disorder

Present illness:	1. No 2. Probable 3. Definite	Duration of present illness:	_____ (weeks)	Age at first episode: ___	Previous episode followed by remission:	1. No 2. Probable 3. Definite

A through C are required.

A. Obsessions or compulsions which are defined as recurrent or persistent ideas, thoughts, images, feelings, impulses or movements which generally are accompanied by a sense of subjective compulsion and a desire to resist the event which is usually recognized by the individual as foreign to his personality or nature, i.e., "ego alien."

Contrary to the standard definition of a compulsion, the definition here includes all repetitive behavior, even if not "ego alien" if it meets the following criteria[5]: it is purposeful, rather than just a series of movements; it is usually performed in accordance with rules or in a stereotyped fashion; it is not an end in itself but is designed to bring about or prevent some future state of affairs; and the activity is not connected to the state of affairs it is designed to bring about by a rational justification (in the view of the observer). Note, certain activities that are inherently or potentially pleasurable, even when ego alien, such as compulsive eating, sexual behavior, picking at hair, or skin, gambling or drinking should not be included here.

True obsessions, as distinguished from obsessive brooding or rumination, are usually stereotyped, repetitive words, ideas or phrases, the content of which is seemingly meaningless to the patient. In contrast, obsessive brooding or rumination usually takes the form of organized thinking about real or potentially unpleasant circumstances or events. The fact that the patient recognizes that his obsessive brooding is disproportionate to the circumstances does not make the disturbance in thinking a true obsession.

B. The obsessions or compulsions, or reactions to them, are a major part of the clinical picture during some phase of the illness being considered.

---

[5] Largely from Valerie J. Walker, *British Journal of Psychiatry,* Vol. 123, 1973.

C. The condition has resulted in either impairment in social functioning, at work, taking medication, or seeking help from someone.

Patients with probable or definite Major Depressive Disorder, Schizophrenia or Schizo-affective Disorder who manifest prominent obsessive or compulsive symptoms do not receive the additional diagnosis of Obsessive Compulsive Disorder for the same period of illness if the obsessive or compulsive symptoms largely overlap temporally with those of the other disorder. However, some patients may have a period of illness that meets the criteria for more than 1 of the following conditions: Panic Disorder, Phobic Disorder, or Obsessive Compulsive Disorder. In such instances more than 1 diagnosis should be made.

For certain purposes, it may be useful to distinguish 2 groups of patients with this disorder: those with predominantly obsessive symptoms, and those with predominantly compulsive symptoms.

19. Phobic Disorder

Present illness:	1. No 2. Probable 3. Definite	Duration of present illness: _____ (weeks)	Age at first episode: ____	Previous episode followed by remission:	1. No 2. Probable 3. Definite

A through C are required for episode of illness being considered.

A. Persistent and recurring irrational fears of a specific object, activity, or situation which the patient tends to avoid. Usually the avoidance is recognized as unreasonable. In some cases, however, patients with Phobic Disorder avoid situations because they anticipate overwhelming anxiety or some other strong emotion, and thereby claim their avoidance is rational. Irrational fears without a tendency to avoid specific situations are not phobias, e.g., most "cancer phobias."

B. The phobic symptom(s), reactions to them, or behavior to avoid them are a major part of the clinical picture at some phase of the period of illness being considered.

C. The condition has resulted in either impairment in social functioning at work, taking medication, or seeking help from someone.

Patients with probable or definite Major Depressive Disorder, Schizophrenia, or Schizo-affective Disorder who manifest prominent phobic symptoms do not receive the additional diagnosis of Phobic Disorder for the same period of illness if the phobic symptoms largely overlap temporally with those of the other disorder. However, some patients may have a period of illness that meets the criteria for more than 1 of the following conditions: Panic Disorder, Phobic Disorder, or Obsessive Compulsive Disorder. In such instances, more than 1 diagnosis should be made.

For certain purposes Phobic Disorder can be divided into the following subtypes: agoraphobia, social phobias, and specific non-social phobias.

20. Unspecified Psychosis

| Present illness: | 1. No 2. Probable 3. Definite | Duration of present illness: _____ (weeks) | Age at first episode: ___ | Previous episode followed by remission: | 1. No 2. Probable 3. Definite |

This category includes patients who might otherwise be labeled as Paranoid State, Hysterical Personality, Gross Stress Reaction, etc. In some cases, at a later evaluation the criteria for one of the other psychoses will be met.

A and B are required for episode of illness being considered.

A. Does not meet the criteria for either Schizophrenia, Schizo-affective Disorder, Manic Disorder, or Major Depressive Disorder.

B. At least 1 of the following is present:

   (1) Delusions.
   (2) Hallucinations.
   (3) Incoherence (as defined in this manual under Formal Thought Disorder).
   (4) Grossly bizarre behavior (e.g., takes off clothes in public, unprovoked shouting and yelling at passers-by).

21. Other Psychiatric Disorder

| Present illness: | 1. No 2. Probable 3. Definite | Duration of present illness: _____ (weeks) | Age at first episode: ___ | Previous episode followed by remission: | 1. No 2. Probable 3. Definite |

This category is for psychiatric conditions which cannot be classified in any of the previous categories as either Probable or Definite. Among the more common reasons are:

(1) The clinical picture does not suggest any of the specific diagnoses listed in the RDC (e.g., Anorexia Nervosa, Paranoid Personality)

(2) 1 or more of the specific diagnoses is suspected but the symptoms are too minimal to meet the criteria for either probable or definite

(3) Inability to determine the chronology of important symptom clusters, e.g., alcoholism, and hallucinations and lack of knowledge of which came first

(4) Inadequate information to establish a definitive diagnosis

(5) A likely known organic etiology, such as alcohol abuse, amphetamine intoxication, ingestion of a hallucinogen, or fever

For a disturbance in mood, thinking, or behavior to be considered Other Psychiatric Disorder it must meet at least 1 of the following:

(1) Sought help from someone

(2) Took medication (other than occasional night-time hypnotic for insomnia)

(3) Caused impairment in functioning socially, with family, at home, or at work

It is possible for a patient to have a period of illness which is considered Other Psychiatric Disorder followed by or preceded by an episode which can be diagnosed as one of the other specific diagnoses.

22. Borderline Features

Present illness:	1. No 2. Probable 3. Definite	Duration of present illness: _____ (weeks)	Age at first episode: ____	Previous episode followed by remission:	1. No 2. Probable 3. Definite

This category is used to qualify another diagnosis (including Other Psychiatric Disorder).

Despite a large literature on the borderline patient, syndrome, personality, state, or condition, and ambulatory, pseudoneurotic or latent schizophrenia, there is no consensus on how to define these groups, and it is unlikely that they represent a distinct condition. On the other hand, the criteria offered here do permit the identification of patients whose episodes of illness or whose usual personality functioning are characterized by features frequently cited in the literature as seen in these conditions.

A and B are required.

A. Has never met the criteria for Schizophrenia (but may have met the criteria for all other diagnoses including Major Depressive Disorder or Other Psychiatric Disorder).

B. At least 1 of the following:

(1) Recurrent periods of dissociation, depersonalization, or derealization (other than during anxiety attacks).

(2) Odd, bizarre, or eccentric behavior or ideation not commonly seen in simple depressive, manic, phobic or obsessive compulsive disorders, and not due to alcohol or drug abuse.

(3) Ideas of reference, extreme suspiciousness, paranoid ideation, suspected delusions or hallucinations, other than during an episode of Manic Disorder, Major Depressive Disorder, or Schizo-affective Disorder.

(4) Extreme social isolation for the last 2 years not explainable by depressed mood.

(5) Persistent difficulty distinguishing fantasy from reality.

(6) Recurrent self damaging impulsive behavior (e.g., self-mutilation, quitting

jobs, suicidal behavior, rage reaction) not accounted for by any other specific diagnoses.

23. Not Currently Mentally Ill

1. No   2. Probable   3. Definite

This category is for individuals who, at the time of evaluation, do not have sufficient symptoms or other signs of disturbance to warrant being given any of the previous specific diagnoses, including Other Psychiatric Disorder, as a present illness. Note: they may have recovered from a previous episode of diagnosed illness, such as a patient with recurrent affective illness who is in remission.

24. Never Mentally Ill

1. No   2. Probable   3. Definite

This category is for individuals who never had sufficient symptoms or other signs of disturbance to warrant being given any of the previous specific diagnoses, including Other Psychiatric Disorder.

DISCUSSION

Uhlenhuth: Would you comment more explicitly on the comparison between your diagnoses using the research criteria and Dr. Gurland's diagnoses using DSM-II? It appears that two very good diagnosticians using two different systems show a strikingly good comparison. Maybe one of the conclusions that we ought to draw here is that reliability of diagnosis is more a function of the skills of the diagnostician than it is of the system used.

Spitzer: There are many problems here. First, the reliability that was obtained between the pairs using the RDC still is significantly better than between me and Dr. Gurland. But I would maintain that if we had Dr. Gurland and people of his calibre using the RDC, the reliabilities would be very much better. The other question is, can we, by using the RDC, more quickly take a person who is not that well trained, or do we have to wait 5 or 10 years to have a Dr. Gurland? I certainly don't mean to imply that a large part of the problem is not training, but I think the RDC would very greatly aid that training.

Uhlenhuth: It would be useful if in further work you could begin to partition out the amount of agreement or disagreement that you might be able to attribute to the systems used and the amount that you might be able to attribute to the skill of the diagnostician.

Spitzer: The other part of the problem is that it just so happens that Dr. Gurland's orientation and mine are rather similar and that is why we happen to have come to this rather good reliability. One could take a very well-trained clinician with a different orientation and show a very poor agreement between his diagnoses and the RDC. The advantage of the RDC is that it makes an orientation explicit and then it can be accepted or rejected.

Blackwell: What happens if you and Dr. Gurland both put on a DSM-II hat and rate 120 patients and then you both put on your RDC hat and rate 120 patients?

Spitzer: I can't put on a DSM-II hat and, in a sense, Dr. Gurland can't really either. Perhaps I should have shown you the DSM-II definition of schizophrenia. It is so general as to not really be a different definition. It is just a general statement and it doesn't tell you how to make the diagnosis, what to do with borderline cases, etc. The DSM-II is not really a different system. The DSM-II was written to offend as few people as possible and to give the general outlines of how different conditions contrast. In a sense, because the DSM-II doesn't really give the specifics, Dr. Gurland is only using DSM-II *categories*. If you asked Dr. Gurland to write out what his notion is of schizophrenia, it probably would not be that different from what we have written in the RDC.

Blackwell: It still seems to me that the only appropriate validity check for the system would be to take the same group of clinicians and give them the same training in both systems and then ask them to rate either the same or different patients.

Spitzer: I thought of that subsequent to hearing some of the criticisms you have made and that Dr. Gurland made, by the way, of this work. Originally, we thought of contrasting DSM-II with RDC, which obviously we did not do. It would be interesting to first give a group of cases to clinicians, tell them to use DSM-II, and then have them use RDC and see whether it changed. We couldn't do it the other way around, because in that case they have already been given specifics. That is a study that perhaps we should do.

Blackwell: One of the things the U.S.–U.K. project showed quite nicely is that the trouble with notes is that the data base is there, whereas with a videotape interview, people trained differently notice different things. They don't just label them differently.

Spitzer: That is quite true. What our approach does is really ignore the problem of the interaction of the interviewer with the patient and, as you point out, how various things are perceived. However, the case records do not obscure different interpretations. For example, it was very clear in going over the case records that Dr. Gurland would very often ignore a statement that the patient was hallucinating, because he decided that it was a hysterical type of hallucination and not a real hallucination, whereas an American or an Eastern-oriented person would more likely take that seriously. On the other hand, you're quite right that the diagnostic process consists of more than just the diagnostic criteria. Our main point is that most studies have shown that the major source of unreliability still is the criteria and not the perception and not even the interaction with the patient. We have done other work in developing interview schedules that try to minimize that variability. In the specific collaborative project that I mentioned, we have a whole structured interview schedule which is very similar to the Present State of Examination of Dr. John Wing. We have also recognized that we have to give examples for many of the concepts that are in the RDC, such as the phrase "obvious overt thought disorder." We have to define that, because there is such a tremendous disparity on what is considered thought disorder. The concept of bizarre or fantastic delusions is another concept which is very important for us, because that's the way to get into either schizo-affective, manic, or depressive. The most common way of getting out of a major depressive illness and into schizo-affective is the presence of fantastic or bizarre delusions. We know we have to give examples of that. This thing kind of gets a momentum of its own and we want to avoid making up a whole glossary of psychiatric terms, although we know we have to do some of that.

Fink: Why is it that the program either ignores or does not widely use physiologic measures of diagnosis? For one thing, you have two facts that would help. Either the historical fact that the patient was previously treated and either responded or not to treatment, or the fact that there are a host of laboratory tests such as sedation threshold, methyl mecholyl, and others which have historical value and provide you with diagnostic criteria.

Spitzer: The reason we are not including response to treatment is that we regard it as validity data, which is, in a sense, external to the system and is the kind of data that we want to test. We want to test whether or not these categories predict treatment response. We couldn't, therefore, include treatment response in the definition of the category. Similarly, if there is schizophrenia in the parents, we don't take that information as part of making the diagnosis of schizophrenia for the same reason. We want to study the genetic variables and how they relate to these categories. As far as the biological tests are concerned, I have been going on the assumption that there were no biological tests that were that reliable or that valid in predicting these conditions.

Fink: To use your kappas 0.54 or 0.35, the methyl mecholyl test will have a kappa of 0.7, the sedation threshold will have a kappa of 0.8. These are very reliable tests.

Spitzer: The reliability is not the question. The question is what its validity is for making these diagnoses. My impression was that they were not that well established. And even if they were established, I guess I would still feel conceptually that these are external validity criteria which we are trying to study. We would certainly hope that other research people would be interested in the clinical criteria and then may want to modify them by, perhaps, including other variables in them.

Whitehead: In the calculation of kappa, you have an extraction for the probability of agreement for two observers by chance. How do you arrive at that and what were those values in your studies?

Spitzer: They are calculated by multiplying the base rates of the condition in question by the two pairs of raters. If one makes the diagnosis of schizophrenia, say 40% and the other one 30%, then the chance expected rate is 0.12.

Zung: Basically, we are talking about agreements, about correlations or r values and then if we square that, the variance. What would you say would be the r value and, consequently, the r^2 of expected disagreement between clinicians, based on your experience and from your going over all the data? In other words, what is the actually observed r and the r^2 of agreement in diagnoses using whatever kinds of data you would like to use? Second, how did you get the fudge factor for the chance alone? And then lastly, what would be the value that, in terms of the r value for prediction, you would like to see to judge as to whether the r number is fair, good, or poor?

Spitzer: These are not r values. They are not, strictly speaking, correlations, because correlations are between continuous variables. These are nominal categories. As I understand it, it is possible to convert a kappa (which is percent of agreement) into a proportion of variance. In fact, Joe Fleiss, our statistician, has written a paper on this in which I think he proved that they are roughly equivalent. That is, a kappa of .8 is roughly equivalent to an r^2, or a .8 proportion of variance. It is not clear to me why people seem to be bothered or do not understand how we calculate kappa or chance corrected agreement. Is it not a fudge factor?

Zung: All I want to know is if you were asked, "What is the correlation or agreement of diagnosis for affective disorders among a group of us?" what kind of figures would you expect here in terms of kappas from your knowledge of the area of diagnosis; how do you figure out this change; and what is the ideal predictive kappa that you would like to actually see that would help further psychopharmacology?

Spitzer: What kind of a predictive value or what kind of a correlation in any kind of research is good? This obviously depends upon what the research question is, how much error you can tolerate, what is the size of your samples. When I stated that generally I would consider a kappa of .7 pretty good, that would also mean that a proportion of variance of .7 is pretty good. Very often in our field, we have to be content with explaining 10 or 20% of the variance, but we obviously would like to explain more. I would like 1.0, but I am very happy if we can get above 0.7 in diagnosis. I would assume that the people in this room not using the RDC but using the standard, would do about as well as people in other studies on reliability of diagnosis of affective illness. I reported this in the summary of six studies and it went in a .3 to .6 range.

Domino: I wonder if you could defend your position with regard to the research development classification of nonaffective schizophrenia? This term is a misnomer. Intuitively, I know what you're getting at. That is, in depression we are dealing with a quantitative disturbance in affect, but in schizophrenia we are talking about quite a different story with regard to flat affect. It seems to me that the term nonaffective schizophrenia is a terrible term.

Spitzer: It is. As I mentioned, we've actually dropped it. We now have schizophrenia, schizo-affective disorder (we don't even call it schizo-affective schizophrenia, because that's the question that everybody's interested in — is schizo-affective disorder really schizophrenia?), and affective illness. In other words, we are trying to apply labels that leave questions open, and that don't pretend that an answer has been found. We only initially used the phrase nonaffective to indicate that it was not schizo-affective disorder, but the concept is schizophrenia in the absence of a major depressive syndrome. It does not exclude schizophrenics who can be quite depressed, but as long as they don't have the whole depressive syndrome, we are happy with the diagnosis of schizophrenia.

Fink: In trying to assess a new compound in 1975, how is one going to select the population? Is this method useful or do you suggest that some other method be used in the selection of patients?

Spitzer: I think that the RDC is a good place to begin to define populations. The approach that we have taken is to look at major categories and then look at subtypes. If the question is for depression, we have actually three types of depression. We have the major depressive syndrome or major affective illness, minor dysphoric illness, and what we call dysphoric personality for people who, throughout their life, seem to react to stress with symptoms of dysphoric mood. The research evidence, and also a kind of clinical intuition, suggest that this is a good place to start with three groups. Within those groups, there are of course subtypes. The bipolar and unipolar distinction is an important one. The psychotic-neurotic distinction is another way of looking at it, although we avoid the use of the term psychotic-neurotic because it is so muddled. We use the phrase incapacitating depression and then we also have a reality-testing-impairment depression. The main advantage that our system has is that it permits communication about what we're dealing with. To say, for example, that we're dealing with a group of mixed, anxious-depressive neurotics really says very little, because within that group will be included some people who have the full endogenous depressive syndrome, some who just have a dysphoric personality and not a real endogenous type of depression, and some who have just an episode of depression. Since there is good reason now to know that those are different types, we think that the RDC is a useful way and we'd be delighted if people started applying it. Although there will be future modifications, the RDC, added as an appendix to our chapter, will at least permit anybody to look at what it looked like at a given point in time. I think the difficulty with using the DSM-II categories is that DSM-II doesn't really give very specific criteria. In identifying patients, if you use the RDC criteria, you will really be giving a much more comprehensive description of what criteria were applied than if you merely said we used the DSM-II categories.

Fink: In relation to using those three classes, how many cases would fit and how many would go undiagnosed?

Spitzer: Most of our experience has been with an inpatient group. We don't have much experience with outpatients. With an inpatient group, about 5% of the patients will be undiagnosed; that is, their present illness would not meet any of our 20 major categories. In our particular inpatient service, about half are schizophrenic and only about 25 or 30% have an affective illness of any type, which is almost always a major depressive illness. There are very few people who are admitted to an inpatient service with a chronic dysphoric personality. I am sure that with an outpatient group you would have a much larger incidence of what we call minor depressive illness and dysphoric personality. We would be delighted if anybody who has access to an outpatient unit would find out what are the distributions of these cases.

Blackwell: I think there is a real paradox in all this. If you go back and read what Kuhn said when he first discovered imipramine, you get a very beautiful description of the type of patient who is, in fact, helped by such antidepressants. However, that is not the group of patients in which they are mostly used. The people in whom they are mostly used are anxious, mixed, affective disorders in outpatients and there is very little evidence, if any, that in these patients those drugs are (a) more effective than placebo, or (b) more specifically effective than any of the other antianxiety agents, such as diazepam or meprobamate. The reason why pharmaceutical industries have such a hard time getting patients is that they stick with Kuhn's original criteria of retarded apathetic vital depressions and when you go to outpatients, of course, those kinds of patients simply aren't there. If you want to prove that a drug is very effective in what Kuhn said these drugs were effective, you have to stick to that kind of patient. If you're content to show that a drug works in anxious outpatients, that is a different thing altogether.

Gershon: I think you are moving toward touching on a problem as to whether there is any drug specificity at all. If there is, then you have to worry about homogenous groups. And if you do worry about homogenous groups, the concern is whether any of the methods proposed this morning will give you homogenous groups. But if they don't apply to homogeneous groups, that would be a very important issue to get an answer to, so that life would be easier for everybody. At the moment, I think we have a series of questions without very good answers and, therefore, the issue of prediction that we're here to address has really not yet been resolved.

Domino: By implication, you have been talking to us with regard to adult psychiatric diagnosis. I wonder if you would comment regarding the whole issue of child psychiatric diagnoses of these categories in children?

Spitzer: You're quite right. The RDC is oriented toward adult diagnoses. As chairman of the APA Nomenclature Committee, I know that we have a real problem with child nosology, but I don't know the answer to it.

Gershon: Apart from how they are labeled, there is a problem in children, whether the pattern of the illness is the same in the child that we're making the analogy to in the adult. This is in no way clearer than it is in manic-depressive disease. We have looked at the children of all of our patients in long-term follow-up and if we use the analogue of what mania or depression looks like in the adult, we don't see these analogues up to the age of 16 in the children. It could well be that we're looking at the wrong thing, that the manifestations are different, that we are not sophisticated in child behavior and, therefore, we're not seeing what we're supposed to. But if we use the adult analogue of this aberrant behavior, then it isn't there, so there is a much bigger problem with child psychiatry.

Predictability in Psychopharmacology: Preclinical and Clinical Correlations,
edited by A. Sudilovsky, S. Gershon and B. Beer. Raven Press, New York,
© 1975.

The Diagnosis of Depression: A Dialectical Dilemma

William W. K. Zung

Duke University Medical Center and Veterans Administration Hospital, Durham, North Carolina 27705

In a previous publication (Zung, 1973), I had examined and discussed the diagnosis of depressive disorders using an epistemologic approach, emphasizing the diversity of the diagnostic process. In this chapter, I attempt to emphasize convergence of the diagnostic process as it is related to depressive disorders. Further, I hope to demonstrate by this approach that the present state of confusion referable to the diagnosis of depressive disorders is more apparent than real.

The following conversation between Dr. E (the expert) and Dr. N (the novice) is a good example of the possibilities for confusion in the diagnosis of depressive disorders.

Dr. N: You should see the new patient who was admitted today. He says that he's blue all the time, down in the dumps, and feels as low as anybody can get. He has crying spells for no reason at all, when ordinarily he never cries. He can't sleep, and keeps waking up in the night. He feels tired in the morning, which is also the worst part of the day for him. He's completely lost his appetite, and lost about 30 pounds in the last two months. Says he doesn't have any interest in sex anymore. In fact, he says he's lost interest in just about everything. He feels knocked out all the time, just no energy. He doesn't enjoy anything, and just feels hopeless about everything. He says that he has trouble thinking clearly, and has trouble making up his mind, even about little things. He feels really worthless and that people would be better off if he were dead.

Dr. E: Sounds like he has a psychotic depression.

Dr. N: During the entire interview, it looked like he never moved. He just sat there like a lump of clay. He talked so slowly that I felt like I had to drag every word out of him.

Dr. E: Sounds like he has a retarded depression.

Dr. N: Funny thing, several months before he came into the hospital, it sounded like he had a period when he felt on top of the world, on cloud nine. He said that he had boundless energy, and could go without sleep for days. He was doing all kinds of things, and felt that the world was going around too slowly for him. From what he says, he must have spent a fortune in buying all kinds of gadgets for his hobby.

Dr. E: Sounds like he has a bipolar depression.

Dr. N: I asked the patient if he knew of anything that brought all this on. He said no, that there hadn't been any changes in his life. He hasn't had any deaths in the family or anyone close he knew. His business is good. He and his wife were getting along fine, and no problems with the children, who all live at home. Nobody's been sick and there just doesn't seem to be any reason for why he should feel the way he does now.

Dr. E: Sounds like an endogenous depression.

Dr. N: He doesn't seem to present with any other psychiatric problems, and he's never had any emotional problems before this.

Dr. E: Sounds like a primary depression.

Dr. N: Dr. E, in your opinion, what do you think is the diagnosis of this patient?

Dr. E: Sounds like he has a major affective disorder, manic-depressive illness, circular type.

Here then is our dilemma: Does the patient have a psychotic depression? A retarded depression? A bipolar depression? An endogenous depression? A primary depression? Or a manic-depressive illness of the circular type? In fact, the patient's present illness can be called by any of these, and they are all applicable. The "correct" diagnosis is dependent on at what stage we listened to the conversation between Dr. N and Dr. E.

Figure 1 is a representation of the pathways by which patients are diagnosed and from which treatment decisions are made for their affective disorders. Starting with the patient in 1–#1 (numbers indicate "Fig. 1, geometric cell # 1"), the patient is examined by a physician who listens to the patient's chief complaint and present illness. During this examination, the physician accumulates information which is sorted out into psychiatric signs and symptoms (1–#2). If we for the moment limit our diagnostic process to affective disorders only, then the physician has to decide whether or not the patient has or does not have depression (or mania) using a set of diagnostic criteria (1–#3). One such example of an operational definition of a depressive disorder is found in Table 1 (Zung, 1965). If the answer is no, then the patient does not need treatment and the flow diagram terminates at 1–#4.

If the answer is yes, then the practicing physician must make a decision as to treatment which was the *raison d'être* for the diagnosis. Here the paths diverge. One pathway for the physician to pursue is to decide on a global basis if the patient has, in addition to his depression, any other psychopathology. Using this clinical global impression, he may then decide to treat the patient with antidepressant, antimanic, antianxiety, or antipsychotic modalities (1–#5), without further recourse to any dialectic on diagnosis.

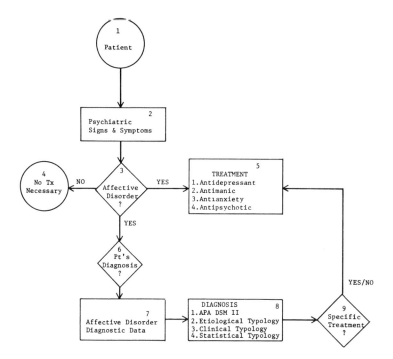

FIG. 1. Diagnosis and treatment of affective disorders based on different dimensions.

These treatment measures can span from pharmacologic agents, to psycho-therapy, to other somatic and psychologic methods.

An alternate path for the physician to pursue at this time is to ask: "What is the patient's diagnosis?" (1–#6). In order to carry out this procedure, the physician will need additional data about the patient (1–#7). We will return to the nature and content of this information after we have examined the various diagnostic procedures.

If we list the most often used nomenclature for depressive disorders, we can see that these can be divided into four basic categories: (1) The American Psychiatric Association, Diagnostic and Statistical Manual, 2nd Edition (1968) or DSM II, (2) labels that are presumed to have etiologic implications, (3) labels that are clinical descriptions of the patient's present illness, and (4) typologies that are statistically derived (1–#8).

Let us examine the DSM II nomenclature closely to see how it is used. Figure 2 is a flow diagram of the decision making processes involved in the DSM II.

2–#1 (PT Affective Disorder) (all #s refer to cells in Fig. 2). We start with a patient who is considered to have an affective disorder with component features of depression and/or mania.

2–#2 (PPT Factor). The first decision made regards whether a precipitat-

TABLE 1. *Criteria for the diagnosis of depressive disorder*

I. Pervasive affect
   1. Depressed, sad
   2. Tearful
II. Physiologic disturbances
   1. Diurnal variation
   2. Sleep: early and frequent waking
   3. Appetite: decreased
   4. Weight: decreased
   5. Libido: decreased
   6. Fatigue, unexplainable
   7. Constipation
   8. Tachycardia
III. Psychomotor disturbances
   1. Agitation
   2. Retardation
IV. Psychologic disturbances
   1. Confusion
   2. Emptiness
   3. Hopelessness
   4. Indecisiveness
   5. Irritability
   6. Dissatisfaction
   7. Personal devaluation
   8. Suicidal rumination

---

ing factor was present or absent. If there is an absence of a precipitating factor, we go on to

2-#3 (Major Affective Disorders). The manual states that the onset of the mood disturbance in this group of disorders does not seem to be related directly to a precipitating life experience (DSM II, pp. 35–36).

2-#4 (Previous Episode?). This is the second decision to be made. Has the patient ever had a previous episode of affective disorder? If the answer is yes, we proceed to #7, but if the answer is no, we go on to

2-#5 (Age: >45 y/o). This is the third decision. If the patient has had no previous episode, what is his present age?

2-#6 (Involutional Melancholia). This is a disorder occurring in the involutional period (>45 y/o) and is distinguishable from manic-depressive illness by the absence of previous episodes, and the disorder is not due to some life experience (DSM II, p. 36).

2-#7 (Manic-Depressive Illness). Patients are given this diagnosis when (1) there is a history of previous episodes, (2) there is no previous history of affective disorder, and the patient is not in the involutional period of his life (DSM II, p. 36).

2-#8 (Mania Only?). Does the patient's present illness consist exclusively of manic episodes?

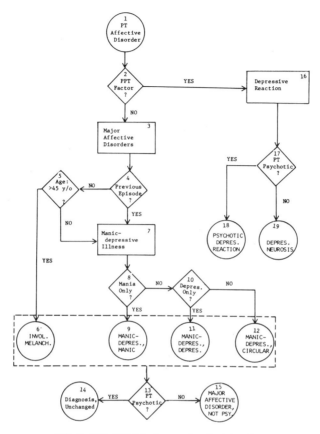

FIG. 2. APA DSM-II diagnostic decision tree.

2-#9 (Manic-Depressive Illness, Manic Type). If the answer to 8 is yes, then the patient is diagnosed as this (DSM II, p. 36).

2-#10 (Depression Only?). Does the patient's present illness consist exclusively of depressive episodes?

2-#11 (Manic-Depressive Illness, Depressed Type). If the disorder consists exclusively of depressed episodes, then this is the appropriate diagnosis (DSM II, pp. 36–37).

2-#12 (Manic-Depressive Illness, Circular Type). If in the present illness the patient has had at least one attack of both a depressive episode and a manic episode, then this is the correct diagnosis (DSM II, p. 37). Some confusion has resulted in using the above labels since they are all listed under the psychoses, and obviously not all patients are psychotic. Therefore, we next ask:

2-#13 (Pt Psychotic?). Psychosis is defined in the manual as when the mental functioning of a patient is (1) sufficiently impaired to interfere grossly with his capacity to meet the ordinary demands of life, (2) when there is a serious distortion in reality testing, (3) when hallucinations and delusions are present (DSM II, p. 23, 38).

2-#14(*Diagnosis Unchanged*). If the patient is psychotic, the diagnosis remains as is.

2-#15 (*Major Affective Disorder, Not Psychotic*). If the patient's diagnosis is one of those in the dotted box (6, 9, 11, 12), but the degree of disturbance is not psychotic, then the manual stipulates that the qualifying phrase *not psychotic* or not presently psychotic should be used (DSM II, pp. 23, 3–4).

Returning to 2-#2:

2-#16 (*Depressive Reaction*). When there is a precipitating factor, the manual recognizes the affective disorder as a reaction to an identifiable event or conflict (DSM II, p. 36).

2-#17 (*Pt Psychotic?*). The same criteria here is applied as in #13 as to whether or not the disturbance of the present illness is or is not of psychotic proportion.

2-#18 (*Psychotic Depressive Reaction*). If the patient's impairment is considered to be psychotic, this is the diagnosis (DSM II, p. 38).

Finally, 2-#19 (*Depressive Neurosis*). If the patient is not psychotic, this is the correct diagnosis (DSM II, p. 40).

Of the other typologies listed in 1-#8, the presumed etiological and clinical are the most often used. These labels represent a shorthand for telling someone else about a patient in a minimum number of words, since underlying each label is a common reference or meaning. Of the etiologic typologies, the endogenous-reactive are the most often used and their diagnostic criteria are listed in Table 2.

Table 3 lists the attributes which have been reported by Perris (1966) of the unipolar and bipolar patients with affective disorders.

Other etiologic typologies are those proposed by Van Praag, Uleman, and Spitz (1965) and by Pollitt (1965). Van Praag et al. (1965) divided the depressions into vital and personal. Vital depressions are primarily affective in sphere in the presence of endoreactive dysthmia with somatic concomitants of the affect. Personal depressions are primarily in sphere of psychic feeling and the existence of the depression is experienced as something rational by the patient. Pollitt suggested a classification of depression based on physiologic disturbances. These include the *S* or somatic type, where symptoms are called collectively, the functional shift, and result from alterations in biologic rhythms, metabolism, and autonomic balance. The second or *J* type is a justified type, where the illness is understandable in terms of the patient's predicament.

Of the various clinical typologies that are used, the psychotic-neurotic

TABLE 2. *Characteristic diagnostic distinctions between endogenous and reactive depressions*

Endogenous depression	Reactive depression
1. Age: older, 40 and over	Younger
2. Family history of depression	No family history present
3. Premorbid personality: normal	Neurotic: inadequate, hysterical, obsessional
4. Precipitating factor: absent	Present
5. Affect: pervasive depression	Less severe or as pervasive
6. Physiologic symptoms A. decreased appetite B. decreased weight C. decreased libido D. increased fatigue	Fewer symptoms, less severe
E. sleep disorder: middle of night and early A.M. wakings	Difficulty in falling asleep
F. diurnal variation: present, depression worse in A.M.	Diurnal variation: absent, depression worse in P.M.
7. Psychomotor activity: retardation, agitation	Less severe
8. Psychologic symptoms: A. loss of interest in life	Less severe
B. self-reproach, guilt, remorse	Self-pity, less guilt
9. Response to ECT: yes	Response to ECT: no

severity continuums are the most often used. Table 4 is a summary of their characteristics.

The agitated-retarded depression typologies focus on a single manifestation of the disorder which is psychomotor activity and readily observed clinically.

TABLE 3. *Characteristic distinctions between unipolar and bipolar psychoses*

Variable	Unipolar psychoses	Bipolar psychoses
1. Affective disturbance	Characterized by recurrent depressions (or manias) of stereotyped symptomatology, and without phases of the opposite polarity	Characterized by the occurrence of both depressive and manic phases
2. Median age at onset	About 45 yr	About 30 yr
3. Family history	Specific heredity for the same form of illness and low for the other within each group More dominant in bipolar than unipolar	
4. Premorbid personality	Predominance of substable or syntonic personality Active, social	Predominance of subvalid or asthenic personality
5. Precipitating factor	No significant differences	Tendency to more frequent "somatic" factors
6. Clinical ratings	No significant differences in anxiety or depression	

TABLE 4. *Characteristic diagnostic distinctions between psychotic and neurotic depressions*

Psychotic depression	Neurotic depression
1. Mood disturbance: pervasive, severely depressed	Minimal, mild, or moderate
2. Physiologic functions (appetite, weight, libido, energy, sleep): markedly decreased	Fewer symptoms, less severe
3. Psychomotor activities: severe retardation or agitation	Minimal, mild, or moderate
4. Psychologic functions: markedly disturbed, may appear to be organic with decreased intellectual and cognitive functions	Fewer symptoms, less severe
5. Loss of capacity to meet ordinary demands of life	Less severe
6. Reality testing: disturbed	Usually intact
7. Delusions, hallucinations: may be present	Absent

The primary-secondary depression classification proposed by Woodruff, Murphy, and Herjanic (1967) could be considered as clinical typologies. A primary depression is defined as a depressive episode occurring in a patient who (1) has a previous history of being well psychiatrically, or (2) had a previous episode of mania or depression and no other psychiatric illness. A secondary depression is defined as a depressive episode occurring in a patient who has had a pre-existing, diagnosable psychiatric illness other than a primary affective disorder (such as organic brain syndrome, schizophrenia, or personality disorders). Thus a primary depression could be thought of clinically as a "pure" depression (or mania), whereas a secondary depression would present clinically as a "mixed" depression.

Other clinical typologies could include anxious, mixed, and masked depression.

The last typologies that are used in the published literature on depressive disorders are those that have been generated from statistical models using multivariate analyses on data from rating scales. Examples of statistical typologies are those published by Overall and Hollister (1964) and Silbermann (1971).

Regardless of which of the typologies one uses in the diagnosis of depressive disorders, there are (1) a basic core of signs and symptoms which the physician uses to determine the presence of the disorder (see Table 1), and (2) additional pieces of information which are necessary for the particular typology. I have summarized the additional data necessary to classify patients using the typologies discussed in Table 5. This is called the Affective Disorder Diagnostic Sheet (ADDS).

These variables represent information about the patient in terms of: (A) demographic data, (B) present illness, (C) past medical history, and (D) family history. Armed with this information, the physician then can diagnose his patient according to almost all of the different ways he chooses. To illustrate this, Table 6 summarizes the different pieces of information

TABLE 5. *Affective Disorder Diagnostic Sheet*

A. DEMOGRAPHIC DATA
    1. Age: _____ years.   Date of Birth: _____.
    2. Sex: male   female
    3. Race: Caucasoid   Negroid   Mongoloid   Other
    4. Marital Status: Single   married   separated   divorced   widowed
    5. Years of education: _____.
    6. Occupation (patient or head of household): _____.
                                                      (Class: 1   2   3   4   5   6   7   8)
B. PRESENT ILLNESS
    1. Precipitating factor: YES, definite   YES, probable   NO
       If YES, what? _____.
    2. Symptoms of depression?   YES   NO
    3. Symptoms of mania?   YES   NO
    4. Severity of illness: Not Psychotic   Psychotic
       If Psychotic:
          1. Loss of reality testing (ex.) _____.
          2. Loss of functional capacity (ex.) _____.
    5. Duration of present illness: _____.
    6. Previous treatment for P.I.?   YES   NO
       If YES, where? _____.
            what? _____.
            and response? _____.
C. PAST MEDICAL HISTORY
    1. Premorbid personality: Normal   Abnormal
       If abnormal, what? _____.
    2. Previous treatment for mental illness: YES   NO
       If YES:
       A. Previous episodes of depression?   YES   NO
       B. Previous episodes of mania?   YES   NO
       C. If previous episode not depression-mania, what? _____.
       D. Number of hospitalizations for mental illness?   0   1   2   3   4   5   or more
       E. For each episode (treatment, hospitalization):

	When?	Where?	Treatment?	Response to Treatment?
1.				
2.				
3.				
4.				
5.				

       F. Age at onset of first manifestation of mental illness? _____ years old.
D. FAMILY HISTORY

	Mother	Father	Sibling
1. Depression-Mania			
2. Schizophrenia			
3. Alcoholism			
4. Other: _____			

that various diagnostic typologies actually use. Conceptually, this is the "Chinese Menu" approach, with the variables obtained from the ADDS listed in their four columns (A, B, C, D) as the bill of fare. Each diagnostician can then, depending on his preference of classification, pick and choose the necessary variables from columns A, B, C, or D to complete his diagnostic

TABLE 6. Diagnosis of depressive disorders by typology using the Affective Disorder Diagnostic Sheet

Affective Disorder Diagnostic Sheet	APA DSM II	Etiological typology		Clinical typology		Statistical typology
		Endogenous-Reactive	Unipolar-Bipolar	Psychotic-Neurotic	Primary-Secondary	
A. DEMOGRAPHIC						
1. Age	x	x	x			x
2. Sex						x
3. Race						x
4. Marital status						x
5. Education						x
6. Occupation						x
B. PRESENT ILLNESS						
1. Precipitating factor?	x	x				x
2. Sxs of depression?	x	x	x	x	x	x
3. Sxs of mania?	x		x		x	x
4. Psychotic?	x	x		x		x
5. Duration of P.I.?						x
6. Previous tx for P.I.?						x
C. PAST MEDICAL HISTORY						
1. Premorbid personality		x	x			x
2. Previous psychiatry hx?	x				x	x
a. Depression?	x		x		x	x
b. Mania?	x		x		x	x
c. Other dx?					x	x
d. Hospitalization?						x
e. Previous tx?						x
f. Age initial onset?						x
D. FAMILY HISTORY						
1. Depression-Mania?		x				x

process. For example, the diagnostician who prefers the DSM II will choose one variable from column A, four from column B, and three from column C. The statistical typologist, on the other hand, will in all probability order and consume everything on the "menu."

For those who want to be the complete diagnostician, we could propose a hypothetical comprehensive code for depressive disorders that would include all typologies. In Table 7, I have listed all the labels and grouped them into their respective origins (DSM II, etiological, clinical, statistical) and proposed a four-digit code. Thus, for our patient who was seen by Dr. N, he could be called a 411X, or a 444X, depending on the diagnostican's personal preference.

The fourth digit or X is what we need to call our attention back to, since it represents a hypothetical typology to be generated by statistical models. This brings us back to our theme, that of predictiveness in psychopharmacology. If we return to Fig. 1, decision box #9, the crucial question is: Can

TABLE 7. *Proposed comprehensive code for depressive disorders*

Diagnostic Code for Depressive Disorders (XXXX)

APA DSM-II (XOOO)
  1. Involutional melancholia
  2. Manic-depressive, manic
  3. Manic-depressive, depressed
  4. Manic-depressive, circular
  5. Psychotic depressive reaction
  6. Depressive neurosis
  7. Other major affective disorder
  8. Cyclothymic personality
  9. Schizophrenia, schizo-affective type
Etiologic typology (OXOO)
  1. Endogenous
  2. Reactive
  3. Unipolar
  4. Bipolar
  5. Vital
  6. Personal
  7. Somatic
  8. Justified
Clinical typology (OOXO)
  1. Psychotic
  2. Neurotic
  3. Agitated
  4. Retarded
  5. Primary
  6. Secondary
  7. Anxious
  8. Mixed
  9. Masked
Statistical typology (OOOX)

we prescribe a more specific and beneficial treatment to a specific patient knowing now all the names by which his malady can be called? Or is the predictiveness of the right treatment for him no better than chance alone, using the old-fashioned clinical global impression?

The science of prediction in psychopharmacology has been considerably advanced by several parallel developments. In the area of mathematical models, the accessibility of computer facilities has made it possible to perform outcome predictions on specified variables. An example of this has been the use of multivariate analysis such as linear discriminate function analysis to predict suicidal behavior (Zung, 1974). In the area of biologic techniques, such studies as sedation thresholds, all-night sleep electroencephalographic recordings, waking EEG frequency analysis, blood enzyme levels, and bioassays for blood levels of psychotropic drugs have all contributed to approaching the goal of predictiveness in psychopharmacology. An example of the combination of mathematical models and biologic data is our work on all-night sleep EEG and the application of the Markov chain process to predict the effects of sleep deprivation (Zung, Naylor, Gianturco, and Wilson, 1966).

To paraphrase Lewis Carroll's *Through the Looking-Glass:*

"The time has come," the Walrus said,
"To talk of many things:
Of shoes–and ships–and sealing-wax
   Of cabbages–and kings
And why the sea is boiling hot
   And whether pigs have wings."

Let us hope that the information in this book—of diagnostic criteria, and statistical principles, and research strategies, of behavioral evaluation, and indoles, and EEG indices—will help to resolve our dialectical dilemma and give us one giant step toward the predictiveness we search for in psychopharmacology.

REFERENCES

Diagnostic and Statistical Manual of Mental Disorders (1968), 2nd edition. American Psychiatric Association, Washington, D.C.

Overall, J. E., and Hollister, L. E. (1964): Computer procedures for psychiatric classification. *JAMA,* 187:583.

Perris, C. (1966): A study of bipolar (manic-depressive) and unipolar recurrent depressive psychoses. *Acta Psychiatr. Scand.,* 42:1–189.

Pollitt, J. D. (1965): Suggestions for a physiological classification of depression. *Br. J. Psychiatry,* 111:489–495.

Silbermann, R. M. (1971): CHAM: A Classification of Psychiatric States. *Excerpta Medica,* Amsterdam.

Van Praag, H. M., Uleman, A. M., and Spitz, J. C. (1965): The vital syndrome interview. *Psychiatr. Neurol. Neurochir.,* 68:329–346.

Woodruff, R. W., Murphy, C. E., and Herjanic, M. (1967): The natural history of affective disorders: 1. Symptoms of 72 patients at the time of index hospital admission. *J. Psychiatr. Res.,* 5:255–263.

Zung, W. W. K. (1965): A self-rating depression scale. *Arch. Gen. Psychiatry,* 12:63–70.

Zung, W. W. K. (1973): From art to science: The diagnosis and treatment of depression. *Arch. Gen. Psychiatry,* 29:328–337.

Zung, W. W. K. (1974): Index of potential suicide: A rating scale for suicide prevention. In: *The Prediction of Suicide,* edited by A. T. Beck, H. Resnik, and D. Lettieri, pp. 221–249. Charles Press, Maryland.

Zung, W. W. K., Naylor, T., Gianturco, D., and Wilson, W. (1966): Computer simulation of sleep EEG patterns using a Markov chain model. In: *Recent Advances in Biological Psychiatry,* edited by J. Wortis, Vol. 8, pp. 335–355. Plenum Press, New York.

DISCUSSION

Domino: I would like to follow up the point that Dr. Max Fink made earlier, because it's very crucial that one introduce as soon as possible research information when one comes to classifying depression or schizophrenia or any other psychiatric illness. There is sufficient information that at least certain depressed cases have low cerebral spinal fluid 5HIA and have low homovanillic acid (HVA). I wonder if the time isn't here today to insist that some of this kind of information be included in any diagnostic procedure? Maybe the day has come when a patient with depression should have a cerebrospinal fluid tap and some of these agents measured.

Zung: Actually, you touched upon my real interests. The development of the depression rating scales is only an adjunct to the clinical neurophysiologic investigations which we have been conducting for the last 15 years. As you know, I am doing sleep EEG studies and developing that kind of a parameter, to be able to correlate it with the patient's depression. So I agree with you. This is really the necessary approach in terms of research strategy, to utilize multivariate analysis. To take laboratory data such as sleep EEG and choose those aspects of it which seem to be clinically and heuristically of value, such as shifts between stage of sleep time and percent time spent in sleep stages one, four, and so forth, as really the fundamental dependent variable and the ratings of depression being the independent variable.

Ayd: I have a problem and I thought for a long time it should be brought to the surface again. Namely, I have never seen a depressed patient who hasn't said to me, "I am depressed because . . ." Now, it is very difficult sometimes to know whether that really is the truth and it is the precipitating factor or it is not. Yet most people do use it as a means of saying this is a neurotic versus a non-neurotic depression. That's the first thing that bothers me and I wish there was some way we could work out a decision among ourselves as to whether or not that is a good way of separating these individuals. Secondly, it depends on at what stage of the illness you see a patient as to whether you would say the symptoms are mild, moderate, or severe. This is sometimes a very important factor in regard to where you finally pigeonhole the patient. Last, but not least, we have now reached the point where we have to factor in the impact of any medication that the patient is taking, not necessarily for the depression, but which may be contributing to the depression or which may be altering the symptoms. For example, I have just finished comparing patients seen 20 years ago with depression versus patients seen last year with depression. Twenty years ago, the vast majority of the patients I saw had, in fact, weight loss. That is not true today and even though they have anorexia, they don't necessarily lose weight. Sometimes, this is because of medication they are taking for other purposes and, although they're taking an inadequate dose of an antidepressant, by the time they get to me, that is enough to change some of the clinical symptoms which would affect how some patients would be categorized. This is important, because ultimately people end up saying a drug is good for *this* type of depression, but not *that* type of depression and that's not necessarily consistent at all with what is really happening in the clinic.

Zung: Your first point is about using a precipitating factor yes/no. One of the reasons we ascertain this is that it has to do with our therapy to the patient, so if the answer is yes, we are going to do psychotherapy along the lines of working through the precipitating factor. But if we look at it also in terms of typology we can, in fact, "through research" find out whether this does or does not make a difference with respect to final outcome, treatment choice, and so forth, and it may be that if you hold that variable and parcel it out, it may or may not be important, depending upon the drug. In terms of the time course and how we rate it, that would be in the Affective Disorder Diagnostic Sheet (ADDS), where we do find out how long the duration was of the present illness. We do try to build it into our ratings and eventually we can do combination prospective-retrospective ratings for the patient. In terms of changing pictures of symptomatology, this simply says that when we come to our typologies and variables, we are going to have to put new weights as we develop them. It is going to be a kind of constant updating process of our variables and the weights for each variable in the psychometric scales that are commonly used and that are available.

Spitzer: Dr. Zung has performed a real service to us by presenting in a flow-chart fashion exactly what DSM-II does. I have never seen it done quite that elegantly and I think it is absolutely correct. But, at the same time, we should realize by examining it what are the assumptions built into that system and whether they really make sense. Dr. Ayd's question really is, does it make very much sense? He is talking about the reliability of the question of whether or not there are precipitating events. There is another very real problem and that is whether it is true that so-called typical endogenous depressions (that is, typical in the sense of the clinical picture) are not associated with a precipitating event. The research answer is that very often they are, so that the notion that precipitating events are mutually exclusive with the clinical picture of endogenous symptomatology is just not correct. DSM-II does say that the major way that you should divide up depressions is by precipitating events. Dr. Zung is quite right. I think that's a very bad way to divide up depressions. The first question should be, are you dealing with the full depressive syndrome, or the so-called endogenous clinical picture, or are you dealing with someone who is very depressed but doesn't have either physiologic or other disturbances? We call the first one major depressive illness, the second one, minor depressive illness. I think you have to teach the DSM-II system to residents and this is a good way to do it, but they should be taught that this is really a mythology in many ways and we should not build into our classification system concepts which have not really yet been demonstrated. That's why we are, in a sense, moving backwards to a simpler system. Is there a full depressive syndrome? And within that, does it make all the various distinctions that Dr. Zung has mentioned? I might also mention that in your four types of classifications, very often you are going to have a problem in that they are not really mutually exclusive. So it doesn't quite fit into those four digits as nicely as Dr. Zung wants. Within our system we have all of the types that Dr. Zung mentioned and we end up with about a dozen of them. They are all non-mutually exclusive and it is a research question as to which of those are going to be valid and which of them are quite trivial.

Weinryb: It's been said that we live in an age of depression and I assume that this is because a greater proportion of patients are being diagnosed as depressed now, relative to some years ago. Does this bias tend to be eliminated by use of the RDC system?

Spitzer: RDC gives explicit criteria and tells people how to apply them. I don't know if I understand exactly what you mean by the bias. There would be a bias only if, in fact, less people were depressed now. I am not aware that there are any serious studies showing this.

Ayd: It is a fact that we do have an increase in depression which is both factual and real, partly because doctors are diagnosing depression more. But I think we have to factor in that we have more people living in an age group where depression is more likely to occur. We certainly are not only living in that age group but we have people with various psychologic or physical disorders which have associated a rather high incidence of depression, for example, cardiovascular disorders. We are also living in an era where there is an epidemic of licit drug taking and a large number of these compounds are, in fact, depressogenic for some individuals. We have to factor in that as the use of certain antihypertensive agents, certain steroids, certain estrogenic preparations, and so forth, increases, we are bound to see an increase in the incidence of depression. And last, but not least, more people are seeing doctors. In some countries, for example, where national health insurance went into effect and more people therefore started going to see psychiatrists, the incidence of depression automatically went up.

Zung: Another alternative is that depression is always underdiagnosed. So even if we now had the same population, the same pool, and nothing else of what Dr. Ayd has enumerated, that alone will make depression higher in terms of epidemiology.

Gershon: This dilemma is something that plagues the pharmaceutical industry because they're told, and it's epitomized by the comment that you made, that there is a large and increasing population of people diagnosed as depressives and when they go out to try their new experimental agent on this large and increasing population of depressives, they could not get a population of depressives to do the study anywhere. There are logical explanations for this, but it is a dilemma that they're faced with.

Uhlenhuth: We have to ask the question, "Is there more depression compared to what?" The only piece of data I have on that is from a general population survey that we did in the city of Oakland where, if you speak in a very non-specific way about depressive complaints, you do find that people report more depressive mood than they do anxious mood. That's as of 1971. There are no prior data to compare that with in reference to the question, "Has there been a change?" On the other hand, in my own clinical work as head of an outpatient department, I have noticed in a sample from recent years in Chicago and in another from the early 1960s at Hopkins, that there really does appear to be less anxiety available for studies if one looks for such patients. I have heard this from others as well and the assumption that I make about it is that the antianxiety agents have, in fact, exerted a significant effect in making it possible to control that group in general practice, so that they don't land in a university psychiatry clinic.

Whitehead: Your system appears to give us a very large number of possible diagnostic categories. What does that add to predicting outcome and selecting samples for studies?

Zung: I was not proposing any system. I was putting this thing together as a way of presenting the available methods for diagnosing patients and I only did this as a dialectical discourse, as a method of teaching to this group. It's not a method whatsoever. In terms of selecting patients, we collect the information on the ADDS, because from that we can then type the patient in any way that is known. Based upon those data, we can tell, in whatever language you want to speak, what the diagnosis is. That is one thing we do. In terms of selecting patients for drug studies, another thing that we do is to use a physician clinical global impression scale, with a cutoff number between one and seven, and a self-rating instrument of some kind with also a cutoff number there. If the patient has a score of certain value, then he can come into the study. As much as I think self-ratings are good for following patients and in terms of looking at data, I think that the doctor's ratings in terms of clinical global impression are best for selecting patients.

Predictability in Psychopharmacology: Preclinical and Clinical Correlations,
edited by A. Sudilovsky, S. Gershon and B. Beer. Raven Press, New York,
© 1975.

Prediction of Clinical Activity of Psychoactive Drugs: Application of Cerebral Electrometry in Phase-I Studies

Max Fink

*Health Sciences Center, State University of New York at Stony Brook, Stony Brook,
New York 11790*

New psychoactive compounds are usually developed by the manipulation of known active chemical structures and are identified as psychoactive in animal screening tests which define properties that are the silhouettes of known compounds. Occasionally, active compounds are identified by serendipity in clinical trials. These methods are time-consuming and expensive and, in early human trials, subject the first volunteers to risks that are difficult to justify.

As the number of compounds for testing has increased, we have become more concerned with the safety of our studies in man, particularly with the possible interference with the rights of the subjects. Our naturalistic methods of assay in man are increasingly restricted, and new safe methods of assay are needed.

To improve our prediction of psychoactive properties of treatments, we and others have applied quantitative measures of brain functions. These methods are derived from classic electroencephalography, but differ so significantly from the usual clinical practice of this art that we have suggested cerebral electrometry as a name for the systematic measurement of cerebral electrical activity by digital computer methods (Fink, *in press*).

The methods derive from the view that disorders in brain function underlie many emotional illnesses. In the absence of a confirmed etiology and a specific therapy, the amelioration of many abnormal mental conditions depends on inducing changes in brain function. In attempting to understand the processes in pharmacotherapy, convulsive therapy, and other "biologic" therapies, it was necessary to develop a heuristic classification of known psychoactive drugs and treatments. Such classification schemes based on changes in brain function in man were developed during the past decade. This chapter describes one scheme and explores two applications of cerebral electrometry: the prediction of clinical activity of putative psychoactive compounds, and as a measure of CNS equivalence and bioavailability. The technical issues of recording, analysis, and classification of electrical activity, the selection of subjects, and the systematic nature of the experiments required for these studies will not be described. The interested reader is referred to methodologic summaries in Fink, Itil, and Shapiro (1967), Fink (1974), Shapiro and Glasser (1974), and Fink et al. (*this volume*).

DEVELOPMENT OF A CLASSIFICATION SCHEME

The recording of changes in the electrical activity of the brain from the intact scalp of man was achieved slightly less than 50 years ago. The initial publications found the electroencephalogram (EEG) to change with wakefulness, performance of tasks, and altered metabolism. The EEG also responded to changes in oxygen, carbon dioxide, and glucose in the blood, and with many drugs. By 1954, it was possible to relate drug effects, EEG, and behavior such that "shifts in the pattern of the electroencephalogram in the direction of desynchronization occurred in association with anxiety, hallucinations, fantasies, illusions, or tremors, and in the direction of synchronization with euphoria, relaxation, and drowsiness" (Wikler, 1954).

To test this hypothesis was tedious and highly subjective, since descriptions of the EEG were limited to visual identification of pattern changes or to manual measurement of frequencies and amplitudes. The development of analogue frequency analyzers and amplitude integrators allowed more systematic analyses of some aspects of the EEG.

Barbiturates induce a sharp increase in 18 to 24 Hz beta activity in a spindling pattern. This effect was considered characteristic and was used by Shagass and others to measure the cerebral response to amobarbital in the "sedation threshold" test. It was relatively easy to distinguish the decrease in beta activity and the increase in slow waves following chlorpromazine from this barbiturate type of activity.

To separate the effects of chlorpromazine from imipramine was more difficult but, by using an analogue frequency analyzer and rigorous control over daily dosages, we were able to separate these two drugs from each other and from placebo (Fink, 1961, 1963b, 1965). Chlorpromazine increased delta (3.0 to 4.5 Hz) and theta (4.5 to 7.5 Hz) activities and reduced beta activity (13.5 to 33.0 Hz), whereas imipramine decreased alpha (8.0 to 12.0 Hz) activity and increased fast beta (22.0 to 33.0 Hz) and theta (5.0 to 7.5 Hz) activities. Placebo use was associated with an increase in theta activity.

We next studied the phantastica and were able to distinguish two classes, deliriants and hallucinogens (Fink, 1960; Itil and Fink, 1966). Ditran, atropine, diethazine, and benactyzine—potent central anticholinergic drugs—elicited increases in both theta and fast beta activities with a reduction in alpha activity. These drugs stimulated the illusory symptoms, motor restlessness, and decreased consciousness characteristic of deliriants. The hallucinogens lysergide (LSD-25) and mescaline also increased fast frequencies, but slow waves and alpha activity decreased. Although the sub-

TABLE 1. EEG patterns of psychoactive drugs

Class	EEG pattern	Frequency (Hz)						Amplitude		Bursts		Example
		Δ (0–3.5)	Θ (3.5–7.5)	α (7.5–13)	β_1 (13–22)	β_2 (22–33)	Var.	Int.	Var.	ΔB	sp	
Ia	Slowing	+	++	±	0	−	−	+	0	+	+	Chlorpromazine
Ib	Slowing with inc. alpha	+	++	++	0	±	−	+	−	0	0	Butaperazine
Ic	Slowing with inc. seizure	0	+	−	0	0	±	+	−	+	+	Reserpine
IIa	Fast activity, inc. ampl.	0	0	0	++	+	+	+	+	0	−	Amobarbital
IIb	Fast activity, dec. ampl.	0	−	−	+	++	+	−	+	−	+	Amphetamine; LSD
IIIa	Fast and slow activity	++	+	−	+	++	+	−	+	−	±	Ditran, atropine
IIIb	Fast and slow activity, inc. seizure	+	++	−	+	+	+	−	+	+	0	Imipramine
IVa	Alpha variation, increase	0	0	+	0	0	−	+	+	±	0	Morphine, alcohol
IVb	Alpha variation, decrease	0	0	−	0	0	+	−	0	0	0	Iproniazid

Inc.: +, increase; 0, no effect. Dec.: −, decrease; ±, variable.
Var.: variability; sp, spikes; ΔB, change in burst activity; Int., integration.
(From Fink, 1969a.)

jects exhibited illusory sensations and anxiety, they did not show the ob-
tunded consciousness or the motor restlessness of the deliriants (Fink,
1959, 1960, 1963a; Itil and Fink, 1966).

Although these observations were interesting and seemed consistent
with the initial EEG-behavioral hypothesis, the EEG pattern of only a few
substances had been characterized by 1961. In a symposium at the World
Congress of Psychiatry in Montreal, the participants reported data for a
variety of antipsychotic drugs and minor tranquilizers that seemed consistent with, and extended, this hypothesis (Fink, 1963a). Because the
known antidepressants were so diverse, however, they did not fit these
observations and a more useful formulation was published eight years
later (Fink and Itil, 1969b).

In 1967, as part of a 10-year review of impact of psychopharmacology
on psychiatry (Efron, Cole, Levine, and Wittenborn, 1969), we reviewed
the data of many studies of the scalp EEG and psychotropic drugs in man.
More than 600 reports were published from 1951 to 1962 (Fink, 1964).
Although much data was poorly quantified or described incompletely, it
was possible to find reports where dosages of established compounds were
within the usual therapeutic ranges for psychiatric patients, and the EEG
changes were described in sufficient detail to allow a classification based on
nine patterns of drug effects in the alert EEG (Table 1). These patterns
were based chiefly on hand and eye measurements of frequency, frequency
variability, amplitude, amplitude variability, delta bursts, and spikes,
supplemented by analogue power spectral data (Fink, 1969a,b).

Using this classification, we reviewed the available EEG data for each
clinically used drug and assigned each drug to an appropriate class. We
found drugs with similar EEG effects to have similar clinical effects (Table
2). Whereas we could have been victims of circular reasoning — we have
used a set of data to define the classification scheme, and then allocated
the same data into the classes — the data provided hypotheses which could
be tested both by studies of known clinically active drugs not used in the
classification, and by studies of new drugs not previously classified.

We applied this classification scheme to two immediate problems. Examining the variety of clinically active antidepressants, we found that they
did not fit a single electrographic type (Fink and Itil, 1969b) (Table 3). We
were able to distinguish four classes of these compounds, which were also
distinguishable from the effects of convulsive therapy (Volavka, Feldstein,
Abrams, and Fink, 1972). This diversity in the neurophysiology of the
available antidepressant treatments was consistent with the diversity in the
classification of depressive illnesses and in opinions as to the relative
efficacy of the treatments.

Examining the known phantastica, it was possible to separate four classes
of neurophysiologic effects, which provided a continuum from the indole
hallucinogens to the anticholinergic deliriants (Fink and Itil, 1969a) (Table

TABLE 2. Classification of drugs by EEG criteria

Class I: Increased slowing of EEG frequencies

Ia.	Ib. Increased alpha	Ic. Increased seizure activity
chlorpromazine	butaperazine	reserpine
chlorprothixene	fluphenazine	
(fluphenazine)	perphenazine	(amitriptyline)
haloperidol	thioproperazine	(bemegride)
pinoxepin	trifluoperazine	cycloserine
thioridazine		diphenhydramine
thiothixene		prochlorperazine
trifluperidol		promazine
triflupromazine		(promethazine)
(bromides)		
(lithium)		

Class II: Increased fast activity

IIa. Increased amplitude	IIb. Decreased amplitude
amobarbital	amphetamine
chlordiazepoxide	bemegride
diazepam	dimethyltryptamine
ethchlorvynol	di-ethyltryptamine
fenfluramine	epinephrine
glutethimide	lysergide (LSD-25)
meprobamate	mescaline
methylpentynol	methamphetamine
pentobarbital	methylpenidate
phenobarbital	phenmetrazine
secobarbital	psilocybin
thiopental	

Class III: Increased slow and fast activity

IIIa. Maximum amplitude decrease	IIIb. Little amplitude decrease
atropine	amitriptyline
benactyzine	cyclazocine
diethazine	imipramine
Ditran	levomepromazine
(phencyclidine)	nalorphine
scopolamine	promethazine

Class IV:

IVa. Alpha variation, increase	IVb. Alpha variation, decrease
alcohol (ethyl)	(azacyclonol)
heroin	benactyzine
(hydroxyzine)	(deanol)
morphine	iproniazid
methadone	(isocarboxazid)
(sulthiame)	(isoniazid)
	(nialamide)
	pipradol
	(tranylcypromine)

(From Fink, 1969a.) Drugs in parentheses, "classification probable."

4). The parallelism in EEG classification extended to the physical and physiologic effects, to the associated behaviors, and to the types of hallucinatory activity induced.

Thus by 1969 a hypothesis of the relation of EEG and behavioral change

TABLE 3. *EEG patterns of clinically active antidepressants*

	Frequency						Amplitude	
	Δ (0–3.5 Hz)	Θ (3.5–7.5 Hz)	α (7.5–13 Hz)	β_2 (13–22 Hz)	β_2 (22–33 Hz)	Vari-ability	Inte-gration	Vari-ability
I. Tricyclics								
Ex. Imipramine	+	++	−	+	++	+	−	+
II. MAO Inhibitors								
Ex. Iproniazid	0	0	−	0	0	+	−	+
III. Phenothiazines								
Ex. Thioridazine	±	++	0/−	±	−	−	+	0
IV. Stimulants								
Ex. Dextroamphetamine	0	−	−	+	++	+	−	+

+ = increase; − = decrease; ± = variable; 0 = no change.
(From Fink and Itil, 1969*b*.)

had been formulated and assessed against prevailing compounds. The data fit the view, for alert man and particularly for psychiatric patients, that the EEG changes in direct relation to the amount and duration of psychoactive drug administered; and that the accompanying behavioral changes are the result of the cerebral biochemical events which are reflected in cerebral electrical activity:

An increase in the amount of EEG slow wave activity (with or without an increase in amplitude) is associated with decreased perceptual discrimination, slowed motor activity, heightened mood, reduced intensity and rate of thoughts, and decreased recall of learned material.

Increased EEG beta activity with an increase in amplitudes and regularity of rhythms, particularly of the spindling variety, are accompanied by behavioral effects which are similar to those accompanying increased slow wave activity, but with increased duration of sleep and reduced affect, particularly of fear and anxiety. Drugs which develop beta spindling also elicit tolerance rapidly, inhibit seizures, and may be associated with spontaneous grand mal convulsions on rapid withdrawal of medication.

When beta activity is enhanced and amplitudes are decreased, mood is heightened and stimuli are perceived more acutely and more clearly. When frequent and prolonged periods of low voltage recording or loss of frequencies also occur, subjects report illusions or hallucinations, increased psychomotor activity, tremors, fears, and reduced sleep duration.

Delirium, with reduced perceptual acuity and recall and increased psychomotor restlessness, is associated with increases in both beta and slow wave frequencies.

When the amounts or the amplitude of alpha activity are enhanced,

TABLE 4. *Comparison of different classes of phantastica*

	Class of drug			
Variable	Indole (lysergide, mescaline)	Stimulants (dextroamphetamine)	Thymoleptic (imipramine, high doses)	Anticholinergic (atropine)
Behavior				
Consciousness	alert; fluctuating rapid thoughts; difficulty in concentration	alert (hyper-alert)	drowsy; sluggish thoughts; complains of memory loss and confusion	drowsy, stupor to coma; blocked thoughts; memory loss, disorientation, confusion
Perception	colorful visual hallucinations, often pleasant; spatial distortion; altered body image	enhanced brightness, effects similar to indole in toxic doses	illusions, occasionally unpleasant	auditory hallucinations, unpleasant
Mood	euphoria; heightened intensity of experience; occasional panic and fear; decreased irritability	euphoria; increased intensity of experience; irritable	pleasant, occasional dysphoria; irritable	dysphoric, irritable and aggressive; fear of death
Motor	weakness, lassitude; occasional restlessness	restless; increased activity	occasionally restless; increased interaction	agitated, very restless (unless in stupor)
Speech	rapid, voluble	talkative	little change	slurred, impoverished
Physical				
Pupil	dilated	minimal change	minimal change	dilated
Heart rate	increase	increase	no change	increase
Blood pressure	increase	no change	no change	little change
Reflexes	increase	little change	decrease may occur	decrease
Salivation	little change		decrease	dry mouth

TABLE 4 (Continued)

Variable	Class of drug			
	Indole (lysergide, mescaline)	Stimulants (dextroamphetamine)	Thymoleptic (imipramine, high doses)	Anticholinergic (atropine)
EEG				
Alpha abundance	decrease	no change (?)	decrease	decrease
Alpha mean frequency	increase	small increase	no change (decrease)	decrease
Beta abundance	increase	increase	increase	increase
Theta abundance	no change (decrease)	no change (decrease)	increase	increase (in high dosage)
Delta abundance	none (or decrease)	none	small increase	increase (in high dosage)
Amplitude	decrease	no change	small decrease	decrease
Variability	increase	minimal increase	increase	marked increase

(From Fink and Itil, 1969a.)

subjects report increased relaxation, reveries, pleasant fantasies, feelings of well-being, euphoria and heightened mood.

But the methods of classification were still subjective and systematic methods of evaluation were yet to be developed. During this time digital computer methods were applied to the reduction of the extensive EEG data and to the classification scheme (Fink et al., 1967; Fink, Shapiro, Hickman, and Itil, 1968). As we developed a greater facility in data analysis, we turned our attention to applications of the classification scheme. One problem was the prediction of the clinical effects of new drugs using EEG measures in volunteer subjects.

PREDICTION OF CLINICAL ACTIVITY

In an early classification study using digital computer methods, we examined different doses of amobarbital in female volunteers, comparing 50, 100, and 300 mg sustained-release formulations (Fink et al., 1968). We were able to distinguish the three dosage forms and found the principal criterion to be the amount of slow waves. Our sample was small and we thought that the slow waves were probably more directly related to a failure to control the state of vigilance of the subjects than as characteristic of amobarbital.

Fenfluramine

In a replication of this study, we added dextroamphetamine and a chemically related new compound, fenfluramine. In dose-finding studies, single doses of 40 mg of fenfluramine and 10 mg of dextroamphetamine effectively altered the EEG within 4 hr without danger to the adult volunteers and with minimal behavioral effects. The drugs were then given orally in a crossover study (Fink, Shapiro, and Itil, 1971).

We observed changes in the EEG for all drugs. When we contrasted their EEG patterns, we found that both doses of amobarbital were highly correlated (+0.80); dextroamphetamine was poorly correlated with the two doses of barbiturate (−0.05, +0.47); and the changes after fenfluramine were better correlated with amobarbital (+0.69, +0.91) than with dextroamphetamine (+0.55).

The significance of these findings was not immediately apparent for, in 1967, fenfluramine was being tested as an anorexigenic agent with presumed stimulating central effects. As clinical experience developed, however, the behavioral effects of fenfluramine were not those of stimulation, but of sedation. Independent EEG studies of the effects on the all-night sleep EEG also showed fenfluramine to be similar to a soporific-sedative (Oswald, Jones, and Mannerheim, 1968). In retrospect, we had defined an important psychoactive property of fenfluramine in the quantitative EEG assessment.

Cyclazocine

We next studied cyclazocine, a narcotic antagonist undergoing clinical trials in the treatment of opiate dependence. In dosage trials, we observed EEG changes similar to imipramine — an increase in theta and beta activities and a reduction in alpha activity. At the time these examinations were done, the profile method was not yet established and we made judgments of these changes by visual assessment of the records and from analogue frequency data (Fink, Itil, Zaks, and Freedman, 1969).

We were sufficiently impressed by the similarity of the EEG effects of cyclazocine to imipramine to predict that cyclazocine would exhibit clinical antidepressant properties. Clinical trials were undertaken in outpatients and well-defined antidepressant activity was observed at half the dosages used in postwithdrawal narcotic addicts in two separate clinical studies (Abbuzzahab, 1970; Fink, Simeon, Itil, and Freedman, 1970).

Doxepin

In the amobarbital-fenfluramine studies we were concerned that different rates of gastrointestinal absorption may have diffused the drug effects. For our study of another presumed psychoactive compound, doxepin, we elected an intravenous study. We first determined intravenous dosages that elicited distinct EEG effects and minimal behavioral effects. These dosages were then systematically given to male volunteers, with doxepin (0.2 mg/kg), imipramine (0.45 mg/kg), and diazepam (0.15 mg/kg) each given in 2 cc saline in 1 min, compared to 2 cc saline alone. Experiments were done in a latin square design in weekly sessions in male volunteers. The two comparison drugs were selected because doxepin, in laboratory studies, was thought to be an anxiolytic and antidepressant (Simeon, Spero, and Fink, 1969).

We found each compound to elicit a different pattern of EEG effects. Imipramine increased theta (4 to 7.5 Hz) and beta-2 (18 to 22.5 Hz) activities; diazepam had a very rapid effect, eliciting extensive beta activity, decreased alpha (8 to 12 Hz) and some delta (1.1 to 4 Hz) activities; placebo had no effect on any frequencies; and doxepin elicited increases in delta, theta, and beta-2 frequencies, and a marked decrease in alpha activity. In amplitude, all drugs acted similarly. The average frequency increased for diazepam, decreased for doxepin, whereas placebo and imipramine had little effect.

When we examined the EEG patterns across 20 variables, we found correlations of -0.06 for diazepam/imipramine, $+0.76$ for doxepin/imipramine, and $+0.22$ for diazepam/doxepin. We concluded that since the EEG profile of doxepin was most similar to imipramine, it should exhibit active thymoleptic properties. Since this determination, clinical studies of doxepin describe it as an effective antidepressant with sedative qualities.

Experimental Compounds

Based on these experiences, we sought to examine new compounds before or concurrently with their clinical testing. In 1969 we assayed three compounds for their EEG profiles: CP-14,368, S-42,548 (mazindol), and GP-41,299. In dose-finding studies, we determined that 250 mg CP-14,368, 4.0 mg S-42,548, and 75 mg GP-41,299 elicited behavioral effects in volunteers. In our first systematic oral classification study, 12 male volunteers received these compounds and placebo at weekly intervals in a latin square design.

We failed to define significant changes in the EEG variables for CP-14,-368. For S-42,548, we recorded systemic effects of nausea, decreased appetite, insomnia and irritability, and a preliminary pattern on EEG that would classify it with amitriptyline. For GP-41,299, we found decreases in amplitude and alpha activity, and increased theta and beta activities – a profile similar to that of doxepin.

Although we suggested further studies with S-42,548 and CP-14,368, we were not sanguine that a clinical profile would be readily elicited. S-42,-548 has since been marketed as an anorexigenic compound. Anecdotal reports suggest it has stimulant and antidepressant activity, although these have not been systematically assayed. For GP-41,299, however, we believed that clinical trials were warranted in populations responsive to doxepin. One study in anxious outpatients has recently been completed, and antianxiety activity at dosages to 400 mg/day, averaging 200 mg/day, has been reported (Gaztanaga, Abrams, Simeon, Jones, and Fink, 1972).

Between 1971 and 1973, we examined seven additional numbered, presumed psychoactive compounds by the EEG profile method (GPA-1714, U-28,774, AHR-1118, ORF-8063, OI-63, RO-3350, PR-F-36-CL). We have made specific predictions of clinical applications for each of these compounds. Although the clinical data is as yet incomplete for each compound, we are encouraged by the reports. For compounds which exhibited a well-defined EEG profile, an association with the clinical effects has either been demonstrated or is still in assay; and for none for which we have failed to define a profile has a clinical application been accepted (Table 5) (Fink, 1974).

While we have proceeded with these studies, Itil in St. Louis has reported similar EEG assays of 16 presumed psychoactive compounds, using not only the waking EEG but also sleep studies and evoked averaged potentials (Table 5). His assays of molindone, loxapine, and tranxene have already been confirmed by clinical trials and by clinical experience since these compounds have been introduced in practice.

TABLE 5. *Drugs classified by quantitative methods in man since 1967*

Classified and confirmed			Classified, awaiting confirmation		
Antipsychotic	year	author		year	author
trifluperidol	69	3	mesoridazine	72	2
haloperidol	70	2	molindone	70	2
thiothixene	69	1	SQ 11,290	72	2
perphenazine	69	2	P-5227	69	2
fluphenazine	71	2	CI-686	73	2
			loxapine	73	2
Sedative (antianxiety)					
chlordiazepoxide	69	2	chlorazepam	72	2
diazepam	68	1	tranxene	72	2
tybamate	69	1	SCH-12,041	71	2
fenfluramine	71	3	U-31,889	72	2
thiopental	69	3	U-28,774	71	1
			ORF-8063	72	1
			U-31,920	73	2
			bromazepam (RO5–3350)	73	1
Thymoleptic					
imipramine	58	1	GB-94 (mianserin)	72	2
amitriptyline	72	3	MK-940	70	2
protriptyline	73	2	GP-41299	72	1
			cyclazocine	69	3
			OI-77	72	2
			doxepin	69	1
			S42–548 (mazindol)	71	1
Stimulant					
dextroamphetamine	71	3	AHR 1118	71	1
			centrophenoxin	73	4
			A-34,519	73	2
			CP 14,368	71	1
			PR-F-36-CL	73	1
			OI-63	73	1
Antimanic					
			cinanserin	71	2
Euphoriant					
cannabis (THC-Δ-9)	71	1,4	GPA 1714	72	1
diacetylmorphine	70	1			

Authors: 1, Fink; 2, Itil; 3, Fink and Itil; 4, Others.

One recent study is of particular interest, that of GB-94 (mianserin). GB-94 is a new pharmaceutical with antiserotonin activity in pharmacology studies. In an application of the EEG profile method, Itil evaluated GB-94, rapidly reported that it had a profile most like amitriptyline, and recommended a clinical trial as an antidepressant.

We undertook an independent comparison of GB-94 and amitriptyline in our laboratory. The EEG effects of amitriptyline become prominent $1\frac{1}{2}$ to 2 hr after oral administration with a profile at 30 mg single doses which is similar to our earlier observation with imipramine. GB-94 has been tested at five, 10, and 15 mg single doses; the EEG profile is clearly that of the thymoleptic class with increased theta and beta activities and a sharp reduction in alpha activities. These changes are well defined within 40 min of oral administration, reflecting perhaps a high central penetrance for this compound. Our assay clearly confirms the earlier reports of Itil.

Clinical trials of mianserin have been undertaken in a number of laboratories in Europe. In a conference in October, 1973, the data of more than 500 cases were presented, with the initial evaluation confirming the thymoleptic activity of mianserin, a potency and activity similar to amitriptyline with fewer side effects, and a more rapid onset of activity.

Our classification of one novel compound, PR-F-36-CL, is an example of the data available in such a study (Fink et al., *this volume*). We have emphasized the EEG data but, in each study, we examine behavioral variables as carefully. We are impressed with the EEG-behavioral correlations, and accept an EEG classification more readily when concurrent behavioral data are consistent with the EEG data. PR-F-36-CL was studied as an anorexigenic. In the EEG profile study, we sought to contrast its central effects with dextroamphetamine and fenfluramine. The studies, both in EEG and behavior, define its similarity to dextroamphetamine, suggesting a clinical profile dissimilar from fenfluramine.

A MEASURE OF BIOAVAILABILITY

As we studied the EEG-dose relations for barbiturates and psychoactive drugs, we inquired as to the applicability of the EEG measures as evidence of rate of onset, duration, and intensity of drug effects on the brain, as a measure of CNS "bioavailability," or "neurophysiologic equivalence."

CNS Equivalence of Two Doxepin Formulations

Following a profile analysis of doxepin (Simeon et al., 1969), an opportunity arose to assess the EEG profile method as a measure of CNS bioavailability. Doxepin (Sinequan®) received an NDA from the U.S. Food and Drug Administration in 1969. In 1970, a cross-licensing arrangement with another manufacturer allowed the sale of doxepin under another trademark and formulation by an alternate means of manufacture. The question was asked whether the new formulation required extensive clinical evaluations or could an equivalence at the site of action of the two formulations be demonstrated? We undertook a fixed dose study in latin square design in male volunteers (Fink, 1974). Twelve subjects received 25 mg each of doxepin

"A," doxepin "B," and placebo. The EEG was recorded for 20 min before and for two hr after oral administration. We found the EEG effects of the two formulations to be the same as our earlier studies of doxepin—with increases in theta-delta (to 7.5 Hz) and in fast beta (>18.5 Hz), and decreases in amplitudes and in alpha and slow beta (7.5 to 18.5 Hz) frequencies. Variability of frequencies and amplitudes increased, as did the number of artifacts. We thus found the two formulations of doxepin to be equivalent, but we could not answer the question of the sensitivity of the methods.

Doxepin Hydrochloride and Doxepin Pamoate

We next determined the EEG profiles of capsules containing doxepin hydrochloride, and a liquid formulation of doxepin pamoate. In dose-finding studies, the pamoate salt affected the subjects at lower dosages than did the hydrochloride. We examined 10 and 25 mg of doxepin hydrochloride, 10 mg of doxepin pamoate, and placebo. The methods of recording and analysis were comparable to the study of doxepin "A" and "B." Thirteen subjects completed the four sessions of the study (Fink, 1974).

We found doxepin to be readily distinguished from placebo, and the pattern of changes in frequency, amplitude, and variability measures was the same as the earlier doxepin study, indicating that the three doses and two formulations of doxepin showed the same central effects. Comparing the three doxepin doses in regression analyses, we found distinctions for the 10 and 25 mg hydrochloride formulations, but the 10 mg pamoate was not distinguishable from 10 or 25 mg doxepin hydrochloride. The 10 mg pamoate formulation was effective at the same rate as the 10 mg hydrochloride, but the effects persisted beyond those of the hydrochloride. At the end of the 2-hr experiment, the pamoate formulation was still increasing its effect, while that of the two doses of hydrochloride was already decreasing. These differences in rate of onset and persistence suggest that the pamoate had a great efficiency in affecting the CNS, acting perhaps with equal rapidity in onset and with a longer duration than the hydrochloride.

Thiothixene

We examined the central activity of two formulations of thiothixene, a capsule and a liquid concentrate. In dose-finding studies, we recorded measurable EEG change in single doses 2 to 3 hr after ingestion of 10 mg thiothixene. The experiments and analyses were similar to the doxepin studies. Thiothixene elicited decreases in 7.5 to 18.5 Hz, increases in 3.5 to 7.5 Hz activities, and a decrease in average frequency. In the comparisons of regression slopes and intercepts, the two formulations were distinguishable in none of the slope comparisons and in five intercepts suggesting the same effect but a more rapid absorption for the concentrate formulation. Both formulations were readily distinguishable from placebo, with the concentrate exhibiting differences greater than the capsular formulation (Fink, 1974).

Bromazepam (Ro 5–3350) and Diazepam

In a classification study of a novel benzodiazepine (Ro 5-3350, bromazepam), we had the opportunity to examine concurrent blood levels. In the dose-finding study, we observed that single oral 9 mg doses of bromazepam and 10 mg diazepam were well tolerated by the subjects and elicited definable EEG patterns with an onset under 30 min, a peak at approximately 90 min, and a duration of 5 to 12 hr (Irwin, Poinier, Fink, and Feldstein, *in preparation*). In 13 male volunteers, we undertook examinations at weekly intervals with drugs given in a latin square design. We recorded EEG and behavioral data as in other classification studies, with the addition that blood samples were taken before the medication was given, after 30 min, and again at 60 min. In the EEG analyses, we found increases in percent-time frequencies below 5 Hz, decreases in 7 to 13 Hz, and marked increases in frequencies over 18 Hz. In the regression analyses, we distinguished both compounds from placebo, but not from each other. These changes were paralleled by the behavioral data.

We correlated the blood level data with each of the EEG measures, using the mean of the 5 min of EEG most proximal to the blood sample. Correlations are not uniform or random, but are highest for the EEG variables most identified with benzodiazepines' cerebral effects: 18 to 25 Hz, > 25 Hz, and 7 to 13 Hz. We also defined differences in the time course of the compounds.

DISCUSSION

During the past decade, quantitative EEG recording and analytic methods have been developed which provide repeatable measures of changes in cerebral electrical activity from the scalp of man. These techniques have been applied to the classification of psychoactive drugs, the prediction of clinical uses, and the measurement of CNS bioavailability of different formulations of active compounds. We find that clinically active compounds stimulate definable patterns of electrical activity. Based on the clinical changes accompanying the use of the compounds, it has been possible to formulate associations between the EEG profile changes and clinical effects. We have applied these associations to the study of presumed psychoactive compounds and are encouraged that for each new compound for which a definable EEG profile has been elicited—for fenfluramine, cyclazocine, doxepin, and GP-41,299—the association with the clinical effects is verified; and for no compound for which we failed to define a profile has a clinical application been accepted. Our studies parallel investigations using methods similar to those used by Itil, who has reported EEG profiles for many new compounds. We are most encouraged that our recent studies of GB-94 confirm his findings.

What are the practical applications of these observations? In five European laboratories electrophysiologic recordings are part of the phase-I screening of new compounds either concurrent with the initial toxicology screening or in parallel studies. Three laboratories have developed their own capability for data reduction and analysis and two are sending tapes to the U.S. for reduction and analysis. In two laboratories, and in two additional laboratories in the United States, efforts are under way to develop similar screening programs in animals using the data reduction and analytic methods of cerebral electrometry. Emphasis is on trials in dogs or monkeys in the anticipation that their metabolism is closer to man's and that their behavior can be controlled sufficiently to provide artifact-free records. This effort to replicate the classification and prediction studies of man in animal species is an important effort.

While the methods are being applied to studies of new drugs, it is the study of bioavailability and neurophysiologic equivalence that deserves special attention now. Dependence on biochemical measures in animals for estimation of processes in man is fraught with the hazards of metabolic, age, body size, and absorption differences. The methods of cerebral electrometry provide an independent, safe, and atraumatic assay of the biochemical effects of compounds in the brain. True, the measures are gross today, and only large segments of brain function are assayed at each examination. Yet the data seem as reliable and as interesting as blood and urine studies — fluids which can only reflect the changes in the CNS through the blood-brain barrier and the hepatic-renal filter system.

What are the principal drawbacks of these prediction methods? They depend on systematic studies in volunteer subjects, and both the experiments and the equipment are complex and expensive. Our laboratory is equipped with an IBM 1800 process control system. Other laboratories have found DEC PDP-12, PDP-15, and the Hewlett-Packard computer systems useful. With appropriate peripherals, the system may cost from $150,000 to $200,000. For some interested in evaluating these methods, however, there is a less expensive approach. By using a data recording system compatible with the analysis system in an established laboratory, one can manage one's own experiments and, at a small cost, use these systems for analysis. The large initial outlay for equipment can be deferred until the method is proven and its use too extensive for outside sources to provide service.

In our experiences with cerebral electrometry, we find the techniques to be sufficiently well developed to define the CNS activity of drugs, and to measure the equivalence of different dosages and formulations of effective compounds. We believe techniques are applicable to phase-I clinical studies of presumed psychoactive drugs. In the same dose-finding and initial toxicity studies in volunteers, the concurrent recording of EEG and quantitative assessment will provide a basis for the confirmation or correction of preclinical judgment. Indeed, we are concerned that too limited a view is usually taken of the variety of data available in the initial acute and chronic toxicity studies in volunteers. Cerebral electrometry seems to provide a safe, relevant, independent method of predicting target populations for presumed psychoactive drugs, and further development of the method is warranted.

ACKNOWLEDGMENTS

This work was aided in part by grants from the National Institute of Mental Health, MH 13358, 15561, and 24020.

REFERENCES

Abbuzzahab, F. S. (1970): The antidepressant properties of cyclazocine. *AJCR*, 1:9–15.
Efron, D., Cole, J. O., Levine, J., and Wittenborn, T. R. (Ed.) (1969): *Psychopharmacology—A Review of Progress, 1957–1967*, Washington, D.C., Government Printing Office.
Fink, M. (1959): EEG and behavioral effects of psychopharmacologic agents. In: *Neuropsychopharmacology*, edited by P. Bradley, P. Deniker, and C. Radouco-Thomas, Vol. 1, pp. 441–446. Elsevier, Amsterdam.
Fink, M. (1960): Effect of anticholinergic compounds on post-convulsive EEG and behavior of psychiatric patients. *Electroencephalogr. Clin. Neurophysiol.*, 12:359–369.
Fink, M. (1961): Quantitative electroencephalography and human psychopharmacology: Frequency spectra and drug action. *Med. Exp.*, 5:364–369.
Fink, M. (1963a): EEG and human psychopharmacology. (Abstracts of Proceedings of Symposium at Third World Congress of Psychiatry, Montreal, 1961). *Electroencephalogr. Clin. Neurophysiol.*, 15:133–137.
Fink, M. (1963b): Quantitative electroencephalography in human psychopharmacology. II: Drug patterns. In: *EEG and Behavior*, edited by G. Glaser, pp. 177–197. Basic Books, New York.
Fink, M. (1964): *A Selected Bibliography of Electroencephalography in Human Psychopharmacology 1951–1962. Electroencephalogr. Clin. Neurophysiol.*, Suppl. 23:68.
Fink, M. (1965): Quantitative EEG and human psychopharmacology III: Changes on acute and chronic administration of chlorpromazine, imipramine and placebo (saline). In: *Applications of Electroencephalography in Psychiatry*, edited by W. P. Wilson, pp. 226–240. Duke University Press, Durham, North Carolina.
Fink, M. (1969a): EEG classification of psychoactive compounds in man: Review and theory of behavioral associations. In: *Psychopharmacology—A Review of Progress, 1957–1967*, edited by D. Efron, J. Cole, J. Levine, and J. R. Wittenborn, pp. 497–507. Washington, D.C. Government Printing Office.
Fink, M. (1969b): EEG and human psychopharmacology. *Ann. Rev. Pharmacol.*, 9:241–258.
Fink, M. (1974): EEG applications in psychopharmacology. In: *Psychopharmacological Agents (Vol. III)*, edited by M. Gordon, pp. 159–174. Academic Press, New York.
Fink, M. Cerebral electrometry: Quantitative EEG applied to human psychopharmacology. In: *Proceedings CEAN*, edited by H. Künkel and G. Dolce *(in press)*.
Fink, M., and Itil, T. (1969a): Neurophysiology of the phantastica. In: *Psychopharmacology—A Review of Progress, 1957–1967*, edited by D. Efron, J. Cole, J. Levine, and J. R. Wittenborn, pp. 1231–1239. Washington, D.C., Government Printing Office.
Fink, M., and Itil, T. (1969b): EEG and human psychopharmacology: IV. Clinical antidepressants. In: *Psychopharmacology—A Review of Progress, 1957–1967*, edited by D. Efron,

J. Cole, J. Levine, and J. R. Wittenborn, pp. 671–682. Washington, D.C., Government Printing Office.

Fink, M., Itil, T., and Shapiro, D. M. (1967): Digital computer analysis of the human EEG in psychiatric research. *Compr. Psychiatry,* 8:521–538.

Fink, M., Itil, T., Zaks, A., and Freedman, A. M. (1969): EEG patterns of cyclazocine, a narcotic antagonist. In: *Neurophysiological and Behavioral Aspects of Psychotropic Drugs,* edited by A. Karczmar and W. P. Koella, Chapter 4, pp. 62–71. C. C. Thomas, Philadelphia.

Fink, M., Shapiro, D., Hickman, C., and Itil, T. (1968): Quantitative analysis of the electroencephalogram by digital computer methods III: Applications to psychopharmacology. In: *Computers and Electronic Devices in Psychiatry,* edited by N. S. Kline and E. Laska, pp. 109–123. Grune & Stratton, New York.

Fink, M., Shapiro, D. M., and Itil, T. (1971): EEG profiles of fenfluramine, amobarbital and dextroamphetamine in normal volunteers. *Psychopharmacologia* (Berl.), 22:369–383.

Fink, M., Simeon, J., Itil, T., and Freedman, A. M. (1970): Clinical antidepressant activity of cyclazocine — A narcotic antagonist. *Clin. Pharmacol. Ther.,* 11:41–48.

Gaztanaga, P., Abrams, R., Simeon, J., Jones, T., and Fink, M. (1972): Clinical evaluation of GP-41299: An antianxiety agent of the doxepin type. *Arzneim. Forsch.,* 22:1903–1905.

Itil, T., and Fink, M. (1966): Anticholinergic drug-induced delirium (experimental modification, quantitative EEG and behavioral correlations). *J. Nerv. Ment. Dis.,* 143:492–507.

Oswald, I., Jones, H. S., and Mannerheim, J. E. (1968): Effects of two slimming drugs on sleep. *Br. Med. J.,* 1:796–799.

Shapiro, D. M., and Glasser, M. (1974): Measurement and comparison of EEG – Drug effects. In: *Psychotropic Drugs and the Human EEG,* edited by T. Itil, pp. 327–349. S. Karger, Basel.

Simeon, J., Spero, M., and Fink, M. (1969): Clinical and EEG studies of doxepin: Interim report. *Psychosomatics,* 10 (Part 2):14–17 (May-June).

Volavka, J., Feldstein, S., Abrams, R., and Fink, M. (1972): EEG and clinical change after bilateral and unilateral electroconvulsive therapy. *Electroencephalogr. Clin. Neurophysiol.,* 32:631–639.

Wikler, A. (1954): Clinical and electroencephalographic studies on the effects of mescaline, N-allylnormorphine and morphine in man. *J. Nerv. Ment. Dis.,* 120:157–175.

DISCUSSION

Wade: Can the EEG predict the relative potency of a drug?

Fink: Yes, if you mean dose equivalence. It is possible to take multiple doses and determine the amplitude or the amount of EEG effect. If you are willing to extrapolate and say that the more the EEG effect is like a standard or the larger the dose the greater the EEG effect, then you can make some statement about potency. We have made a statement about GB-94 in the following way: We obtain an EEG profile with 2.5 mg of GB-94. On the other hand, in order to find an EEG profile with amitriptyline, we have to give 10 mg in the same subjects. (We find very little with 2.5 and 5 mg.) There is also a time difference, the peak effect for GB-94 is between 40 and 60 min; the peak effect for amitriptyline was between 90 and 120 min. We could, therefore, say that GB-94 at half the dose was at least twice as fast in having the peak effect, and predicted that the clinical dose for GB-94 will be between one-half and one-quarter that of amitriptyline. This is indeed what is happening in the clinical population. The clinicians have settled on a ratio of approximately one-third against amitriptyline as being the appropriate dose for GB-94 (between 100 and 120 mg).

Lee: Since you only include for evaluation subjects with alpha wave, and we don't know too much about subjects related to alpha activity, wouldn't your sample be biased?

Fink: Most of our work has been done with homogeneous populations. After all, we do a complete study on 10 to 14 subjects and if you are working with a small N you try to reduce the variability to begin with. One of the variables that we control is sex. We use only males. Body weight is held constant to a narrow range to insure fixed doses. Age is held from 21 to 28 years. Alpha activity has to be above 45%. We have settled on these control values to reduce variability in our small samples. We've also done a study with a low alpha group. The changes are slightly different, but you can see the same dose effect with a low alpha group as with a high alpha group. It is easier with a high alpha group, so we start that way. With GB-94, for example, investigators in Holland collected a group of EEGs, did the profiles, and then showed them to me and it was easy to see that even with low alpha the subjects have the same theta increase and the same beta increase as we get with high alpha. However, it is a little harder to see, so their N has to be a little greater, but you can get the same results, if you start with a homogeneous group. This methodology does not limit itself to high alpha. We have used high alpha for tactical reasons. If one starts with a heterogeneous sample, the sample size will have to be increased, and we are faced with a kind of cost-benefit decision as to total expenses of the study.

Blackwell: Are your volunteers selected even further, maybe to the extent that these are people who show specific drug responses?

Fink: We make no selection according to their responsivity to drugs. The volunteers are students at the university or they were medical students who heard about our work and then volunteered. We pay a fixed fee per hour for their participation. Initially, we know nothing about their drug responsivity. We do occasionally find a subject in whom our calculated dose has no effect. This is often matched by a subject who, with the same dose, shows a large effect. Occasionally we are fooled by the over- or the under-reactor, but these experiences even out — even in small studies.

Uhlenhuth: Do you have a notion about the peak effect time of oral chlorpromazine from your studies in man?

Fink: About $1\frac{1}{2}$ to 2 hr.

Uhlenhuth: Would that be liquid administration?

Fink: Yes. We use liquid formulations to be able to more easily test small incremental dosages.

Blackwell: Have you looked at any subjects in terms of responders and nonresponders?

Fink: That's very difficult for me at the present time, because I do not have good control of a patient population. The most difficult thing in clinical studies is to find patients who have only had one drug. When we've had patients under our treatment alone, and we gave them only one drug, we could and did assess EEG characteristics of responders and nonresponders.

In a study that Itil and I did in Missouri with a group of therapy-resistant schizophrenics, the patients had been in the hospital an average of 9 yr. They were moved to a research ward, and all drugs were discontinued for periods of 3 to 6 mo. Most were able to tolerate being drug free. They were then studied and compared as far as drug reactors and nonreactors. There were some relations to EEG — poor reactors were alpha stable with high percent time even when drug free. He treated some with drugs, including ditran followed by chlorpromazine, or LSD followed by phenothiazines; some improved, and showed an EEG response. They became "reactors" on this so-called "provocation therapy." (See Itil et al., *Comprehensive Psychiat.* 7:488–493, 1966).

Bass: Would you comment on the state of the art in diagnosing different types of psychoses?

Fink: Many workers have examined quantitative resting EEG for the classification of the mentally ill. None of these studies have been replicated enough to say that the method is good. One problem with the resting EEG as a classification measure is that most patients at the time of study were already receiving medications. To become drug free, they have to go through various periods of withdrawal. This difficulty aside, there are now some publications which suggest that we can distinguish depressives from so-called normal people; or psychotic patients from normals and other psychotic schizophrenics; or "anxious neurotics" from the other groups by resting EEG criteria. A much better classification device was developed a decade or so ago, using the cerebral reaction to a stressor, whether a barbiturate, a psychoactive substance of another class, or a stimulant. When I moved to New York in 1967, we considered using EEG as a diagnostic predictor. But we have had to develop methods of data reduction, classification, and recording and it has taken us about seven years to accomplish what we have today. We have been less interested in diagnosis than in bioavailability, which I think is the next step for my work. Itil, however, is studying EEG criteria in the diagnosis of schizophrenic children and the mothers of schizophrenic children. Volavka and Mednick are assessing the EEG correlates of genetic typologies (as XYY). Others, (e.g., Shagass and Lipshitz) are examining cerebral responsivity for diagnosis using evoked potentials or the contingent negative variation. We need more studies of the barbiturate response, however. This is the state of the art today.

Taylor: Since electroconvulsive therapy has a profound effect on both depression and schizophrenia, are there any studies that compare the EEG effect of ECT with that of the antipsychotic drugs or the antidepressant drugs?

Fink: The EEG effects of ECT have been well documented, going back to the early 1940s. Some authors were able to show that the therapeutic effects of ECT were well correlated with the amount of induced slow waves. The characteristic thing about ECT is that the slow waves and the decrease in fast activity go hand in hand, which is exactly the same as for an antipsychotic drug, but different for the thymoleptics. The process of improvement with thymoleptic drugs in the treatment of depression appears to be a different process than the process of ECT. One study, by Exner and Murillo, is now in progress and compares the EEG effects of ECT and drug therapy.

Knill: Do you ever see a biphasic effect based on dose?

Fink: Yes, this has been shown with a number of drugs. The best example in our studies has been trifluperidol. Trifluperidol is a drug that has one EEG profile at low dose and another at high dose. This puzzled us very much, until we found out that at low doses we were seeing a dopaminergic effect and at high doses, a certain amount of anticholinergic (antiparkinson) effect as well. We think that the EEG dose response for trifluperidol is related to both its therapeutic activity and the difficulty that the profession has had in accepting it as a therapeutic agent. Another example is ORF-8063, a benzodiazepine. In the clinical work, some effects are seen early and then it takes a week or 10 days before the therapeutic effects come on. Some clinicians were very upset that the drug effect didn't come on right away. When we examined its EEG effects, we found the changes better related to blood levels of the metabolite than the first substance, and this may explain some of the delay. For some drugs we seem to have a step-function—a level at which the EEG and be-havioral effects are not measurable; a level where therapeutic effect and an EEG sig-nature are measured; and a "toxic" level, where behavior is not salutary and the EEG effects are quite different.

Goldberg: Since antidepressants have a delayed onset of action in depression, I'm wondering whether the EEG profile is different in normal volunteers after single drug administration than after repeated administration.

Fink: What is the correlation of the profile done in volunteers against the profile in patients on the chronic dosage? For three or four compounds, there is no question about the direct correlation. With the benzodiazepines, what you see in the volun-teers is what you see with a chronic dose in patients, if you are careful about your dosage. If your patient takes very big doses, then of course you exceed what you do in the volunteer because you can only give the volunteer threshold doses. With anti-psychotic drugs, the chronic administration and the effects of the single dose are equivalent. Opiates are complicated by tolerance development and what you see in the acute subject disappears after some days or weeks, depending on the drug you are studying. This is also true for LSD and mescaline, but not for the deliriants, ditran and atropine.

If you examine imipramine in an acute study, you get a certain profile. If you examine imipramine in the patient, if you're testing the first 3 hr, you get the same profile, but then it disappears. If you test a subject with a single dose after 8 to 12 hr, you have nothing. However, after about 10 to 14 days, we find a persistent theta increase and the decrease in alpha activities remains with the patient, which is ex-actly the part that remains in the treatment of psychosis. Three wk later, the imipra-mine patient is not identical to the acute, but close enough, taking into account the probable effect of tolerance.

Goldberg: Does amitriptyline produce effects like imipramine?

Fink: Yes. Amitriptyline has also been examined in chronic and acute administra-tion. Amitriptyline is a little faster acting, and may produce more slow waves than imipramine. Tolerance to amitriptyline in EEG seems to develop after about 10 days.

Wade: What information can you gather from the animal EEG effects of drugs?

Fink: There has been an extensive amount of study of the animal EEG. A big problem with these studies is that we cannot control the behavior of the animal. The EEG is highly responsive to set, to movement, eye-opening, eye-closure, and to varying states of vigilance. The only reason we can do careful studies in man is because we can train a man to keep his eyes closed, his head still, and be quiet while you're collecting lengthy samples of EEG. It is difficult to train an animal to the same criterion. So when we study the EEG of animals we wait for periods of sleep. But most drug effects on EEG are wiped out during sleep, except after massive doses.

A second difficulty with animal classification studies is species specificity. Drug effects may or may not be similar between man and an index species. Two decades ago, when the rabbit was the animal of choice, the discrepancies between EEG classification studies in rabbits (as by Himwich and his co-workers) and those in man were considerable. We now know that the metabolism of many psychoactive sub-stances in the rabbit differs from that in man. The same is true for the cat. Some scientists have found more similar metabolism of drugs in some species of dog, and in monkeys and apes, suggesting that EEG studies could be done in these species.

I know of two laboratories in Europe and one in the United States that are specifically looking at the EEG of dogs and monkeys under controlled conditions. In one study, the monkey is in a seat, given a task to perform. Part of his task is to keep his eyes closed for 40 to 60 sec. The EEG is collected during that period. Then the monkey is given a reward and, after a few minutes, the process is repeated. This provides epochs of 1 to 2 min duration for study. I have seen some EEGs done in this way in Holland and they are very good. They should show a dose-response curve which may be comparable to studies in man. If we apply the methods of quantification to suitable species and control the animal's vigilance, my own prediction would be that, in a few years, human EEG profiling will become only confirmatory. At the moment, however, human EEG studies are the only useful ones we have.

Domino: For me, perhaps the most significant part of your presentation is the emphasis on the tremendous waste of current Phase I studies and for the classification of the mentally ill that are going on throughout the world in view of the failure to look at a lot of physiologic variables. The message that I am certainly getting from you is of the necessity for looking at physiologic variables. I think we ought to look at a lot more than we are currently. The whole issue of evoked potentials, for example, is one that hasn't been well studied. I like your statements concerning GSR and so on, but it seems to me that sleep studies are also extremely important. Even though many of the drugs show a richness of change in the awake EEG, the richness of the sleep EEG is also significant.

Fink: For special purposes, it is very valuable. Dr. Domino and his coworkers published the first quantitated EEG study of cannabis in the world literature. It was a very nice, clear, systematic study of volunteers who smoked cannabis. We replicated that study and showed that one can apply the same methodology to drugs that are not ordinarily classified as psychoactive from the therapeutic point of view. We have done the same profiling now for drugs of abuse, like the opiates, hallucinogens, etc. There's not much question that the application of quantitative EEG to sleep was really one of the main thrusts for EEG as well as for sleep research and many researchers are doing it, including yourself. My own interest starts from a specific premise: the correlation of EEG changes and changes in mood, affect, and thought processes, as occur following drugs in man. From that point of view, the sleep EEG, except for the soporific drugs, is a weak tool. We should pick the right tool for the right purpose. EEG is a very powerful measure for other purposes, but for classification of a psychoactive drug, the sleep classification is difficult, and at the moment has not gotten as far as the alert EEG classification.

Gershon: My questions are all argumentative. The first one is very simple. You've got GPA 1714 and I think we did some work with that and it was absolutely inert. Is that the correct number and compound? It was proposed as an antidepressant.

Fink: No. It was proposed as a compound that had some effects on dopamine. It was supposed to be a dopamine-blocking agent and we were able at that point to do a profile. The important thing is that some profiles are very easy to get and some profiles are difficult. GPA 1714 was a difficult one to classify. I put it in the scheme with a question mark, but I think that's where it belongs. All it did was increase the alpha activity of our subjects. We have never done any clinical studies with it and neither has the manufacturer.

Gershon: The other question is again the same sort of thing, but even more tongue-in-cheek. If lithium is an antimanic and haloperidol is an antimanic, shouldn't they both have the same profile?

Fink: Yes, if their therapeutic effects were similar and using the same mechanisms. Lithium has been classified in the table on the basis of Itil's work as increasing slow waves. I think that lithium ought to be in the class of antipsychotic drugs, as I read his notes. But there is also a report from your laboratory (Johnson, Gershon, Maccario, and others) in which they show the EEG effects of this drug. I have not studied lithium myself so I put it in a separate class only because they did. When we study antidepressants, we know that MAO inhibitors, thymoleptics, and amphetamine, although antidepressant, do so by different cerebral mechanisms — and, incidentally, have different EEG patterns. Perhaps lithium and haloperidol will be found to have antimanic effects by different mechanisms.

Gershon: Chlorpromazine is an antipsychotic and your EEG data would agree that it was, and I think also thioridazine. Now, the study that you and Klein did and the data derived from that study which I think are quite meaningful (I'm not prepared to dismiss those data, although you might want to in retrospect), would tend to suggest that it's a perfectly effective antidepressant. Hollister did a sort of similar study with thioridazine and said it also looks like an antidepressant. Isn't there disparity?

Fink: No, the answer to that is seen in Table 3. There is not much question that we can distinguish imipramine from chlorpromazine and thioridazine. Chlorpromazine and thioridazine would fit in the same class. It is the clinician who tells us that under certain conditions these drugs are antidepressant. In the study that Klein and I did, in which we compared placebo, imipramine, and chlorpromazine in 144 subjects and which Klein replicated a few years later in another 150 subjects, the antidepressant activity of chlorpromazine was limited to a small group of depressives, a group which he has subsequently reported as having special characteristics. Perhaps the differences in clinical results match the differences in EEG effects. Also, our study was labeled a comparison of imipramine and chlorpromazine-procyclidine mixture. Every patient in that study received chlorpromazine plus procyclidine. There was 1,200 mg of chlorpromazine and 15 mg of procyclidine. When we studied the EEG, it was not the EEG of chlorpromazine alone but of the combination, and this may have contributed to the EEG class.

Predictability in Psychopharmacology: Preclinical and Clinical Correlations,
edited by A. Sudilovsky, S. Gershon and B. Beer. Raven Press, New York,
© 1975.

EEG Classification of a Novel Anorexigenic: PR-F-36-CL

Max Fink, Peter Irwin, and Patrick Sibony

*Department of Psychiatry, Health Sciences Center, State University of New York at Stony
Brook, Stony Brook, New York 11790*

The classification of new psychoactive drugs is difficult. Theories relating chemical structure or pharmacologic profile to behavior are not sufficiently specific. We usually depend on a new drug exhibiting a profile in animal studies similar to existing compounds. Another model for identifying psychoactive drugs is derived from the particular relations of EEG changes to human behavior. The many observations that psychoactive drugs affect not only the behavior of subjects but also the scalp-recorded EEG provide the basis for an EEG profile method to classify psychoactive drugs. Because the changes associated with psychoactive drugs do not appear related to a specific mental disorder, we believe their effects may be defined in normal subjects as well as in the mentally ill. Using these ideas, we have studied established psychoactive compounds (thiothixene, amobarbital, thiopental, dextroamphetamine, diazepam, imipramine), new drugs (doxepin, cyclazocine, fenfluramine), and experimental numbered compounds in normal adult volunteers. In these studies, a method of defining the EEG profile for an orally administered psychoactive drug using digital computer techniques has evolved (Fink, 1969, 1974). Some applications of this method include the following.

1. The definition of cyclazocine, an established narcotic antagonist, as a clinical antidepressant, and its clinical verification
2. The finding that doxepin has an EEG profile more like imipramine than like diazepam. In clinical trials its antidepressant features have been described
3. The definition of fenfluramine as a sedative compound with more similarity to amobarbital than to dextroamphetamine. In clinical trials fenfluramine is reported to be anorexigenic with sedative properties

During the past two years, we have examined the EEG profiles of various experimental numbered compounds in phase I human trials. Of these, we were able to define an EEG profile for three compounds (GP-41299, AHR-1118, U-28774) which are now in clinical trial. Interest in other compounds waned, usually because of inadequate additional data including the lack of a specific EEG profile (CP 14,368, GPA 1714), and a low therapeutic index (S-42, 548).

In animal screening tests, PR-F-36-CL demonstrated a profile suggestive of an anorexigenic compound. In preliminary human trials it inhibited appetite and its use was accompanied by weight reduction. Subjects reported drowsiness, euphoria, restlessness, insomnia, headache, and nausea as associated symptoms (Oliver, 1974).

There are two putative types of anorexigenic compounds — those related to amphetamine and associated with central nervous system (CNS) stimulation, and a lesser number of "sedative-type" agents, represented by chlorphenteramine and fenfluramine. Although the definition of the latter class of compounds is in some dispute, both as to their anorexigenic potency and sedative effects, there is sufficient interest and data to warrant continued use of this classification for further study.

There were two goals of interest regarding PR-F-36-CL: the definition of its EEG profile, and a determination of whether it is similar to either of the two classes of anorexigenic compounds.

The activity of PR-F-36-CL on systems other than the CNS appeared minimal and, in the doses recommended for assay, the effects in man seemed to be restricted to the CNS. In some subjects, however, tachycardia and decreased blood pressure were evinced on chronic dosage. In single dose studies in volunteers, the minimal effective dose was 200 to 250 mg, and the maximum tolerated dose was between 350 and 600 mg. The anorexigenic dose was 50 to 75 mg/day in two or three doses. From these data, it was thought probable that single doses to 250 mg would be well tolerated.

The sedative qualities of fenfluramine were defined in an EEG screen in 1966. In that study, fenfluramine (40 mg) was compared to dextroamphetamine (10 mg) and amobarbital (50 and 100 mg) in female volunteers. Both the EEG profile and the associated symptoms of fenfluramine at this dose were found more similar to 50 mg amobarbital than to 10 mg dextroamphetamine.

With this experience in mind, the EEG study of PR-F-36-CL was planned in two steps: (1) a dose-finding study with preliminary definition of an EEG effect, and (2) a classification study, which would combine the comparison of PR-F-36-CL with placebo and with the two anorexigenic agents, dextroamphetamine and fenfluramine.

In the dose-finding study, single doses of PR-F-36-CL elicited consistent behavioral effects at doses of 300 mg and above. Onset of effects occurred approximately 1 hr after drug ingestion; peak and duration of effects varied. The data suggested that it was similar to amphetamine, "with increased blood pressure, increased alertness, anorexia, and insomnia the prevalent symptoms." The EEG profile was obscure. In doses below 300 mg, effects were variable and difficult to distinguish from our experience with placebo.

Data of the classification study are summarized here. It was undertaken in the Department of Psychiatry laboratories at New York Medical College between January and May, 1973. A dose of 350 mg PR-F-36-CL was chosen as an identifiable comparison dose against 10 mg dextroamphetamine, 40 mg fenfluramine, and a placebo. EEG, heart rate, blood pressure, continuous performance, and subjective state data were collected.

METHODS

Volunteers were selected who were 21 to 29 years of age, 130 to 185 pounds in weight (59 to 84 kg), had no evidence of recent medical or mental illness, and no familial history of congenital disease. In addition, a resting, eyes-closed EEG had to be within normal limits with greater than 30 percent-time alpha activity. The nature of the study was described and an informed consent obtained from each acceptable volunteer.

An initial single-blind placebo trial was used to orient these volunteers to the setting and exclude those unusually sensitive to the experimental conditions. Subjects were assigned to a morning or afternoon schedule, one session per week. Morning trials began at 9:30 A.M., and afternoon sessions started at 1:30 P.M. Subjects were instructed to abstain from drugs for at least 72 hr and to obtain a good night's sleep before each session. They were also asked not to eat during the 2 hr immediately preceding a session, and prior to that only a light meal (e.g., breakfast equivalent to one cup of coffee, a small glass of fruit juice, and two slices of bread). Subjects were asked to telephone on the following weekday to report aftereffects, if any. All sessions proceeded on a prescribed schedule.

Approximate time (min)	Procedures
0–25	*Preparation and initial measures:* machine calibration, electrode placement, initial interview, blood pressure (BP 1)
25–45	*Predrug EEG with continuous alerting task:* eyes closed, supine, eye-opening for 40 sec every 5 min with alertness self-assessment
45–54	*Baseline measures:* BP 2, Abramson Symptom Questionnaire (ASQ 1)
54–55	*Drug administration:* by EEG technician
55–82	*Time to allow for drug absorption and distribution:* subject permitted to sit up, read, or converse
82–85	*Heart measure:* BP 3
85–175	*Post-drug EEG with continuous alerting task:* eyes closed, supine, eye-opening for 40 sec every 5 min with alertness self-assessment and symptom report
175–190	*Final measures:* BP 4, ASQ 2, Irwin Form
~ 24 hr	*Telephone report:* aftereffects

Sessions were conducted double-blind by an interviewer. The study required each subject to participate in five sessions—the initial adaptation session in which he received placebo, and four trials in which he received three capsules containing dextroamphetamine (10 mg), fenfluramine (40 mg), PR-F-36-CL (350 mg), or placebo. Compounds were sequenced in a latin square design and numbered consecutively. Upon completion of data collection, the numbers were grouped under a letter code corresponding to the drug represented, and analysis to discriminate the compounds proceeded. Drug codes were not broken until analyses were concluded. Specifics of each data-collecting procedure are described below.

Initial Interview

An initial interview was conducted while the instrumentation was being prepared and the electrodes placed. Questions were asked about the time and duration of the previous night's sleep, time and content of the latest meal, and recent drug use. Room temperature was noted. Means were calculated by drug and t-tests used to assess differences.

Physiologic Data

Electroencephalogram and Heart Rate

Electrophysiologic data were collected using a Grass Model VII polygraph with 7P511 amplifiers. Electrodes were placed according to the International Federation's 10–20 system. Derivations recorded on strip-chart were O_1–O_2, F_3–F_4, O_1–F_3, O_2–F_4, O_1–Cz, O_2–Cz, and R ear-chest (for heart rate). The O_1–F_3, O_1–Cz, and heart rate lead pairs were additionally recorded on Scotch Model #871 tapes. Sessions included a 20 min pre- and 90 min postdrug EEG and heart rate sampling, during which subjects remained resting with their eyes closed. Eyes were opened only during arousal periods interspersed at 5-min intervals. Data of these periods were rejected from subsequent analyses.

Tapes were replayed for analogue-to-digital conversion at $\frac{1}{4}$ real time. Analogue data were processed through a 60 Hz[1] notch rejection filter and a Krohn-hite Model 3750 filter set at 1.1 to 40.0 Hz[1] band pass. Digital conversion was done at a rate of 320 samples[1]/sec in 20-sec[1] epochs, with 3.5-sec[1] interepoch intervals for calculations. Primary wave period analysis was performed, which portrayed percent time in each of the following frequency bands (represented by their upper limits): 3.5, 4.5, 6.0, 7.5, 9.0, 11.0, 13.0, 15.0, 18.0, 21.0, 24.0, 27.0, 30.0, 33.0, 40.0, and above 40.0 Hz. In addition, average relative amplitude, its deviation, average baseline

---

[1] Real-time equivalents.

cross-frequency, and its deviation were derived and a counter tabulated heart rate.

A trained EEG technician examined all EEG records for noncerebral activity ("artifacts"). Epochs subjectively determined to have more than 5% of distinct artifact or more than 10% of probable artifact were identified and omitted in further statistics. The average and standard deviation of the predrug epochs and the average for each 5 min of the postdrug period were calculated for each variable in each record. The postdrug 5-min averages were then transformed into z-scores using the predrug mean and standard deviation. The z-scores were used in a quadratic regression analysis which further reduced the data to four components for each drug: intercept (mean level of activity), linear (direction and degree of change), quadratic (curvi-linearity of response over time), and standard error of estimate [SEE] (variability of response). t-Tests were used to compare these components between drugs for each variable. Multivariate randomized t-tests were used to examine the legitimacy of the profiles of differences obtained (Shapiro and Glasser, 1974).

A second model applied to these data was a multiple stepwise linear regression analysis, after Cohen (1968). Questions asked were if the drugs differed from placebo and from each other, if the effects differed over time, and if the effects could be related to other variables (buzzer releases, heart rate, or artifacts). This analysis allows the investigator to examine independent variables sequentially in accounting for the variance associated with a dependent variable. For these analyses, the EEG data were reduced to 15-min means, and the postdrug measures were treated as dependent variables. Dummy coding, as described by Cohen, was used to express the nominal data of subject, time period, drug, and interactions. The analysis proceeded using predrug measure, (latter 15 min), mean of the subjects, age, weight, time periods, drugs, and drug-by-time period interactions as independent variables. Specific analysis of the average amplitude, 6 Hz, 9 Hz, and 24 Hz measures by time period used predrug measure, subjects, drugs, non-EEG variable, and drug-by-non-EEG variable interactions as the independent variables.[2]

Blood Pressure

Using a standard cuff and gauge, the EEG technician measured resting blood pressure at the outset of the session, prior to drug administration, and before and after the postdrug EEG period (approximately 30 and 120

---

[2] A drawback of this analysis is the tendency to pose more questions than the sample size justifies. Although the p-level can be adjusted, criteria may not be adequate to select the appropriate adjustment. Recognizing this difficulty, our reports include no adjustment for the number of analyses performed, but may be accepted as a reflection of the most prominent indications, rather than of an absolute p-value of less than 0.05.

min following drug administration). The Wilcoxon matched-pairs signed-ranks test was used to evaluate these data.

Behavioral Data

Continuous Alerting Task

A continuous alerting task was used to maintain subjects in a more uniform state of attention during their EEGs. Subjects were asked to hold down a resilient button which retained a buzzer in an open contact position. Release of the button closed the contact and the buzzer sounded loudly, signaling the subject to resume pressure on the button. Registrations of the buzzer were automatically noted on the EEG strip-chart by an event marker. These were summed by 5-min epochs and displayed in tables and graphs. Drug differences were determined by t-tests.

Alertness Self-Assessment

Subjects were asked to evaluate their relative degree of alertness using the scale presented below, with their state at the onset of the session as their "0" point. Assessment was made upon inquiry at each 5-min interval pre- and postdrug. Results were displayed in tables and graphs, and the Wilcoxon test was used to ascertain interdrug differences.

```
-6    -5    -4    -3    -2    -1     0    +1    +2    +3    +4    +5    +6
I----I----I----I----I----I----I----I----I----I----I----I----I
Less alert                         No change                        More alert
```

Abramson Symptom Questionnaire

A modified Abramson symptom questionnaire was administered by a research assistant prior to and 2 hr following drug ingestion. It consists of a check-list of 40 symptoms. On the predrug questionnaire, subjects were requested to give a present evaluation. On the postdrug questionnaire, subjects were requested to summarize postdrug changes. Symptoms were assessed on an "absent," "slight," "moderate," or "marked" basis. A sign test was used to evaluate pre- to postdrug changes among the four compounds.

Subjects' Voluntary Reports

During session

At 5-min intervals throughout the EEG recording, subjects were requested to open their eyes for 40 sec. During each period, the research assistant recorded the subject's response to the question, "Do you feel any change?" Responses were probed for details, and observations by the research assistant were included on the record. These data were summarized in tables across subjects and a sign test was performed on drug-placebo differences. Frequency of report of a symptom was used as a measure of relative degree.

Aftereffects

Subjects were asked to telephone the next weekday morning following each session to report the presence or absence of any aftereffects. These data were added to the record and summarized in tables.

Irwin Form

The Irwin Form contains specific and summary questions concerning changes in physiology, mood, or thought perceived by the subject and has been developed for these studies. Subjects answered the questions in a final interview at the conclusion of each session. Responses were assessed with a sign test.

RESULTS

This report summarizes the data of 13 volunteers, ranging in age from 21 to 27 years (mean 23), and weighing 62 to 76 kg (mean 69). A 14th subject selected to participate withdrew from the study after his first session in which he received dextroamphetamine. The reason he gave was that he did not like the setting. Two of the subjects had to repeat their PR-F-36-CL sessions: one because he felt ill during the session and it had to be discontinued, the other because he later admitted to having had alcohol the night before.

The average dose by weight of each drug administered was 5.05 mg/kg PR-F-36-CL, 0.58 mg/kg fenfluramine, and 0.14 mg/kg amphetamine. Six subjects came on a morning schedule and seven subjects on an afternoon schedule. The laboratory setting was the same for all sessions.

Initial Interview Data

Volunteers averaged 8 hr sleep prior to their sessions with a mean within-subject range of 1.7 hr. No subject reported less than 6 hr sleep before any session. Subjects were awake an average of 1.8 hr preceding a morning session and 4.5 hr before an afternoon session. The mean within-subject range was 1.5 hr. All subjects had abstained from food for at least 1 hr preceding their sessions. Mean time since the previous meal was 2 hr with an average within-subject range of 1 hr. No volunteer reported taking any drug within 60 hr of his session. Mean room temperature was 77°F with an average within-subject range of 4°F.

Multiple t-tests were performed comparing uncontrolled variables across drugs. Differences suggested were: (a) less sleep the night before fenfluramine sessions than the night prior to amphetamine sessions, and (b) more recent drug use previous to PR-F-36-CL sessions than to fenfluramine sessions.

Physiologic Data

EEG and Heart Rate

The quadratic regression model was applied to the data in two analyses, one involving the full 90-min postdrug period, and one dividing the postdrug period into two blocks of 43 and 47 min.[3] The divided analysis was performed because behavioral observations in the pilot study suggested that the effects of PR-F-36-CL did not have their onset until the second hour after ingestion.

Results of the full 90-min analysis indicate a difference between PR-F-36-CL (350 mg) and placebo in the linear component. At this dose, the drug increases heart rate and percent time 11 to 13 Hz activity and decreases the percent time in beta frequencies above 18 Hz during the session. It differs from fenfluramine (40 mg) in the quadratic component but is indistinguishable from dextroamphetamine (10 mg) by any component. In the divided analysis, PR-F-36-CL differs from placebo in intercept for the second portion of the session in a lesser percent time 18 to 33 Hz activity. PR-F-36-CL differs from fenfluramine in intercept for the second portion and from dextroamphetamine in the first section in the SEE component (Table 1).

Dextroamphetamine is distinguished from both placebo and fenfluramine in intercept and SEE components, with a decrease in frequency deviation and percent time 4.5 to 6 Hz and +21 Hz activities, an increase in 9 to 13 Hz frequencies, and less variability in the EEG measures. Dextroamphetamine additionally differs from placebo in the linear component and from fenfluramine in the quadratic component over the total 90 min of a session. Fenfluramine is not distinguishable from placebo by any component in either analysis.

In sum, EEG effects of PR-F-36-CL are not discerned in the first hour after administration but may be distinguished from placebo and fenfluramine (40 mg) in the second hour. The EEG effects are similar to those of dextroamphetamine, and are distinguishable from placebo and fenfluramine at the onset of our EEG sampling (30 min after drug administration). No

---

[3] One subject was eliminated from the split analysis because of an interruption in one of his sessions for micturition and technical difficulties with the EKG record in another session.

TABLE 1. Significant differences in EEG regression components

Variable	Intercept			Linear			Quadratic			Standard error of estimate		
	1–9[a]	10–20[b]	1–20[c]	1–9	10–20	1–20	1–9	10–20	1–20	1–9	10–20	1–20
DA vs. PR	.06	—	—	—	—	—	—	—	—	.001	—	.08
DA vs. PL	—	.001	.001	—	—	.001	—	—	—	—	.001	.02
DA vs. FE	.02	.04	.001	.08	—	—	—	—	.02	.02	.02	.001
PR vs. PL	—	.02	—	—	—	.04	.11	—	—	.08	—	—
PR vs. FE	—	.02	—	—	—	—	—	—	.02	—	.11	—
PL vs. FE	—	—	—	—	—	—	—	—	.11	—	—	—

Table of probabilities $< .11$ (multivariate randomized t-test of 20 EEG variables). PR = PR-F-36-CL, 350 mg; PL = placebo; DA = dextroamphetamine, 1 mg; FE = fenfluramine, 40 mg.
[a] 13 subjects; time periods 1 through 9 (approximately 43 min).
[b] 12 subjects (subject 14 excluded); time periods 10 through 20 (approximately 47 min).
[c] 13 subjects; time periods 1 through 20 (90 min).

differences are found between PR-F-36-CL and dextroamphetamine in the second half of the sampling period or between placebo and fenfluramine throughout the sampling period (Table 1).

As the graphs of the EEG data reflected a biphasic image with a possible delay in onset of effects of PR-F-36-CL, we inquired whether another statistical approach might not clarify these effects. Using the stepwise linear regression model (page 93) we found placebo associated with decreased heart rate and percent time alpha and beta-1 (up to 15 Hz) and increased percent time in other slow and fast frequencies. Relative to the effect of placebo, PR-F-36-CL decreases amplitude and frequency variability, decreases percent time beta frequencies above 15 Hz, increases heart rate, and decreases artifacts. Dextroamphetamine decreases amplitude and frequency variability, decreases percent time in frequencies below 7.5 Hz (especially 3.5 to 6 Hz), increases alpha and beta-1 (especially 9 to 13 Hz), and decreases beta-2 frequencies above 21 Hz. It increases heart rate and decreases artifacts. Fenfluramine increases amplitude variability and decreases artifacts.

PR-F-36-CL and dextroamphetamine differ from fenfluramine in the same measures that they differ from placebo, but to a greater degree. They differ from each other in the theta frequencies and in 9 to 18 Hz activity (PR-F-36-CL elicits more of the former and less of the latter). All three compounds differ from placebo in reducing the number of artifacts. The most significant difference between the compounds is in amplitude variability. PR-F-36-CL and dextroamphetamine decrease this measure, while fenfluramine increases it (Table 2).

Prior to account for differences due to drugs, the second and third 15-min means are distinct from the remaining sampling periods in having less alpha and more percent time in frequencies below 6 and above 21 Hz. Interaction

TABLE 2. *Multiple stepwise linear regression analysis of drug differences*

Dependent variable	(F) Drug set	DA vs. PL	PR vs. PL	FE vs. PL	DA vs. PR	DA vs. FE	PR vs. FE
Ave. ampl.						2.37	
Dev. ampl.	20.87	−4.46	−3.16	2.77		−7.45	−6.09
Ave. freq.			−2.25		2.56		−2.27
Dev. freq.	6.08	−3.63	−2.32			−3.45	−2.15
3.5 Hz		−2.30				−2.35	
4.5 Hz	3.39	−2.59			−2.53	−2.77	
6 Hz	6.99	−3.97			−3.47	−3.80	
7.5 Hz					−2.17	−2.37	
9 Hz		2.38					
11 Hz	7.75	3.94			2.96	4.44	
13 Hz	6.23	3.29			2.12	4.19	2.07
15 Hz	3.51	2.17			2.10	3.15	
18 Hz	3.65		−3.00		2.80		−2.24
21 Hz	4.90		−2.86				−3.57
24 Hz	4.62	−2.65	−2.89			−2.26	−2.72
27 Hz	6.99	−2.89	−2.77			−3.22	−3.22
30 Hz	5.03	−2.43				−3.38	−2.25
33 Hz	5.83	−2.56				−3.24	−2.70
40 Hz	7.51	−3.43	−2.05			−4.13	−2.63
+40 Hz	7.92	−3.76			−2.07	−4.15	−2.07
Artifacts	6.00	−3.37	−3.87	−2.12			
Heart rate	15.40	3.38	4.11			5.19	5.77

Independent variables accounted for previous to drug set include predrug measure, subjects set, age, weight, and time period set. Significant *F*-test and *t*-test values, $p < .05$. PR = PR-F-36-CL, 350 mg; PL = placebo; DA = dextroamphetamine, 10 mg; FE = fenfluramine, 40 mg.

variables were not found to contribute significantly as a group. However, PR-F-36-CL stands out in decreasing the percent time +21 Hz and increasing heart rate throughout the last 45 min of the session. In this analysis, PR-F-36-CL exhibits an onset delay of 60 to 75 min, rather than a biphasic effect, with a peak in the range of 75 to 90 min postadministration.

To relate EEG and non-EEG measures we selected average amplitude, 6, 9, and 24 Hz EEG measures as dependent variables of interest. No association was found between heart rate or artifacts and any of these measures, although artifacts are directly related to 6 Hz and inversely related to the 9 Hz measure in the last 15 min of the sessions. Buzzer releases are directly related to percent time in the 4.5 to 6 Hz band and inversely related to the 7.5 to 9 Hz band throughout the experiment.

Blood Pressure

An increase in systolic blood pressure was observed 2 hr after dextroamphetamine and PR-F-36-CL. The increase was not in evidence 30 min postdrug and did not occur with placebo or fenfluramine.

TABLE 3. *Variations in blood pressure (means) with different drug treatments*

Pressure and treatment	Dextroam-phetamine	PR-F-36-CL	Placebo	Fenflur-amine
Systolic BP				
Predrug 1	120	120	119	119
Predrug 2	119	118	118	119
Postdrug 30 min	119	118	118	117
Postdrug 120 min	130[a]	129[b]	118	117
Diastolic BP				
Predrug 1	74	74	72	73
Predrug 2	72	73	70	72
Postdrug 30 min	75	76	75	72
Postdrug 120 min	78	81	76	75

[a] $p < .05$.
[b] $p < .01$.
Wilcoxon matched-pairs signed-ranks test versus placebo – drug 3; two-tailed test.

Comparison of pre- versus postdrug values showed the systolic increases in blood pressure to be significant for both dextroamphetamine and PR-F-36-CL. These increases were correlated with increases in heart rate. The diastolic increases following dextroamphetamine, PR-F-36-CL, and placebo were not significant (Table 3).

Behavioral Data

Continuous Alerting Task

The mean number of postdrug button releases per 5-min epoch was adjusted by predrug means to reflect the average change from "pre-" to "post." Change scores were then tested for differences between drugs. Significantly fewer releases occurred after dextroamphetamine than after fenfluramine. No other interdrug differences were significant. We reviewed the number of button releases and number of subjects releasing the button at each 5-min interval and found the fewest releases after dextroamphetamine. More button releases followed fenfluramine than placebo, whereas PR-F-36-CL was similar to fenfluramine during the first half of the sessions, but showed fewer releases (similar to dextroamphetamine) in the second half (Table 4).

Alertness Self-Assessment

The difference between drugs in alertness assessment totals was tested. A significant decrease in alertness was found associated with fenfluramine as compared against placebo. No other interdrug differences reach significance. Plots of the data suggest that placebo and dextroamphetamine are indistinguishable by this measure. PR-F-36-CL appears to have a biphasic effect, decreasing alertness in the first 75 min, but increasing it during the last 45 min. Fenfluramine uniformly decreases alertness after the first 40 min (Table 5).

TABLE 4. *Continuous alerting task: Total number of button releases*

Subject no.	Dextroam- phetamine		PR-F-36-CL		Placebo		Fenflur- amine	
	Pre	Post	Pre	Post	Pre	Post	Pre	Post
1	3	19	0	26	0	9	0	70
2	2	6	5	42	2	23	4	21
3	0	3	0	1	0	0	0	1
4	0	0	0	0	0	0	0	4
5	0	0	0	0	0	0	0	3
6	3	12	1	2	0	5	2	16
7	0	0	0	1	0	0	0	3
8	1	5	0	6	0	1	0	4
9	0	0	0	0	0	0	0	0
10	0	0	0	3	0	34	1	14
11	0	0	0	1	0	1	0	1
13	1	0	0	14	10	51	2	20
14	0	1	0	11	0	10	0	2
Mean	0.8	3.5[a]	0.5	8.2	0.9	10.3	0.7	12.2

[a] $p < .05$; t-test versus Fe; two-tailed test.

TABLE 5. *Alertness self-assessment: Totals across time*

Subject	Dextroam- phetamine		PR-F-36-CL		Placebo		Fenflur- amine	
	Pre	Post	Pre	Post	Pre	Post	Pre	Post
1	0	−10	0	−7	−1	−3	−1	0
2	0	−4	−2	−18	0	8	0	0
3	−1	−2	0	9	−3	0	0	0
4	0	−1	0	13	0	12	0	1
5	0	−2	0	4	0	−3	0	−7
6	3	−5	−2	−18	−3	−8	−2	−26
7	0	0	0	1	0	0	0	−1
8	−6	−55	−4	−11	−1	−24	−7	−52
9	0	13	0	6	0	−8	0	−27
10	0	2	0	0	0	0	0	0
11	−1	−15	0	−5	0	−4	0	−3
13	0	0	0	−1	−6	−8	0	−5
14	−3	0	−2	−12	0	0	2	−3
Mean	−0.6	−6.1	−0.8	−3.0	−1.1	−2.9	−0.6	−9.5[a]

[a] $p < .05$; Wilcoxon matched-pairs signed-ranks test versus placebo; two tailed test.

Abramson Symptom Questionnaire

Symptoms most commonly associated with each drug as compared against placebo at these doses in this setting, are as follows:

1. PR-F-36-CL—aware of heart beat (8Ss), heart beat faster than usual (4Ss), increased salivation (4Ss), tense (4Ss), anxious (4Ss), restless (5Ss), dizzy (4Ss), and fatigue (4Ss);
2. Dextroamphetamine—aware of heart beat (5Ss);
3. Fenfluramine—drowsy (8Ss) and hot (5Ss).

Subjects' Voluntary Reports

During session

According to informal reports volunteered by the subjects, PR-F-36-CL (350 mg) and dextroamphetamine (10 mg) have similar profiles as compared to placebo. Both compounds are associated with cardiovascular symptoms (esp., aware of heart beat), limb symptoms (esp., tremors and twitching with PR-F-36-CL), and head symptoms (esp., lightheadedness). Fenfluramine (10 mg) was solely distinguished by visual symptoms.

Aftereffects

PR-F-36-CL (350 mg) had a mean duration of effect of 10 hr (11Ss). According to spontaneous reports, the most commonly persisting symptoms were sleep disruption (8Ss) and anorexia (4Ss). All other aftereffects following PR-F-36-CL or the other three compounds were reported by fewer than four subjects.

Placebo was distinguished by the largest number of asymptomatic reports (9Ss). Mean duration of those effects reported (4Ss) was 3 hr, as compared with 5+ hr following 10 mg dextroamphetamine (8Ss) and 3 hr following 40 mg fenfluramine (7Ss). Euphoria (2Ss) was the most distinguishing feature after dextroamphetamine, whereas sedation (3Ss) was most prominent after fenfluramine.

Irwin Form

Drug versus placebo comparisons suggested similar profiles for dextroamphetamine (10 mg) and PR-F-36-CL (350 mg) and no differences between fenfluramine (40 mg) and placebo. Global change, physical change, and a faster sense of time were common to PR-F-36-CL and dextroamphetamine. In addition, thought change and expression difficulty were associated with PR-F-36-CL, whereas mood change followed dextroamphetamine.

In their overall evaluations 140 min postdrug, nine subjects identified placebo as inactive. PR-F-36-CL and dextroamphetamine were judged inactive by two subjects each, and fenfluramine was considered a placebo by six subjects. PR-F-36-CL had the most definite effects, being mainly characterized as a stimulant with some initial sedative properties. Dextroamphetamine was predominantly classed as a stimulant, and fenfluramine was classed as a sedative or inactive.

DISCUSSION

With one caveat, the goals set for this study have been successfully fulfilled: (a) an EEG profile for PR-F-36-CL has been defined in our setting in a select population at a 350 mg dose over a continuous time course from $\frac{1}{2}$ to 2 hr postdrug ingestion, and (b) PR-F-36-CL (350 mg) is more similar to dextroamphetamine (10 mg) than to fenfluramine (40 mg) or to placebo in these measures. A range of onset and duration of PR-F-36-CL activity has been determined, a behavioral profile has been elicited, distinguishing features have been characterized, and a correspondence in the time course of behavioral and physiologic changes has been observed. The caveat is the single dose, which leaves open the possibility that similarities between dextroamphetamine and PR-F-36-CL and differences from fenfluramine may be dose-related.

Some support for the generality of these findings comes from our experience with placebo in 44 similar subjects in 55 placebo sessions in five previous studies. Both the physiologic and behavioral profiles of placebo in this study fall within the range of changes found associated with placebo on those studies.

The sensitivity of behavioral measures in distinguishing these drugs is encouraging. In light of the acknowledged vagaries of subjective reporting and the wealth of experience documenting placebo reactors, we might have expected individual variability to obscure systemic effects. The factors, other than chance, which affected these results are many. The set in these studies is more stringently controlled than in the usual behavioral studies, since EEG measurement requires strict stability of the sensory environment. Our volunteers are college-level and graduate students, who are verbal, well motivated, and cooperative for economic and social reasons. They also appear sophisticated regarding drug effects, in part a result of the increased popular use of psychoactive compounds.

SUMMARY

A study in 13 volunteers compared physiologic, EEG, and behavioral effects of single doses of PR-F-36-CL (350 mg), dextroamphetamine (10 mg), fenfluramine (40 mg), and placebo. An EEG profile of PR-F-36-CL was defined and found similar to dextroamphetamine at these doses. The onset of effects was delayed for 75 min. Duration averaged 10 hr. Chief symptoms were increased systolic blood pressure, increased heart rate, nervousness, lightheadedness, and sleep disruption.

Dextroamphetamine was associated with increased systolic blood pressure and increased heart rate. Its effects were initially observed at 30 min and lasted 5+ hr. Chief effects of fenfluramine were drowsiness and temperature sensitivity.

ACKNOWLEDGMENTS

This work is aided in part by grant number MH 24020 and 13358 from the National Institute of Mental Health. We are indebted to the assistance of Leslie Stanton, Carolyn Poinier, Ira Snapper, and Steven Kahn.

REFERENCES

Cohen, J. (1968): Multiple regression as a general data-analytic system. *Psychol. Bull.,* 70: 426–443.

Fink, M. (1969): EEG and human psychopharmacology. *Ann. Rev. Pharmacol.,* 9:241–258.

Fink, M. (1974): EEG applications in psychopharmacology. In: *Psychopharmacological Agents,* Vol. III, edited by M. Gordon, pp. 159–174. Academic Press, New York.

Oliver, J. T. (1974): Anorectic activity of 4-chloro-2'-(methylamino)methyl benzhydrol HCl (PR-F-36CL). *Arch. Int. Pharmacodyn.,* 212:139.

Shapiro, D., and Glasser, M. (1974): Measurement and comparison of EEG-drug effects. In: *Psychotropic Drugs and the Human EEG,* edited by T. Itil, pp. 327–349. S. Karger, Basel.

Predictability in Psychopharmacology: Preclinical and Clinical Correlations,
edited by A. Sudilovsky, S. Gershon and B. Beer. Raven Press, New York,
© 1975.

Diazepam: Efficacy and Toxicity as Revealed by a Small Sample Research Strategy

E. H. Uhlenhuth, M. Stern, C. R. Schuster, and D. Domizi

Department of Psychiatry, University of Chicago, Chicago, Illinois 60637

Most recent efforts to increase the sensitivity of drug evaluation have employed ever larger samples (Rickels and McLaughlin, 1968). In contrast, our strategy sought to: (1) identify and measure certain potential sources of variability, and (2) reduce extraneous variability by structuring a more closely controlled test situation with a small number of subjects.

Diazepam was chosen for study as a well-established antianxiety agent (Garattini, Mussini, and Randall, 1973). Effects on three psychomotor performances and on subjective mood were measured. Possible sources of variability in response selected for study were (1) medication dose, and (2) contingencies associated with task performance.

METHOD

Subjects

Subjects were six carefully selected, paid volunteers solicited through an advertisement in the university newspaper. All were white male university students, full or part time, aged 21 to 28. Screening procedures included complete physical and psychiatric history, including details of drug intake during the past month and routine physical examination. No subject had any current physical or psychiatric problem or took any drug or alcohol more than twice weekly. One subject had had some depressive symptoms several months earlier in association with a marital separation and another subject described a somewhat eccentric family background, but there were no other indications of possible psychopathology in any subject. All subjects were right-handed.

General Design

Each subject participated in seven sessions, generally at weekly intervals, although three subjects had one session after a 2-wk interval because of an equipment failure and later had two sessions in 1 wk to make up the time

TABLE 1. *Experimental design*[a]

Session no.	Medication
1	placebo
2	placebo
3	diazepam, 5 mg
4	placebo
5	diazepam, 10 mg
6	placebo
7	diazepam, 20 mg

[a] Contingency: First half, no reinforcement; second half, reinforcement.

lost. The experimental conditions were the same for all six subjects at each session, as shown in Table 1.

Procedure for Each Session

The subject presented himself for each session at the same hour of the day, at least 8 hr postprandial, and the order of procedure was as follows:

1. Subject completed Profile of Mood States (POMS) (McNair, Lorr, and Droppleman, 1971).
2. Technician administered medication dose.
3. Subject completed Hopkins Symptom Checklist[1] (Derogatis, Lipman, Rickels, Uhlenhuth, and Covi, 1974).
4. Subject waited until $1\frac{1}{2}$ hr after ingesting medication.
5. Subject completed POMS.
6. Technician administered visual tracking[1] (Holzman, Proctor, and Hughes, 1973) and performance tasks.
7. Technician administered debriefing interview.
8. Physician measured nerve conduction velocity[1] and recovery time[1] in selected sessions.

Performance Tasks

Three different performance tasks were selected to emphasize somewhat different aspects of function ranging from muscular speed and coordination through attention to cognition and short term memory. Stimuli were administered and responses were recorded and timed by means of a laboratory computer equipped with a cathode ray tube (CRT), whistles, and a

---

[1] Not included in this report.

response board. Attached to the response board were three metal plates $3\frac{1}{4} \times 3\frac{1}{4}$ in. arranged at the angles of an isosceles triangle with a base measuring $14\frac{3}{4}$ in. and legs measuring 18 in. The response board lay on a table so that the base of the triangle was nearest the seated subject. The CRT and whistles were on the table facing the subject at a distance of about $4\frac{1}{2}$ ft from the subject.

Two-Point Tapping

At the word "START" on the CRT, the subject alternately tapped the two metal plates nearest him with the right index finger until the word "STOP" appeared, accompanied by a whistle. Each trial lasted 5 sec from the first tap, and there were five trials, the first discarded as practice.

Lift-Off Reaction Time

At the word "START" on the CRT, the subject placed his right index finger on one of the nearest plates. After a randomly varied interval ranging from 1 to 5 sec, the word "GO" appeared on the CRT accompanied by a whistle, and the subject moved his finger to the distant plate as rapidly as possible to turn off the stimuli. Latency before lift-off was measured. There were five sets of five trials, the first set discarded as practice.

Memory Scan

This procedure was adapted from Sternberg (1966). At the word "START" on the CRT, the subject placed an index finger on each plate nearest him on the response board. A series of digits ranging in length from one to six were displayed on the CRT sequentially for 1.2 sec each. After 2 sec the word "READY" appeared on the CRT for 2 sec, immediately followed by a single test digit accompanied by a whistle. The subject lifted his right index finger to indicate that the test digit was a member of the preceding series or his left index finger to indicate that it was not. A correct response turned off the stimuli. There were seven sets of 12 trials, the first set discarded as practice.

The stimulus sets were designed so that each series length occurred twice in random order within each set of trials, once with a test digit in the series (positive trial) and once with a test digit not in the series (negative trial). The location of the test digit in the series varied at random in positive trials.

Contingencies

Two contingency conditions were associated with each task. After every set of trials, the CRT displayed for 10 sec a score in dollars and cents reflecting the speed and accuracy of the subject's performance. During the first three (or four, for the memory scan) sets of trials, only this feedback was provided. During the final two (or three, for the memory scan) sets of trials, the subject was paid in accordance with the scores shown.

Scores were computed on the basis of experience with each subject so that he could earn an average of about $15.00 per session in addition to his "base pay" of $5.00 per session. The computation for the memory scan included a deduction of 25¢ for each error. Subjects were informed of the penalty and told that the most profitable strategy was to work as fast as possible while maintaining accuracy. All earnings were paid only after the series of sessions was completed.

The actual formulas for computing the scores for each set of trials were:

$$\text{Score (TAP)} = \$0.90 + (N_t - C) \times 0.2,$$
$$\text{Score (RT)} = \$1.40 + (C - \overline{L}) \times 50,$$
$$\text{Score (MEM)} = \$1.94 + (C - \overline{L}) \times N_c - 0.25 \times (12 - N_c),$$

where N_t was the number of taps, N_c the number of correct trials, $\overline{L}$ the mean latency from signal to lift-off, and C an estimate of the subject's performance on the basis of past experience. Initially, C was set equal to the mean performance of normal young adult males for each procedure.

Medications

All subjects received diazepam orally, 5 mg at session three, 10 mg at session five, and 20 mg at session seven, with one exception: the smallest subject appeared so drowsy after the 10-mg dose that he was given 2.5 mg at session seven as his "low dose." (In retrospect this was an error, but no effort to compensate was made in calculating the results.) Medications were administered in liquid form in two different flavored syrup bases containing quinine. The two different bases were employed at random in different sessions.

Data Analyses

The following results were computed for each subject at each session under nonreinforced and reinforced conditions separately: (1) mean number of taps, (2) mean lift-off reaction time (latency), (3) total errors on memory scan, and (4) slope of latency versus series size on memory scan. The slope on memory scan was computed by fitting a line to the latencies for correct trials at each series length (one to six). The slope of this line is said to reflect the time required to scan an element in active memory during error-free performance (Sternberg, 1966).

The POMS at each session was scored to reflect six factored dimensions of mood (McNair et al., 1971): anxiety, dejection, anger, vigor, fatigue, and confusion.

In further calculations, the results of session one were discarded as practice. Each measure of performance listed above was treated similarly. For each subject, a line was fitted to the three results in each condition: nonreinforced/placebo (sessions two, four, six), nonreinforced/diazepam (sessions three, five, seven), reinforced/placebo (sessions two, four, six), and reinforced/diazepam (sessions three, five, seven). Two indices of response were derived from the fitted line in each condition. (1) The estimated value of the measure at session five was taken as an index of overall response. (2) The slope of the line was taken as an index of time-related effects and, in the drug conditions, dose-related effects as well. The nonreinforced/placebo condition was regarded as a control condition for the effects of time and repetition. Every possible pair of conditions was compared by means of a one-sample *t* test applied to the mean of the differences between conditions.

The POMS measures were analyzed in a similar way, but there were only two conditions (placebo, diazepam) to compare.

RESULTS

Performance

Table 2 shows the mean results over the six subjects in each condition, as well as the comparisons between pairs of conditions. Tapping decreased reliably (5 df, $p < 0.05$, 2-tailed) under diazepam, as measured by the difference between the diazepam and the control conditions and by the difference between the diazepam and the reinforcement conditions in the estimated number of taps at session five. This effect of diazepam was reliably related to dose, as measured by the difference between the slopes of the lines fitted to the diazepam and the control conditions. In the presence of reinforcement, however, diazepam did not reliably decrease the number of taps (Fig. 1).

Lift-off latency tended to increase under diazepam ($p < 0.10$), and the slowing effect of diazepam was reliably related to dose. Although diazepam seemed to produce a dose-related increase in lift-off latency in the presence of reinforcement as well, this effect was not so marked and was not reliable (Fig. 2).

In the memory scanning procedure, the number of errors decreased reliably under diazepam. This effect was not dose-related (Fig. 3). The scanning time increased reliably under diazepam in the presence of reinforcement. Diazepam also tended to produce a dose-related increase in scanning time in the absence of reinforcement ($p < 0.10$) (Fig. 4).

TABLE 2. Mean slopes and estimates at session five from lines fitted to results from six subjects in four conditions

Condition	No. taps		Lift-off		No. errors		Slope	
	B	$\hat{Y}$	B	$\hat{Y}$	B	$\hat{Y}$	B	$\hat{Y}$
Nonreinforcement/Plac (C)	0.10	29.24	-0.003	0.248	0.54	4.54	-0.003	0.021
Nonreinforcement/Diaz (D)	-0.67	26.19	0.004	0.259	0.50	2.61	0.001	0.023
Reinforcement/Plac (R)	0.37	29.99	-0.003	0.245	0.46	3.29	-0.003	0.018
Reinforcement/Diaz (R/D)	0.64	28.64	0.002	0.254	0.71	3.22	-0.002	0.027
Differences between conditions								
D-C	-0.77[a]	-3.05[a]	0.007[a]	0.011[b]	-0.04	-1.93[a]	0.004	0.002
R-C	0.27	0.74	0	-0.004	-0.08	-1.25	0	-0.002
R/D-C	0.54	-0.60	0.005	0.006	0.17	-1.32	0.001	0.007[b]
R-D	1.04	3.79[a]	-0.007[b]	-0.014[b]	-0.04	0.68	-0.004[b]	-0.004
R/D-D	1.31	2.44[b]	-0.003	-0.005	0.21	0.61	-0.003[b]	0.004
R/D-R	0.27	-1.35[b]	0.005	0.009	0.25	-0.07	0.001	0.009[a]

[a] $p < 0.05$.
[b] $p < 0.10$.
B is the dose/response slope.
$\hat{Y}$ is the effect estimated at session 5.

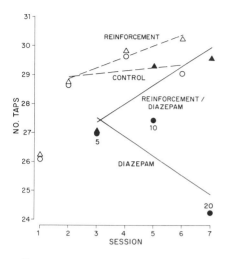

FIG. 1. Mean number of taps for 6 subjects at each experimental session. Subjects received diazepam at sessions 3 (5 mg), 5 (10 mg), and 7 (20 mg). Solid symbols, results under diazepam; triangles, results with reinforcement.

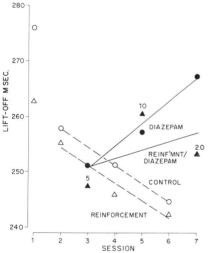

FIG. 2. Mean lift-off reaction time (latency) for six subjects at each experimental session. Subjects received diazepam at sessions 3 (5 mg), 5 (10 mg), and 7 (20 mg). Solid symbols, results under diazepam; triangles, results with reinforcement.

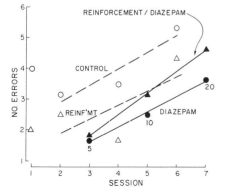

FIG. 3. Mean number of errors on memory scan for six subjects at each experimental session. Subjects received diazepam at sessions 3 (5 mg), 5 (10 mg), and 7 (20 mg). Solid symbols, results under diazepam; triangles, results with reinforcement.

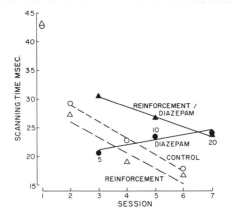

FIG. 4. Mean scanning time per digit in active memory for six subjects at each experimental session. Subjects received diazepam at sessions 3 (5 mg), 5 (10 mg), and 7 (20 mg). Solid symbols, results under diazepam; triangles, results with reinforcement.

TABLE 3. *Mean slopes and estimates at session five from lines fitted to results from six subjects in two conditions*

Condition	Anxiety B	Anxiety Ŷ	Vigor B	Vigor Ŷ	Fatigue B	Fatigue Ŷ	Confusion B	Confusion Ŷ
Placebo	0.01	0.56	−0.21	1.11	0.07	0.49	0.01	0.53
Diazepam	0.03	0.28	−0.11	0.94	0.15	0.86	0.03	0.60
Diaz-Plac	0.02	−0.28[a]	0.10	−0.17	0.08	0.37	0.02	0.07

[a] $p < 0.05$.

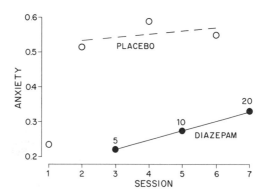

FIG. 5. Mean anxiety scores on the Profile of Mood States for six subjects at each experimental session. Subjects received diazepam at sessions 3 (5 mg), 5 (10 mg), and 7 (20 mg). Solid symbols, results under diazepam.

Mood

Table 3 shows the mean results over the six subjects in the diazepam and placebo conditions, as well as the comparison between the two conditions. Anxiety scores decreased reliability under diazepam, but this effect was not dose-related. Figure 5 shows these results. Although fatigue seemed to increase under diazepam, this effect was not reliable.

DISCUSSION

The observed effects of diazepam on tapping and lift-off latency were entirely in accord with expectation: dose-related impairment in both cases (McNair, 1973). These results document the sensitivity of the procedures, even with the small samples employed. The fact that these results were obtained within the therapeutic dose range of diazepam further supports the sensitivity of the procedures.

A more interesting observation concerns the joint effects of diazepam and reinforcement on the two tasks. Given sufficient reinforcement, subjects largely overcame the impairing effects of diazepam on tapping. A similar interaction effect on lift-off latency was observed, although it was less marked and not reliable.

This appears to be only the second direct demonstration of an interaction between the effects of drug and reinforcing contingencies in humans. Hill, Belleville, and Wikler (1957) showed that the slowing of reaction time by pentobarbital could be reversed in former drug addicts by providing morphine for high performance. The marked individual variability in response to psychotropic medication in therapeutic settings has been discussed in terms of interaction between drug and nondrug effects (Fisher, Cole, Rickels, and Uhlenhuth, 1964). However, these interactions have been very difficult to demonstrate reliably in the clinic (Uhlenhuth, Covi, Rickels, Lipman, and Park, 1972). Motivational factors like those in the present study probably are among the factors that interact with drug effects in clinical practice.

The interaction between diazepam and reinforcement in the memory scan appears to be even more complex than in the tapping and reaction time tasks. Errors *decreased* reliably under diazepam, but not in the presence of reinforcement. Scanning time appeared to increase under diazepam, especially in the presence of reinforcement. These findings might suggest a trade-off between accuracy and speed controlled jointly by drug and reinforcement, although the evidence in the present study is not clear on this point.

The contrasting effects of diazepam on accuracy in the memory scan and on tapping and reaction time may be more understandable in the light of crucial differences in the procedures themselves. Only the memory scan involves discrimination or stimulus control. Anxiety (arousal, emotionality) might be expected to disrupt discrimination more readily than the simpler functions sufficient for tapping and reaction time. Given a state of increased arousal, then, an antianxiety agent might be expected to improve discrimination but not tapping or reaction time.

These are, of course, exactly the conditions observed in the study: The subjects appeared to be stressed and aroused by the procedures. They certainly reported subjective anxiety. Diazepam reduced the reported level of anxiety by 50%, and accuracy (discrimination) improved.

Why did not diazepam produce greater accuracy in the presence of reinforcement? The acquisition of stimulus control requires differential reinforcement (Terrace, 1966) like that provided under the reinforced conditions of this study. Presumably, stimulus control also would be maintained more effectively in the presence of reinforcement. Accuracy did seem to be greater with reinforcement than without, although not significantly. Quite possibly reinforcement maintained discrimination so effectively, even in the presence of arousal, that diazepam could not produce a substantial additional improvement. This would represent an interaction between reinforcement and diazepam with a "ceiling" effect.

Diazepam impaired (slowed) scanning rate, especially in the presence of reinforcement. This effect contrasts with the improved accuracy under diazepam. Sternberg (1966) theorizes that the match-to-sample (discrimination) is a single, distinct operation that follows an exhaustive scan of the entire series of digits stored in active memory. Although others have pointed out the logical inconsistency of his position (Corballis, Kirby, and Miller, 1972), the results of this study do suggest that the memory scanning task includes at least two processes differentially affected by diazepam and reinforcement.

Finally, the subjective reports, in addition to their possible bearing on the performance results, indicate that the experimental procedure was sensitive to the effects of diazepam on anxiety. Given the level of anxiety present in this study, subjects did not report significant sedation under diazepam, even though certain sedative effects on performance were detectable. The subjective experience instead paralleled the improvement in discrimination. The clear-cut reduction observed in anxiety, with minimal subjective sedation and minimal deterioration in performance under conditions of high motivation, certainly exemplify highly desirable properties in an antianxiety agent for clinical application.

The procedures employed in this study permitted the sensitive detection of diazepam's effects on both performance and subjective state, even in a small sample of normal subjects. The study, then, suggests means for more economical and convenient evaluation of the efficacy and toxicity of antianxiety agents in humans.

ACKNOWLEDGMENTS

This study was supported by Contract No. 72–42 from the U.S. Food and Drug Administration and by the Louis Block Fund for Basic Research and Advanced Study.

Professor David L. Wallace provided statistical consultation. Professors Israel Goldiamond, Philip S. Holzman, Victor Laties, and Bernard Weiss provided consultation on experimental procedures and interpretation of results. Dr. Arthur Snapper provided the SKED system for programming behavioral procedures on the PDP-8/e. Miss Elizabeth Grether, Mrs. Betty Raaf, Mrs. Linda Sang, and Mr. Herman Weinreb provided technical assistance.

REFERENCES

Corballis, M. D., Kirby, J., and Miller, A. (1972): Access to elements of a memorized list. *J. Exp. Psychol.*, 94:185–190.
Derogatis, L. R., Lipman, R. S., Rickels, K., Uhlenhuth, E. H., and Covi, L. (1974): The Hopkins Symptom Checklist (HSCL): A self-report symptom inventory. *Behav. Sci.*, 19: 1–15.
Fisher, S., Cole, J. O., Rickels, K., and Uhlenhuth, E. H. (1964): Drug-set interaction: The effect of expectations on drug response in outpatients. In: *Neuropsychopharmacology, Vol. III*, edited by P. B. Bradley, F. Flugel, and P. Hoch. Elsevier Publishing Co., Amsterdam.
Garattini, S., Mussini, E., and Randall, L. O. (Eds.) (1973): *The Benzodiazepines.* Raven Press, New York.
Hill, H. E., Belleville, R. E., and Wikler, A. (1957): Motivational determinants in modification of behavior by morphine and pentobarbital. *Arch. Neurol. Psychiatry*, 77:28–35.
Holzman, P. S., Proctor, L. R., and Hughes, D. W. (1973): Eye-tracking patterns in schizophrenia. *Science*, 181:179–181.
McNair, D. M. (1973): Antianxiety drugs and human performance. *Arch. Gen. Psychiatry*, 29:611–617.
McNair, D. M., Lorr, M., and Droppleman, L. F. (1971): *Profile of Mood States* (manual). Educational and Industrial Testing Service, San Diego, Calif.
Rickels, K., and McLaughlin, B. E. (1968): Sample size in psychiatric drug research. *Clin. Pharmacol. Ther.*, 9:631–634.
Sternberg, S. (1966): High speed scanning in human memory. *Science*, 153:652–654.
Terrace, H. S. (1966): Stimulus control. In: *Operant Behavior: Areas of Research and Application*, edited by W. K. Honig. Appleton-Century-Crofts, New York.
Uhlenhuth, E. H., Covi, L., Rickels, K., Lipman, R. S., and Park, L. C. (1972): Predicting the relief of anxiety with meprobamate: An attempt at replication. *Arch. Gen. Psychiatry*, 26: 85–91.

DISCUSSION

Ayd: What was the time interval between the reward and the non-reward sessions?
Uhlenhuth: Ten sec. In any given procedure (for example, the lift-off reaction time), there was a set of fine trials and then a 10-sec period when the feedback was displayed, followed by the next five trials. The first five trials were thrown away. The second two sets of five trials were under the non-reward condition and the next two sets were under the reward condition. Actually, the procedures are largely

subject controlled. In other words, the machine, as it were, says, "I am now ready whenever you wish," and then the subject activates a given trial by putting his hand down on the initial plate, so it's paced by the subject.

Ayd: Did the subject know whether he was in a non-reward or reward situation?

Uhlenhuth: Yes, he did.

Ayd: What influence would that have, in terms of knowing, "why bother now, the next session is a reward session?"

Uhlenhuth: That's what reward is about—that the subject knows he is going to get paid for doing especially well.

Zung: Maybe Frank Ayd is thinking in terms of practice effect. But if instead you used a random design, a crossover with the reward and non-reward, then you would obviate that problem.

Uhlenhuth: You mean that there is a possible confounding between practice and reward here, in the sense that the latter part of every session was the reward? That is certainly a possibility.

Spitzer: You can see from their behavior that they were acting very differently and it was not just from practicing. It was obvious when the reward period started.

Uhlenhuth: Actually, I meant that in a more general sense. That is to say, once we got this procedure set up this way, people got much more involved in it. It does happen, however, that we did do this without any reward in an earlier set of subjects and we found more of a fatigue effect than a practice effect. With the tapping, for example, the curve runs from the first set up to the second set and from then on it's downhill. Thus, without the reward you will get less tapping.

Ayd: At what time of the day and in what relationship to meals did you give the drug?

Uhlenhuth: It was always at least 8 hr after the last meal. The time of day varied for different subjects, but was constant for a given subject. In other words, every subject was run at the same hour of the day for every session.

Ayd: I am very curious, because usually normal individuals are very sensitive to diazepam, even in the 5-mg dose. You get quite a bit of drowsiness. With an interval of 2 wk, certainly, no tolerance develops, so there should have been a tremendous amount of drowsiness after that 20-mg dose.

Uhlenhuth: There was. What would happen is that the subject would be given the dose of diazepam and would go to the place where he has to wait and then when it was time, $1\frac{1}{2}$ hr later, you'd almost have to wake him up. Actually, they'd stagger down the hallway, they'd drop cigarette butts and ashes on the rug, and they'd get in front of the machine and they'd start right in. It was really dramatic. There is a real interaction between reward and drugs. I think it suggests that if you have to do it, like if you have to get somewhere in the car, you can do it in the face of these drugs. That's the interesting thing about the whole business.

Blackwell: I have two questions. One is a design question and the other is an interpretation question. In terms of the design, what was your reason for not randomizing the drug dosage? I know that you have to incorporate some ways for the repeated placebo administration so that you can get some sequencing, but you also increased the number of sessions that you need to do by doing that. The other question is, what do you think it all means in terms of a therapeutic effect?

Uhlenhuth: The second question is probably harder than the first. We felt this was a simpler thing to do than trying to randomize doses. We've done a second study in which, in fact, we did randomize doses and the results are very similar. One very great advantage in this scheme, by the way, is the presentation, because it makes perfect sense to just show the time curves and it is very easy to understand. You can't do that with the other scheme. You have to use deviation scores from the original data because, if you are going to line up doses (since the doses different people get are different in different sessions and so on), it really ruins the presentation of the thing. This is much easier to do. What does it all mean? I think it means, first of all, that it is certainly possible to use normal subjects to evaluate antianxiety drugs. First of all, you can get antianxiety effects, given the right conditions, and using small numbers. The economy of this kind of an approach impresses me. Secondly, the performance tasks provide at least an approach to toxicologic study, and they certainly indicate that the commonest toxic effect, if you like, of these drugs is highly modifiable by the contingencies. I think the study opens questions that are very interesting in terms of the possible underlying role of the subject's state of arousal being an important factor in how he is going to respond to a particular dose of this drug and whether it's going to have primarily therapeutic effects (as it did here in the subjective measures) or whether it's going to have primarily side effects (as it did not in these subjective measures). We couldn't really demonstrate, clearly at least, any subjective sedative effect, even though we did get some on the performance tests under certain conditions.

Fink: Why do you call it therapeutic? Didn't you have symptom rating scales and, perhaps, see some negative effects at 10 and 20 mg of diazepam?

Uhlenhuth: They didn't. That's the point. They did not report it. What they felt at this level of initial anxiety was relief and not sedation.

Fink: That depends on your inquiry.

Uhlenhuth: No, it doesn't. I'll do again what I intended not to do, and that is to give you the results of the second study in this regard. Again, the subjects took the same mood scale and they started at an anxiety level that was only half as great as it was in this study, that is, their initial anxiety level was equivalent to the anxiety level in the first study on diazepam. In the second study, we were not able to demonstrate any decrease in anxiety. On the other hand, we got highly significant reports of fatigue, decreased vigor, etc.

Fink: Are you presenting this with the idea that it is a predictive device in evaluation of antianxiety agents?

Uhlenhuth: I think it suggests that this kind of an approach would be useful in some of the early investigation of antianxiety agents.

Vukovich: As a follow-up to Dr. Fink's question, if a new potential minor tranquilizer were inactive in this test, would that preclude further testing in patients?

Uhlenhuth: No, certainly not at this point. I think it's too early to say that. We will need to understand, I think, more clearly how the subjective measures respond.

Meyer: I wonder, hypothetically, if you hadn't known that this was diazepam and somebody handed you the drug and said, here is compound X and you had gone through the same exercise and obtained similar results, what kind of summary would you make of this experiment?

Uhlenhuth: I think that it would be difficult for me to outline that right now. I'd like to say that I would have said the same thing, but that's clearly not possible, since I know all the things that you say I shouldn't know. The issue at this point, however, is to be clear that we're trying to develop a procedure and that naturally you have to start with known agents first in developing such a procedure. Not only that, so far we have studied the procedure only with antianxiety agents, so that it is not possible at this time to talk about how a set of results obtained with some other class of agent might contrast with these. This is in the works.

Fink: I think that the extrapolation from a similar study of diazepam and anti-anxiety agents is perhaps premature. We should like to know, for example, what 2, 5, and 10 mg of chlorpromazine would produce.

Uhlenhuth: We would also like to know.

Fink: It is very easy to picture that, without the second contingency, the first contingency that was done would show that a small dose of chlorpromazine will have effects that are not distinguishable in the motor test and in the reaction time test from the effects of diazepam. If one were taking imipramine at equally small doses, one should not be able to distinguish it between these tests. There is extensive experimental evidence for these three compounds and it is very difficult to use test performance to categorize the drugs, whether it be tapping or reaction time.

Uhlenhuth: Or discrimination?

Fink: Discrimination is very complicated, because of which test you use. Of course, it hasn't all been done for all the drugs. The answer to the question of predicting an antianxiety drug effect would have to depend on perhaps the identical experiment being done with an antipsychotic, a thymoleptic, an antiepileptic drug, and perhaps with six or seven compounds all of which have an associated overall "sedative component," whatever that word means, before we can use antianxiety descriptively.

Uhlenhuth: I agree with the kind of reservation you are introducing and it's for that reason that we have, in fact, proposed to do a series of studies using different representative compounds from various classes. I think that what you're suggesting is maybe we ought to even look at different compounds from the same class and see what happens there.

Gershon: The problem is that the various compounds that Dr. Fink listed all have, in his quotes, these "sedative effects," and it may be in this system that the sedative effect is the effect that we are observing and if indeed propranolol, which doesn't have a sedative effect, were used it may not be picked up, because this procedure is picking up non-specific anxiolytic properties of a non-specific group of compounds that have sedation as a part of their effect. Squibb has a compound that might have anxiolytic properties and does not appear to have any sedative effects at all and, therefore, a test like this could "pin it to the wall" if the trials were done with this compound and, let's say, with propranolol. It would be an extreme test of the procedure.

Uhlenhuth: I think that you're addressing not only a methodological point, but also a substantive point which has not yet been resolved by anyone. And that is whether anxiety and sedation are actually on different spectra or not. They may be on the same dimension actually, at opposite ends. That's not impossible. So, there may be no specific antianxiety and non-sedative drug.

Domino: One has to distinguish between the issue of does this compound have human pharmacology as opposed to the issue of, does this compound have a potential or significant therapeutic effect. In this kind of study, you're getting at the issue that diazepam has a human pharmacology in a dose range of 5 to 20 mg. That is very important information if you did diazepam as the first clinical investigator in a Phase I study, because it would allow you to then say that now we're going to do other studies in patients, and since we know that normals in general can take only smaller doses, at least you are giving the dose range in which to begin with. Rather than arguing that this may be a test of value for antianxiety agents, it seems to me you'd be on far firmer ground to argue that here is a test of behavioral pharmacology in man and it may be behavioral toxicity. Nevertheless, you will pick out the effective doses and from that point of view, I'm convinced it's very valuable that a test such as this should be continued. My question is simple. What kind of a mood test are you using?

Uhlenhuth: The test is the POMS, an adjective check list that was developed by McNair and Lorr. It's a fairly standard instrument. It asks people to rate themselves on an intensity scale for each of a series of 65 adjectives and then scores them into groups representing various mood factors.

Blackwell: I am interested to know how many subjects lie behind that statistical significance. In other words, of the six subjects, how many actually showed reduction in anxiety and on how many tested occasions did this happen. When you say "not dose related" do you mean it happened at 10 mg and not at either of the other two doses used, or it happened at all three doses used and just wasn't different, or was there a trend?

Uhlenhuth: No. What I mean specifically is that if you fit a line to the results at the several doses, that line has a slope of zero effectively and it doesn't show any relationship to dose, even though the whole set is moved from the control condition. That is really an interesting question and perhaps we ought to also present results in terms of percent responses.

Zung: Have you done this across populations?

Uhlenhuth: Not exactly the same thing yet, but that again is a contemplated thing. By the way, there is another important issue and that is, what good do single-dose studies do in terms of generalizing to multiple-dose studies? The results are often very different. Here the results happen to be similar to the ones that we did get with subjects in a multiple dose.

Ayd: I would like to see you repeat this, but instead of $1\frac{1}{2}$ hr, you do it in 4 hr when normally you would have the maximum absorption and highest plasma levels of diazepam.

Uhlenhuth: I don't think that's right. We looked at the data about plasma levels before selecting $1\frac{1}{2}$ hr, as a matter of fact, and that appeared to be shortly after maximum. That's why we picked that time.

Ayd: All the data that I'm familiar with would show that approximately 4 hr after an oral dose you get peak effects.

Uhlenhuth: It also depends upon the way you give it. We gave it dissolved in liquid. If you give it as a pill or capsule, that does delay it.

Ayd: I'm aware of that. But even so, when you look at these things from a standpoint of plasma levels, although you may have some difference in the rate of absorption, biochemical formation, and other factors, there's still a delay in maximum peak levels and it's certainly, not generally speaking, at $1\frac{1}{2}$ hr. It would be well worth repeating it just to see. I might make one final comment. Here it is known from clinical experience something about 5, 10, and 20 mg doses of diazepam. If this had been a drug never given to humans before, whether or not subjective tests would be of value without going through a whole lot of dose ranges is highly doubtful.

Predictability in Psychopharmacology: Preclinical and Clinical Correlations,
edited by A. Sudilovsky, S. Gershon and B. Beer. Raven Press, New York,
© 1975.

Behavioral Evaluation of Antianxiety Drugs

Barry Blackwell and William Whitehead

*Department of Psychiatry, College of Medicine, University of Cincinnati, Cincinnati,
Ohio 45267*

The purpose of this chapter is to review selectively some of the con-
temperary methods of "antianxiety" drug evaluation in man and to propose
additional strategies within a behavioral framework. At present, drugs that
affect mood in man are selected on the basis of tests that alter behavior in
animals. Subsequent attempts to demonstrate efficacy usually rely on an
unobservable and poorly defined end state labeled "anxiety." It is difficult
to be sure if this antithetical and inprecise system originates from a cultural
determination to distinguish man from animals or, more simply, that the
prevailing Freudian framework has emphasized emotion over behavior.
Whatever the reason, the influence on new drug development has been
profound. Patients and physicians have been trained to lump together an
array of psychologic, physiologic, and behavioral endpoints under the
common rubric "anxiety." In a procrustean effort to match chemicals with
diagnoses we have named categories of drugs after diseases. The futility
of this practice is illustrated by noting that a recent survey of psychotropic
drug use in five Cincinnati hospitals showed that the use of antianxiety
drugs is ubiquitous across all diagnoses. Table 1 shows that the most commonly used major tranquilizer is given equally often to patients called schizophrenic, depressed, and anxious (Blackwell, Winstead, Anderson, Eilers,
and Buncher, *unpublished data*). In another recent study (Winstead, Anderson, Eilers, Blackwell, and Zaremba, 1974), diazepam was made freely
available to all patients on a psychiatric inpatient service. Table 2 shows
that there was no difference in drug-seeking behavior between diagnoses,
all of which appeared to find the drug useful. By contrast, drug use was
closely correlated with anxiety scores. Irwin (1968) stated this viewpoint
elegantly in his eloquent but overlooked plea for a rational and behavioral
approach to drug development. He states, "The danger with therapeutic
labels of classification, e.g., antipsychotic, antidepressant, or anxiolytic,
is that they become viewed as real entities against which a drug can some-
how act. Nothing could be further from the truth or lead to studies, explanations and experimentation so lacking in relevance."

Given such a lack of precision or specificity in outcome criteria, it is not
surprising that antianxiety drugs are difficult to distinguish from placebo
and impossible to differentiate from each other. Figure 1, based on actual

TABLE 1. *Use of drugs by diagnostic criteria in five city hospitals*

Drug	Patients taking drug (%)		
	Schizophrenia	Depression	All diagnoses
Benzodiazepines	11	33	24
Thioridazine	18	19	16
Amitriptyline	12	26	15

From Blackwell et al., 1974.

TABLE 2. *Drug-seeking behavior for diazepam[a] by diagnosis and anxiety score*

	Percentage of patients		
Drug-seeking index[b]	0	< 0.50	> 0.51
Diagnosis			
Psychosis	25	50	25
Neurosis	38	31	31
Character disorder	18	49	21
Anxiety score			
Low	40	60	0
Medium	30	45	25
High	18	32	50

[a] From Winstead et al., 1974.

[b] Drug seeking index $= \dfrac{\text{no. requests for medication}}{\text{no. days in hospital}}$.

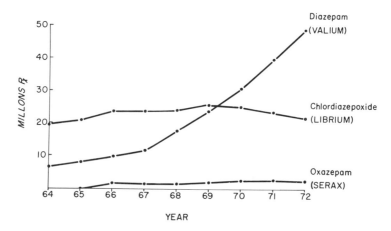

FIG. 1. Trends of use of benzodiazepines.

prescribing of these drugs over eight years, shows that diazepam is a vastly preferred drug to chlordiazepoxide which in turn is used more than oxazepam. Yet no clinical studies have ever shown differences between these drugs in a way that would confirm the wisdom of clinical practice and patient preference (Blackwell, 1973).

In the current system, the failure of animal tests to predict clinical utility is hardly surprising and accounts for many elaborately and expensively tailored failures elegantly named "the Edsels of psychopharmacology" (Goldman, *personal communication*). In order to improve on this performance it will be necessary to identify a conceptual framework of drug action as well as the criteria for an ideal test pathway and an ideal test model.

THE IDEAL CONCEPTUAL FRAMEWORK FOR DRUG ACTION

There are many points at which drugs may act within an organism or in its interaction with the environment. Figure 2 is modified from Irwin's conceptual framework of drug action. Broadly speaking, drugs may alter any of the functions in the diagram. The emphasis in this chapter will be on those aspects of drug action that produce observable and quantifiable endpoints. These include the public manifestations of the intrinsic processes which are shown in the central area of the figure, ranging from arousal to mood states. These external manifestations can be divided into three categories: physiologic function, sensorimotor (or performance) measures, and observations of the individual's behavioral interaction with the environment (along an approach-avoidance continuum). The hopeful thesis of this chapter

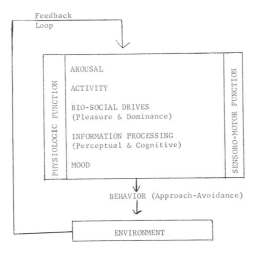

FIG. 2. Conceptual model of sites for drug action. (Modified from Irwin, 1968.)

is that by adopting an observable and behavioral framework for drug evaluation in humans, it may be possible to increase the predictive value of animal tests, improve the sensitivity and reliability of clinical studies, and develop more specific criteria for drug action. It may also become appropriate and possible to rename such compounds after the specific behaviors they alter (without reducing their commercial success).

THE IDEAL TEST PATHWAY

In developing such drugs it would be important to pursue a critical pathway from laboratory to clinic through three separate stages of testing, each designed to predict outcome at succeeding levels of approximation to clinical use. Table 3 suggests that these three levels would be: (1) an animal model in which a specific drug effect occurs, (2) a human test model in normal volunteers which offers a precise analogue to the animal model, and (3) a clinical paradigm that accurately reflects both of the two preceding steps and also the eventual widespread utility within its social and interpersonal context.

Surprisingly, it is possible to illustrate this pathway from within our existing knowledge. The one test which reliably and specifically distinguishes antianxiety drugs from all others is the passive avoidance or conflict model (Geller, 1962). In this situation the animal is punished by shock while engaging in a rewarding activity such as eating. The eating behavior is suppressed. The effect of drugs like the benzodiazepines is to attenuate the suppressant effect of punishment selectively.

Attempts have already been made to translate this model into humans replacing food with monetary reward and retaining shock (to the fingers) as a punishment. There are reasons, however, why this precise extrapolation may be less than adequate, and we believe that it can be improved by use of a procedure described later involving a conflict that is both more appropriate, safe, and consistent. Taking the final step from the volunteer to the clinic poses the vital question of what is the appropriate behavioral endpoint in patients that reflects the preceding test procedures but does so in a social and interpersonal framework relevant to eventual clinical use. We believe that the social analogue of passive avoidance is the situation in which one person fails to engage in dialogue or express appropriate feelings

TABLE 3. *Critical pathway for drug development*

Model	Comment
Animal	Specific to drug category
Human experimental	Analagous to animal model
Clinical	Reflects 1 + 2; predicts eventual use

to another individual for fear of unpleasant consequences. This lack of appropriate assertiveness may be assumed to be a learned behavior based on previous aversive interpersonal interactions. Later we present some data to suggest that this may indeed be an important parameter of drug action with the benzodiazepines and outline a strategy for studying this social dimension.

THE IDEAL HUMAN TEST MODEL

As a preface to considering the physiologic, performance, and behavioral strategies that may be used in studying drugs supposed to affect anxiety it may be helpful to construct an ideal paradigm against which such tests can be evaluated. The features of an ideal test procedure can be listed as follows.

1. *Valid:* Test procedure should reflect drug action in the animal analogue and predict it in the clinical condition.
2. *Sensitive:* The procedure should produce a reasonable range of drug effect and a good drug placebo discrimination.
3. *Observable endpoints:* The criteria of drug action should be capable of external corroboration and measurement.
4. *Reliable:* Effects are reproducible within the same individual and are stable over time.
5. *Practical:* Test procedures should be rapid and inexpensive. If possible, they should be applicable to normal volunteers as well as to patients, and tests should be capable of completion within a single session.
6. *Safe and ethical:* The test procedure should be congruent with the requirements of informed consent.
7. *Economical:* A major shortcoming of existing models that rely on subjective endpoints is a large placebo effect that necessitates unwieldy sample sizes which in turn add both to the expense and insensitivity of the procedures.

PHYSIOLOGIC INDICATORS OF ANXIETY

Physiologic indicators have had a continuing appeal in drug evaluation perhaps because it is by physiologic signs that we recognize anxiety in others outside the laboratory. However, to date most physiologic indicators have been disappointingly unreliable. (1) There are inconsistent findings between different investigators (Lader, 1969). (2) When a physiologic measure does correlate with a subjective measure of anxiety, the correlation is typically below 0.5, which means that less than 25% of the variance in one measure can be predicted from a knowledge of the other. (3) When multiple physiologic measures are taken, they are poorly correlated with one another.

A few of the problems with physiologic outcome measures follow. First, they are technically complicated and expensive to measure. It is worth noting that the physiologic measures which are most easily recognized by the casual observer and by the subject himself (e.g., tremor, voice changes, palpitations, blushing, and hyperventilation) are the most variable in expression. They are also usually the easiest to measure. The physiologic measures which are more reliably associated with anxiety across subjects, e.g., the forearm blood flow measure developed by Kelly (1966) and the rate of habituation of physiologic responses to external stimuli investigated by Lader and Wing (1964), are less accessible to observation and more difficult to measure.

Kelly's forearm blood flow measure correlates only modestly with subjective measures of anxiety (0.24) but shows reliable differences between different diagnostic groups presumed to differ in anxiety (Kelly and Walter, 1968), reliable changes following effective treatment for anxiety (Kelly, Walter, and Sargant, 1966), and consistent changes with stress in normal subjects. Figure 3 illustrates its use in a drug trial of chlordiazepoxide.

The rate of habituation measure used extensively by Lader (1969) also has a modest correlation with subjective report of anxiety (0.46), but shows reliable differences between diagnostic groups presumed to differ in anxiety (Lader and Wing, 1964). The rate of habituation of several physiologic measures is affected by anxiety (Lader, 1969), but Lader reports that the galvanic skin response (GSR) yielded the most meaningful results in his investigations. The chief limitation of the method for drug trials is that within-subject or cross-over designs would be of questionable validity because habituation trials run on one day would be expected to affect habituation rate on subsequent days.

A second problem with the use of physiologic outcome measures is that physiologic changes are multiply determined. Many of them, such as the

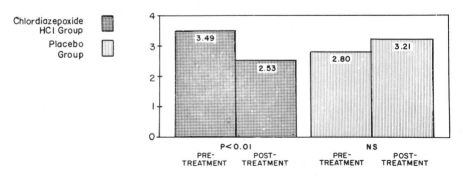

FIG. 3. Forearm blood flow. At rest, mean values in ml/100 ml/min. (From Kelly, Brown, and Shaffer, 1973a.)

GSR and vasomotor activity, subserve temperature regulation and may be substantially influenced by variations in room temperature. Many of these measures may also be influenced by deep breathing (Stern and Anschel, 1968; Sroufe, 1971).

A related problem which occurs when physiologic measures are used to assess pharmacologic preparations is that there may be a direct peripheral drug effect on the physiologic system which either mimics or overwhelms the effects to be expected from anxiety reduction. When this occurs the test discriminates drug from placebo but is not valid because it does not measure anxiety reduction. The experience with the beta-blocker class of drugs is illustrative. These drugs effectively eliminate many of the autonomic physiologic changes associated with anxiety and cause physician ratings of anxiety to go down. However, patients usually report that they are still anxious (Tyrer and Lader, 1973).

Third, we should note that the usual assumption that use of autonomic physiologic indicators will eliminate the placebo effect is not true. Placebo effects have been demonstrated on vegetative responses (Wolf, 1950). Whether drug-placebo discrimination is better or worse than for subjective report has not been clearly established. One report suggests that physiologic measures are poorer drug-placebo discriminators than subjective report measures (Kelly, Pik, and Chen, 1973b), but between-subject sources of variability were not adequately controlled.

SUGGESTIONS FOR IMPROVING PHYSIOLOGIC MEASURES OF DRUG ACTION

In what follows we would like to make some suggestions for improving the usefulness of physiologic indicators in pharmacologic drug evaluation. First, because the possibility of a peripheral drug effect limits the interpretation of the data, we believe drug trials should involve two or more physiologic indicators which are highly correlated under normal circumstances (i.e., functionally equivalent) but which are mediated, peripherally at least, by different neural transmitters. A random selection of physiologic measures, however, is not indicated. An example from the literature on antidepressants follows.

Several investigations have shown that the magnitude of the GSR is reliably reduced in depression. This raises the possibility of using the GSR as a measure of antidepressant drug action. However, the GSR is a cholinergically mediated sympathetic response, and most antidepressants have marked peripheral anticholinergic activity. It has been noted, however, that digital vasoconstriction is a highly correlated sympathetic response which is mediated by an adrenergic neural transmitter. Since the peripheral antiadrenergic effects of the antidepressants are typically less pronounced than the anticholinergic effects, finger vasoconstriction would be a preferred outcome measure which is functionally equivalent to the GSR.

We have not developed comparable pairs of functionally equivalent but chemically distinct physiologic indicators for the antianxiety drugs. Kelly's forearm blood flow measure does not lend itself to this kind of analysis because it is multiply determined by heart rate, stroke volume, and arteriolar resistance (Kelly, 1966). Possibly the GSR and finger vasoconstriction may be useful to assess habituation.

A second suggestion for enhancing the value of physiologic outcome measures relates to the concept of individual response stereotype. What is meant by response stereotype is that in response to stress, subjects will show more reaction in one physiologic response system than in others (for example, more change in heart rate than in respiration), that the same physiologic response system will show maximum change to all stresses in the same individual, and that the physiologic response system showing maximum change is different for different individuals (some subjects will show maximum change in heart rate and others in respiration, etc.). Lacey and his colleagues (Lacey, Bateman, and Van Lehn, 1953) have shown quite convincingly that at least one-third and possibly as many as two-thirds of normal subjects show individual response stereotype. Engel and Bickford (1961) have shown for a group of hypertensives that psychosomatic patients show response stereotype to an even greater extent than normals and that, as expected, maximum change is shown for the symptomatic response.

Obviously, individual response stereotype has contributed substantially to the variance in those drug trials which have used physiologic outcome measures because most of these investigators have assumed that all subjects would show comparable changes in the same physiologic responses when stressed. We propose taking advantage of individual response stereotype by selecting a population of subjects who respond the same way physiologically to stress. This ought to reduce the between-subject variance by eliminating differences in individual response stereotype. It ought additionally to make the outcome measure more sensitive to variations in anxiety since for each subject the variable showing maximum change in response to stress would be used. Finally, it should be possible to avoid confounds with peripheral drug action by selecting a physiologic variable with a chemical mediator known to be relatively unaffected by the drug. Selection of subjects with psychosomatic disorders might be a good method of screening for subjects with specific response stereotypes, that is, subjects with a predictable physiologic response to stress.

PERFORMANCE MEASURES OF ANXIETY

If physiologic measures have been disappointing to date, performance measures have been largely ignored. The usual kinds of tasks that have been studied include vigilance, hand-eye coordination, auditory or visual discrimination, and various intellectual parameters (such as the Wechsler Digit Symbol Substitution Test). With sedative and depressant drugs, performance on these tasks has been used mostly to predict unwanted effects such as drowsiness, incoordination, and ataxia. The tasks themselves are remote from both the animal models and the clinical situation, as well as irrelevant to therapeutic efficacy.

Attempts have been made, however, to make the performance task more relevant to the therapeutic problem. The first advocate of such procedures was Lindsley (1962). His proclivity for reporting seven-year base lines and the remoteness of his experimental task from clinical concerns, however, resulted in his having little impact on the drug industry. The task he used involved having the subject pull a plunger to obtain candy or cigarettes. Only recently has interest in operant-conditioning models of drug evaluation in man revived.

A more promising attempt to quantify the effects of drugs on performance in a clinically relevant way has been to introduce an element of conflict into the procedure. An animal model which has been highly successful in evaluating antianxiety drugs is the conflict or passive-avoidance model developed by Geller (1962). The task of the animal is to press a lever for food which becomes available at variable intervals. A buzzer sounds periodically, at which time the animal is rewarded with food for every lever press but is simultaneously given electric shock, thus creating a conflict. Under nondrug conditions the animal presses very little when the buzzer is on, but drugs such as the barbiturates and benzodiazepines cause the animal to respond despite the shock. This action appears to be specific to the antianxiety drugs.

A version of the conflict procedure was tried in humans by Lehmann, Black, and Ban (1970), and Lehmann and Ban (1971). These investigators required the subject to hold down a telegraph key which caused a continuous train of shocks to occur, and paid the subject for the number of seconds the key was depressed. Minor tranquilizers significantly increased the amount of time the key was depressed, but so did amphetamine; the drug-placebo difference was not large.

We have been experimenting with a type of conflict procedure in which voluntary breathholding is the aversive stimulus. The conflict is between the mounting desire of the subject to breathe on the one hand, and the desire to follow instructions by holding the breath for as long as possible, on the other hand.

Breathholding has particular appeal and relevance as a conflict procedure. First, because prolonged breathholding is experienced as aversive by all people, the conflict is universal. Second, holding one's breath is a learned response that is ordinarily suppressed by its aversive consequences. Viewed in this light, diazepam might be expected to extend the duration of breathholding by reducing the aversiveness of its consequences and releasing this normally suppressed behavior. If monetary reward is added as a reinforcer for extended breathholding, the conflict would be intensified, and one would expect the effects of diazepam to be enhanced.

Breathholding has several advantages over conflict tasks involving electric shock. It becomes highly aversive very rapidly—in less than 2 min for most subjects—and yet it is completely safe. By contrast, the amount of electric shock which is considered aversive varies considerably between human subjects. Moreover, the prospect of receiving electric shock discourages both many subjects from participating in the experiment and many ethics committees from approving the project, whereas the prospect of breathholding is viewed with more equanimity. Breathholding time can vary over a considerable range so that one does not have to resort to frequency measures. Breathholding time can be measured quickly so that pre- and postdrug measures can be obtained in a single session. The task is easily understood by the subject, and the only equipment required is a stop watch. Normal subjects can be used.

In support of the validity of this method Mirsky, Lipman, and Grinker (1946) reported that anxious patients are unable to hold their breath for as long as normals. In a pilot experiment done by us, breathholding time was increased 1 hr after 10 mg oral diazepam and 1 hr after 25 mg oral chlorpromazine.

The presence of conflict in the clinical situation is most clearly demonstrated by phobic behavior in which a person seeks to avoid specific objects or situations. In several investigations (Silverstone, 1973; Razani, 1974) minor tranquilizers have been found to reduce phobic anxiety and to facilitate behavioral therapy directed at the treatment of phobias.

We believe that phobic avoidance behavior will become a powerful method of evaluating antianxiety drugs for the following reasons. (1) The avoidance behavior is stable in the absence of specific therapeutic intervention. It rarely shows spontaneous recovery (Marks, 1969). Thus, the anxiety-related behavior is predictable and requires little interpretation on the part of the observer. (2) It is possible to select groups of patients who exhibit the same avoidance behavior to the same class of stimulus situations. (3) The response can be made publically observable by measuring how close the subject can approach the phobic object (Lang, 1968). There is, in fact, a substantial literature describing the objective measurement of changes in phobic anxiety because of the long-standing interest in evaluating systematic desensitization. Investigators of drug effects on phobia have so far not availed themselves of these techniques but have relied on subjective ratings of phobic anxiety. (4) There are convincing animal analogues of phobic anxiety. In the trace conditioning method (Heise and McConnell, 1961), for example, a complex stimulus sequence signals that shock will occur unless an avoidance response is made. The effect of minor tranquilizers is to delay the avoidance response so that it occurs closer to the shock.

Although the phobic model cannot be applied in normal subjects, there is reason to believe that subjects with common and relatively mild phobias such as phobia of public speaking (Paul, 1966) or of snakes (Lang, Lazovick, and Reynolds, 1965) could be used, as has been done in studies of systematic desensitization. If so, the supply of potential subjects would be large – 1 to 2% of the population (Marks, 1969), and readily available. The measurement of a drug's effects could be done in a single session. Data from the outcome studies of systematic desensitization indicate that good discrimination of effective treatment from placebo can be had in relatively small groups of approximately 10 subjects each (Paul, 1966). Thus, many of the criteria of the ideal test indicator are met by the model of phobic-avoidance behavior. Its only shortcoming is some remoteness from the social situations in which most individuals take drugs.

CLINICAL, BEHAVIORAL, AND SOCIAL ENDPOINTS IN ANXIETY

The evaluation of psychotropic drug effect has focused heavily on changes in mood and thought rather than on observable alterations in behavior. In particular, behavior in relation to social interactions has been almost totally ignored, although most people take drugs in order to effect some dimension of interpersonal behavior. Only when it has proven impossible to measure affect have psychopharmacologists resorted to behavioral measures. Yet when they have done so the results have been rewarding. Obvious examples occur in pediatrics and geriatrics where the reporting of emotions has not yet been learned or has become obscured by senility.

The stimulant drugs, such as amphetamine, have been available for 40 years and despite heavy use as antidepressants in adults their utility remains unproven. In contrast, their efficacy in the behavioral disorders of childhood have been quite rapidly and successfully demonstrated (Sprague and Sleator, 1973). Another example from psychopharmacology and pediatrics concerns the utility of the tricyclic antidepressant drugs. The evidence that they are effective in childhood enuresis is far more consistent and compelling than the comparable data in adult depression (Blackwell and Currah, 1973). A dry bed is a very tangible criterion of drug action.

In the geriatric area patients are often unable to provide accurate assessments of mood, and drug-placebo discrimination is blurred by eagerness to please or the response to attention. In some recent unpublished work (Blackwell, 1972, *unpublished*) on a liquid tonic it was found that self reports of anxiety showed an approximately 70% placebo response and responses to a vague question about feeling "generally better" yielded a 90% affirmative placebo response. Only when a nurse's observational scale of ward behavior was used in later studies was it possible to reduce the placebo response to approximately 50% and produce some drug-placebo discrimination. Another recent example of success in the area of behavioral measurement has been the approval of the drug hydergine for geriatric patients. The research on this agent used behavioral endpoints and the FDA-approved indications are mostly behavioral, including changes in communication, cooperation, and self care.

A review of behavioral rating scales used in psychopharmacology (Salzman, Shader, Kochansky, and Cronin, 1972) reveals the extent of attention paid to such measures by psychopharmacologists in various areas of drug development. As might be predicted, one-third of the available scales are in the geriatric area for reasons already discussed. In the nongeriatric area the great majority of the remaining 27 behavioral scales are designed for use in psychotic inpatients. It is perhaps no surprise that the evidence for efficacy of drugs used in the treatment of schizophrenia is more compelling than drugs used to treat either depression or anxiety. The behavioral manifestations of schizophrenia are often gross and the rating scales used to evaluate drug effect therefore reflect this by including behavioral measures. Such observations are facilitated by the fact that patients are usually admitted to hospital where disturbed behavior is readily observable and measurable. In contrast, patients with the manifestation of anxiety are seldom admitted to hospital and evaluations of drug effect have relied heavily on subjective mood states. Only two of the 27 nongeriatric behavioral scales are suitable for outpatients. Of these, one (Gross, Hitchman, Reeves, Lawrence, Newell, and Clyde, 1961) is designed for psychotic patients, leaving only one scale (Free and Guthrie, 1969) designed specifically for behavioral measures in outpatients with anxiety. In clinical practice it is also clear that the patient is very rarely asked to define or record what behavioral changes are associated with anxiety either causally or coincidentally. Possibly the only psychopharmacologist who has devoted detailed attention to behavioral measures has been Irwin (1968). He has attempted to extend systematic observations of drug effects on animals into a clinical analogue using a variety of behavioral, neurologic, autonomic, performance, and subjective state evaluations. No less than 12 separate rating scales are included in the inventory of drug effects. Some interpretation must be exercised by the rater, but high interrater reliability is reported by Irwin. This method meets many of the criteria of an ideal test model but the procedures are so comprehensive as to be virtually overwhelming. Perhaps for this reason the tests are rarely used outside Irwin's laboratory. Instead we have chosen to focus in detail on a single possibility that appears theoretically and practically to have heuristic value in the assessment of drugs that might affect anxiety. The dimension we propose to examine has the added advantage that it involves not only behavior but social interaction.

During the past two years we have been applying learning theory techniques to an understanding of patients treated on the Psychosomatic Unit at the Cincinnati General Hospital (Blackwell, Wooley, and Whitehead, 1974). As one result, we have begun to define much more precisely the behavioral accompaniments of alterations in mood, particularly anxiety. Since Table 4 shows that two-thirds of the benzodiazepines are prescribed in so-called psychosomatic disorders, our findings may be relevant to drug evaluation in this area. Careful enquiry in patients with anxiety almost always reveals the behavioral stimuli which precede the affect and which may prove to be more precise measures of drug effect.

For example:

> A 25-year-old, single, white girl visited her internist complaining of headaches. After a negative neurologic examination she was given an analgesic. This failed to benefit and when she returned it was found that headaches occurred when she felt "nervous." For this reason, a benzodiazepine was prescribed. This provided only transitory relief. On admission to the Psychosomatic Unit a detailed behavioral history revealed the social stimuli that provoked being "nervous" and the behavioral responses she made in addition to experiencing headache. In response to individuals who either put her down or made unfulfilled promises, the patient felt upset and either exploded angrily or withdrew and sulked. Following this she experienced headache. In this instance, the appropriate measure of drug action would be to explore its effects on the patient's capacity to be appropriately assertive when socially provoked.

This social dimension of assertiveness appears to be the behavior most commonly disturbed in anxious individuals and may be the most appropriate for quantifying antianxiety drug effect. It is also of special interest in the psychosomatic area, particularly in hypertension. Alexander's (1950) original psychoanalytic speculations in this disorder was that patients suffered from a failure to be normally assertive and became hypertensive as a result of stifled aggression. Psychotherapy was directed toward encouraging assertive responses, and was reported to result in reduced blood pressure, although relatives found patients who became more assertive less pleasant to live with.

TABLE 4. *Indications for diazepam (1971–1972)*

Diagnosis	%	Diagnosis	%
Mental disorders	30	Gastrointestinal	6
Musculoskeletal	17	CNS disease	6
Circulatory	16	Genitourinary	3
Geriatric	8	Other	7
Medical/surgical aftercare	7		

Sixty-four percent used in combination with other drugs.

In an attempt to corroborate these speculations we have been reviewing the use of benzodiazepines in the Cincinnati Hypertension Clinic. Approximately one-third of all patients are taking these drugs—a fact of some interest since the population is composed mainly of women and blacks, two social groups with identified problems in assertion. In our few interviews to date, we have attempted to focus specifically on the behaviors that are affected by the benzodiazepines and for which the patient finds drugs are beneficial.

The following is an example:

> A 56-year-old, white, widowed female had been taking diazepam for four years. She stated she took the medication to calm her nerves but did not know its name. When asked to be specific about what made her nervous she described the following situation. When her husband died she had begun a lesbian relationship with a woman who moved into her apartment and dominated her life. She was unable to rid herself of this partner and was totally subservient to her. The only time she was able to assert her own needs was after she had taken diazepam, in which case she could state them with less concern for the consequences.

These speculations are still based on slender data, but we believe that the social dimension of assertive behavior may prove to be the best measure of drug effect for compounds similar to the benzodiazepines. The components of assertive behavior are shown in Table 5. The idea that drugs such as benzodiazepines affect this dimension is particularly attractive for a number of other reasons. First, lack of assertiveness has face validity as the human analogue for passive avoidance, the one test that is highly specific in animals to the benzodiazepines. Psychologists have tended to view lack of assertiveness as a failure to learn. However, we regard it as more likely being a socially suppressed behavior since it is very often specific to certain social and interpersonal situations. For instance, psychosomatic patients are often highly assertive in soliciting caretaking responses but poorly assertive in situations requiring independent activity. With regard to hyper-

TABLE 5. Components of assertive behavior

Expressing personal needs
Expressing personal preferences
Initiating social contacts
Disagreeing openly
Seeking explanations
Talking about self
Accepting compliments
Requesting alternate behaviors
Maintaining direct eye contact

Each of the above may be sit-
uation- or person-specific.

tension, Alexander (1950) pointed out that lack of assertiveness manifested itself at puberty when behavior was suppressed in response to painful social consequences.

A second reason for regarding assertiveness as the appropriate dimension for studying drug effect is the evidence that exists already to suggest that benzodiazepines alter this dimension. Although DiMascio, Shader, and Harmatz (1967) first observed and labeled this effect an unmasking of hostility, others have disagreed and Rickels and Downing (1974) recently suggested that the change noted in anxious outpatients was more appropriately labeled an improvement in healthy assertiveness. In our own study we also believe that there may be indirect evidence that diazepam alters social dimensions (Winstead et al., 1974). For instance, Fig. 4 shows that when diazepam was made freely available to all patients on a psychiatric ward for 6 months, maximum use of the drug occurred at two peak times. These were around lunch and in the early evening, both times of maximum social interaction. Also in this study, Fig. 5 shows that drugs were equally available to all patients but were used more often by women, and it is women who use two-thirds of all minor tranquilizers on a national scale. The conditions of this study eliminate differences due to physician access or prescribing behavior but would support the commonly held view that women have special problems in assertive behavior because of social conditioning in a passive role.

A final pragmatic reason for interest in this behavioral dimension of drug effect is the availability of expertise and measuring instruments. Assertive behavior in particular and social skills in general are becoming increasingly prominent in the psychological literature (Rathus, 1972, 1973). We are currently working to explore this dimension and to modify the existing rating

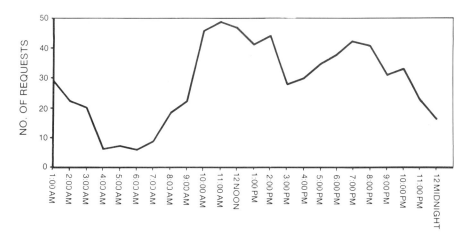

FIG. 4. Use of diazepam by time of day.

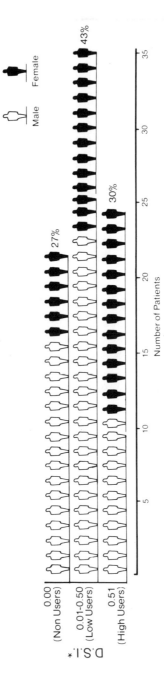

FIG. 5. Diazepam use by sex. *D.S.I.: drug-seeking index = number of requests by a patient/length of stay.

devices so that we can measure the effects of drugs on assertive behavior as well as comparing these effects with various training procedures designed to modify assertion.

CONCLUSION

This selective review of research strategies for evaluating drugs in the benzodiazepine category has stressed the importance of selecting observable behavioral endpoints. In choosing among these it is important to define a logical sequence of testing that links the animal laboratory and the clinical researcher with appropriate social and behavioral dimensions of drug effect in patients. We suggest that these criteria may be satisfied by selecting the passive-avoidance or conflict model in animals and extending it first into normals using a conflict procedure such as breathholding and then into patients measuring changes in either phobic anxiety or assertive behavior.

ACKNOWLEDGMENTS

This work is supported by a generous grant from Hoffmann-La Roche. We are grateful to Mrs. Barbara Klein for typing this manuscript.

REFERENCES

Alexander, F. (1950): *Psychosomatic Medicine*. W. W. Norton, New York, pp. 143–153.
Blackwell, B. (1973): Psychotropic drugs in use today: The role of diazepam in medical practice. *JAMA*, 225:1637–1641.
Blackwell, B., and Currah, J. (1973): The Psychopharmacology of Nocturnal Enuresis. In: *Bladder Control and Enuresis,* edited by I. Kolvin, R. C. MacKeith, and S. R. Meadow. J. B. Lippincott Co., Philadelphia.
Blackwell, B., Wooley, S., and Whitehead, W. (1974): Psychosomatic illness: A new treatment approach. *Cinc. J. Med.,* 55:95–98.
DiMascio, A., Shader, R. I., and Harmatz, J. (1967): Psychotropic drugs and induced hostility. *Psychosomatics,* 10:46–47.
Engel, B. T., and Bickford, A. F. (1961): Response specificity: Stimulus-response and individual-response specificity in essential hypertensives. *Arch. Gen. Psychiatry,* 5:478–489.
Free, S. M., and Guthrie, M. B. (1969): Response to trifluoperazine–amobarbital in outpatients with anxiety. *Dis. Nerv. Syst.,* 30:195–200.
Geller, I. (1962): Use of approach avoidance behavior (conflict) for evaluating depressant drugs. In: *Psychosomatic Medicine,* edited by J. H. Nodine and J. H. Moyer, pp. 267–274. Lea and Febiger, Philadelphia.
Gross, M., Hitchman, I. L., Reeves, W. P., Lawrence, J., Newell, P. C., and Clyde, D. J. (1961): Objective evaluation of psychotic patients under drug therapy: A symptom and adjustment index. *J. Nerv. Ment. Dis.,* 133:399–409.
Heise, G. A., and McConnell, H. (1961): Differences between chlordiazepoxide-type and chlorpromazine-type action in "trace" avoidance. In: *The Third World Congress of Psychiatry,* Vol. 2, p. 917. Montreal, Canada.
Irwin, S. (1968): A rational framework for the development, evaluation and use of psychotropic drugs. *Am. J. Psychiatry, Suppl.,* 124:1–19.
Kelly, D. H. W. (1966): Measurement of anxiety by forearm blood flow. *Br. J. Psychiatry,* 112:789–798.

Kelly, D., Brown, C. C., and Shaffer, J. W. (1973a): Forearm plythysmography as a measure of anxiety. Exhibit at the American Medical Association meeting, Chicago.

Kelly, D., Pik, R., and Chen, C. N. (1973b): A psychological and physiological evaluation of the effects of intravenous diazepam. *British Journal of Psychiatry,* 122:419–426, 1973.

Kelly, D. H. W., and Walter, C. J. S. (1968): The relationship between clinical diagnosis and anxiety, assessed by forearm blood flow and other measurements. *Br. J. Psychiatry,* 114: 611–626.

Kelly, D. H. W., Walter, C. J. S., and Sargant, W. (1966): Modified leucotomy assessed by forearm blood flow and other measurements. *Br. J. Psychiatry,* 112:871–881.

Lacey, J. I., Bateman, D. E., and Van Lehn, R. (1953): Autonomic response specificity: An experimental study. *Psychosom. Med.,* 15:8–21.

Lader, M. H. (1969): Psychophysiological Aspects of Anxiety. In: *Studies of Anxiety,* edited by M. H. Lader, pp. 53–61. Headley Brothers, Ltd., Ashford, Kent.

Lader, M. H., and Wing, L. (1964): Habituation of the psycho-galvanic reflex in patients with anxiety states and in normal subjects. *J. Neurol. Neurosurg. Psychiatry,* 27:210–218.

Lang, P. J. (1968): The mechanics of desensitization and the laboratory study of human fear. In: *Assessment and Status of the Behavior Therapies,* edited by C. M. Franks. McGraw Hill, New York.

Lang, P. J., Lazovick, A. D., and Reynolds, D. J. (1965): Desensitization, suggestibility and pseudotherapy. *J. Abnorm. Psychol.,* 70:395–402.

Lehmann, H. E., and Ban, T. A. (1971): Effects of psychoactive drugs on conflict avoidance behavior in human subjects. *Act. Nerv. Super.,* 13:82–85.

Lehmann, H. E., Black, P., and Ban, T. A. (1970): The effects of psychostimulants on psychometric test performance with special reference to conflict avoidance behavior. *Curr. Ther. Res.,* 12:390–393.

Lindsley, O. R. (1962): Operant Conditioning Techniques in the Measurement of Psychopharmacologic Response. In: *Psychosomatic Medicine,* edited by J. H. Nodine and J. H. Moyer, pp. 373–383. Lea and Febiger, Philadelphia.

Marks, I. M. (1969): *Fears and Phobias.* Academic Press, New York.

Mirsky, A., Lipman, E., and Grinker, R. R. (1946): Breathholding time in anxiety states. *Fed. Proc.,* 5:74.

Paul, G. L. (1966): *Insight versus desensitization in psychotherapy: An experiment in anxiety reduction.* Stanford Univ. Press, Stanford, Calif.

Rathus, S. A. (1972): An experimental investigation of assertive training in a group setting. *J. Behav. Ther. Exp. Psychiatry,* 3:1–6.

Rathus, S. A. (1973): A 30 item schedule for assessing assertive behavior. *Behav. Ther.,* 4:398–406.

Razani, J. (1974): Treatment of phobias by systematic desensitization: Comparison of standard vs. methohexital-aided desensitization. *Arch. Gen. Psychiatry,* 30:291–293. *Am. J. Psychiatry,* 131:442–444.

Rickels, K., and Downing, R. W. (1974): Chlordiazepoxide and hostility in anxious outpatients.

Salzman, C., Shader, R. I., Kochansky, G. E., and Cronin, D. M. (1972): Rating scales for psychotropic drug research with geriatric patients: I. Behavior ratings. *J. Am. Geriatr. Soc.,* 20:209–214.

Silverstone, J. T. (1973): Lorazepam in phobic disorders: A pilot study. *Curr. Med. Res. Op.,* 1:272–275.

Sprague, R. L., and Sleator, E. K. (1973): Effects of psychopharmacologic agents on learning disorders. *Pediatr. Clin. North Am.,* 20:719–735.

Sroufe, L. A. (1971): Effects of depth and rate of breathing on heart rate and heart rate variability. *Psychophysiology,* 8:648–655.

Stern, R. M., and Anschel, C. (1968): Deep inspirations as stimuli for responses of the autonomic nervous system. *Psychophysiology,* 5:132–141.

Tyrer, P. J., and Lader, M. H. (1973): Effects of beta adrenergic blockade with sotalol in chronic anxiety. *Clin. Pharmacol. Ther.,* 14:418–426.

Winstead, D. K., Anderson, A., Eilers, M. K., Blackwell, B., and Zaremba, L. (1974): Diazepam on demand: Drug seeking behavior in psychiatric inpatients. *Arch. Gen. Psychiatry,* 30:349–351.

Wolf, S. (1950): Effects of suggestion and conditioning on the action of chemical agents in human subjects. *J. Clin. Invest.,* 29:100–109.

DISCUSSION

Ayd: Clinically, the patients who have problems with assertion are the obsessive and the obsessive-compulsive individuals. These are the people who will let others walk all over them. They will suppress a lot of the anger that this produces in them, but I have found benzodiazepines to be of no value in these patients over a period of time. A lot of them are getting diazepam or chlordiazepoxide and they take it. But it doesn't really produce a very good clinical effect in these individuals.

Blackwell: It would depend very much on what your measure of outcome was. It would be highly unlikely that the benzodiazepines would significantly affect any excessive compulsive rituals because they seem to be so overlearned and to serve such a useful anxiety reducing function. I always assume that if people continue to take medication they are getting something from it. It may be that what they're saying to you is that the thing that affects them most is their rituals and they haven't gotten rid of the rituals. But, there may still be other dimensions that the drug is affecting that is of some benefit to them.

Ayd: You mentioned that the nurse gave the medicine if she felt it was appropriate. Could you comment on that?

Blackwell: What actually happened is that out of the more than 800 contacts occurring during the course of the study, drug was not given on something like 25 occasions, and, in fact, almost all of these occurred very early in the study. One of the findings, talking about the ward as a whole, was that there was an escalation in drug use during the period of the study. The ward as a whole behaved in a somewhat similar way to the nation as a whole.

Fink: Studies with infusion of epinephrine to induce anxiety show that certain substances blockade it and certain substances don't. Work was done a few years ago by Fitz and Curran with infusions of lactate. The excitation and acute anxiety episodes in anxious patients are treated successfully by diazepam. I wonder if it's not an experimental model that would fit into this paradigm under the physiologic measurements?

Whitehead: The literature suggested that the subjective anxiety effects of epinephrine are pinned very strongly on the setting expectation. Patients with a history of anxiety symptoms tend to report anxiety in response to epinephrine and lactose injections. Under fairly threatening situations they also report anxiety, so that there has been some variability, in fact, in this subjective response to epinephrine injection.

Gershon: Dr. Garfield and I, when we were in St. Louis, did the study comparing epinephrine against yohimbine in a block design. The anxiety-like response induced by yohimbine which was much more consistent, more like real anxiety than that of epinephrine and not dependent on prior conditions, showed a simple drug relationship. You gave the drug and you got the response. Unfortunately, in screening drugs, anything that was a CNS depressant was effective. That may not be such a devastating criticism. It could be that all of the effective anxiety agents known today are CNS depressants, so the system works in provoking the model, but we can't screen out specifics. Again, that isn't that horrible because, as you know, most of the companies that are selling phenothiazines are presenting data that suggest that they may be as anxiolytic as diazepam or chlordiazepoxide. But there is a drug that is better than epinephrine. That's yohimbine. The lactate is dependent on state.

Fink: There's still some question as to whether the lactate is specific or not. It does not induce an anxious response in so-called normal individuals but it does produce response in patients with anxiety.

Whitehead: I think it was an oversight not to mention that in the review.

Fink: The lactate model may have some merit. I think it is an expensive procedure to do and very time-consuming but it has the merit of potentially giving us some idea about the physiology of the anxiety process.

Uhlenhuth: I think one of the most exciting things that you mentioned is the situation you have where people are very closely observed and the notion of using that as a free choice situation where you can see in what circumstances people pick the drug. It seems like an obvious thing that you would look at the curve of drug taking frequency and see what's happening at those times. In a less structured way it can give you a very nice idea of what drugs do and what the people who take them think they do.

Blackwell: We did that for the first time but we hadn't really yet set up an effective system of computerizing our data. Among all the other things we're pursuing, I'd very much like to pursue that general notion because I think it is a very good model for studying some of the social dimensions of drug effect.

Uhlenhuth: That sounds like a new idea too.

Blackwell: Yes. It's in the literature already which is one of the reasons that I didn't emphasize it much today, whereas we have not bounced some of the other ideas off anybody before.

Knill: Were most of the people on the diazepam-on-demand study obese?

Blackwell: No. As a matter of fact, that study was not done on the psychosomatic unit. It was done at the Cincinnati General Hospital in one of our 16-bed acute short-stay psychiatric units and the patients weren't obese.

Knill: I have two other questions. Diazepam is acknowledged as a muscle relaxant. The first question is, what is the interrelationship of muscle relaxation and anxiety? The second is, are anxiolytics bound to be dependence producing agents?

Blackwell: I do have some data on the abuse aspect. One of the concerns that Roche understandably had about us doing that study was that some criticism might be directed at us for making the drug available in a free access way, and we looked very carefully at that by comparing drug use in the first quarter of every individual patient's stay with his drug use in the second, third, and fourth quarter of his hospital stay. There was a significant reduction in use with time. By the time the patients were in the last quarter of their stay they were taking significantly less diazepam, which suggests that the drug may have been taken for appropriate reasons. With regard to your first question, I don't think that anybody has really attempted to tease apart muscle relaxant from antianxiety properties within the same individuals.

Gershon: The issue is that the doses that you are giving in humans do not attain adequate amounts to produce muscle relaxation although in the laboratory you get it.

Goldberg: With respect to association of muscle relaxant effects — I can't speak for humans, but we did a study in animals using several different known metabolites of chlordiazepoxide and found that a derivate had no muscle relaxant or anticonvulsive properties in the appropriate animal models and yet showed every bit the anxiolytic activity in regard to conflict schedules. So I do believe that these things can be totally disassociated.

Domino: Would you comment more from the point of view of categories of antianxiety agents? We're in an age that one might call of benzodiazepine mania while previously we were, or perhaps still are, in an alcoholic and barbiturate age. I keep thinking from a historical point of view that why aren't there more comparisons to our classic antianxiety agents such as ethanol and the barbiturates? I wonder if you could just comment with respect to your review in the specific tests that you have suggested how these more classic antianxiety agents fit in the scheme?

Blackwell: A number of us here in this room were at the NIMH conference that addressed itself to the question, "Are we an overmedicated society?" in which some of the excellent epidemiologic work that has been done by Dr. Uhlenhuth, among others throughout the country, was discussed. One of the things that was looked at was ethanol use as an alternate coping mechanism. Some evidence indicated that young males tended to resort more to alcohol use as a coping mechanism for life crisis and stress. If you question alcoholics, as all of us here have done, about what the use of alcohol does for them, you very frequently get the statements around assertive dimensions: "It allows me to talk more; it makes me more outgoing; I can stick up for myself." Although there are other reasons for drinking alcohol, assertiveness is a very common dimension. In the case of women, my interpretation is that it is socially more acceptable for women to take a pill but that they had more problems with assertion. The whole women's rights movement has to do with the social conditioning of nonassertive behavior in women.

Goldberg: Have attempts been made to correlate the temporal aspects of drug seeking behavior with known circadian rhythms of the biogenic amines and on whether this is in any way an internal cue for anxiety producing situations?

Blackwell: We have looked at this in depression, but we've never looked at it in anxiety.

Predictability in Psychopharmacology: Preclinical and Clinical Correlations,
edited by A. Sudilovsky, S. Gershon and B. Beer. Raven Press, New York,
© 1975.

Effects of Diazepam on Galvanic Skin Response and Conflict in Monkeys and Humans

Bernard Beer and Bernard Migler

The Squibb Institute for Medical Research, Princeton, New Jersey 08540; and Rutgers, The State University, New Brunswick, New Jersey 08903

In an excellent review of the literature on anxiety, Lader and Marks (1971) trace the historical and contemporary definitions of anxiety. According to these authors, the modern concept of anxiety implies a continuum of emotion ranging from situational anxiety or phobic anxiety related to fear where there exists a specific unpleasant state indicating the presence of some danger to the organism to anxiety neurosis (clinical anxiety) or free-floating generalized anxiety, i.e., an apprehension or uneasiness stemming from the anticipation of imminent danger from a largely unknown source. This continuum of affective state suggests that there are no qualitative differences between nonclinical or normal anxiety and that condition called clinical anxiety. The differences, according to Eysenck (1969), are quantitative, like the differences in IQ scores.

It is generally agreed that the symptoms of anxiety may include peripheral autonomic effects, such as sweating, palpitations, tachycardia, pallor, frequent urination, nausea, and abdominal cramps as well as behavioral signs often manifested as a general tendency of the organism to suppress ongoing behavior, particularly that associated with anxiety-provoking events.

Since the physiological and behavioral effects of anxiety are qualitatively similar in all states of anxiety, we have used animals and normal adult humans exposed to experimental environmental situations, which have a great deal of face validity for producing anxiety, and have then tried to reverse these anxiety effects by the administration of diazepam which has clinical utility in anxiety. We feel that this approach, using analogous models between species, is useful in predicting the effects of new chemical agents for clinical anxiety states.

GALVANIC SKIN RESPONSE

Preclinical procedures used to predict antianxiety activity of compounds in the clinic are reviewed by Blackwell and Whitehead in this volume. In their chapter, they mention the Galvanic Skin Response (GSR) as a possible index of anxiety. We consider the GSR to be a convenient measure of the activity level of the sympathetic division of the autonomic nervous system and thus an important measure of anxious states.

The GSR is a recording of the electrical conductivity of the skin, particularly that of the palms and other hairless surfaces. At low skin resistance levels, this resistance varies with the activity of the sweat glands. At high resistance levels, before sweating has reached a critical level, epidermal activities other than sweating may contribute to the GSR (Darrow and Gullickson, 1970). Any pleasant, unpleasant, or novel stimulus is reflected in a reduction of resistance (Gullickson, 1973). The resistance usually returns to the basal level within a few seconds.

The magnitude of the GSR has been shown to be directly proportional to the magnitude of a threatening stimulus (Pirkko, 1969). The GSR has also been used as a measure of therapeutic progress during the treatment of phobias by psychotherapy since the magnitude of the GSR to phobic stimuli was reduced as the treatment was continued (Wolpe, Lazarus, and Fried, 1968).

In animals, there are long-term changes in the basal skin resistance level that reflect the general level of stress or nonstress (Kaplan, 1963). In man, the basal skin resistance level is correlated with clinical ratings of anxiety (Lader and Wing, 1966).

The sensitivity of the GSR to emotional stimuli has resulted in its use as one of the measures in the so-called polygraph "lie detector" (Kugelmass, 1968).

There have been several reports on the effects of drugs on the GSR in man. For example, d-amphetamine was reported to have no effect on the magnitude of the response to electric shock (Lobb, 1968); however, the drug has been shown to retard habituation to a warning stimulus preceding a shock as well as to retard the extinction of the response when shock no longer followed the warning stimulus (Lobb and Kaplan, 1970). On the other hand, ethanol reduced the magnitude of the GSR to electric shock, a result interpreted as due to a reduction in anxiety (McGonnell and Beach, 1968).

The GSR has been studied in some disease states. Hypertensive patients show a heightened GSR to stress as well as to weak neutral stimuli (Richter-Heinrich and Lauter, 1969). In chronic schizophrenic patients, skin resistance is lower than in normal subjects. In these patients there is a greater number of GSRs in the absence of the presentation of specific stimuli (nonspecific responses) and the GSR is slow to habituate (Zahn, Rosenthal, and Lawlor, 1968), suggesting high arousal and fluctuating attention. Lapierre (1974) recently reported on the effects of imipramine and chlorimipramine on the GSR in neurotic patients. Forty-eight hr after chlorimipramine administration the GSR indicated arousal. This effect was not seen with imipramine or placebo.

The physiology of the GSR is not completely understood. Certain brain areas known to be involved in emotional behavior in animals are also involved in control of the GSR. For example, lesions in the amygdaloid nucleus in the monkey cause abnormal social behavior and apparent loss of fear (Klüver and Bucy, 1938). In addition, it has been shown that these lesions also cause a marked reduction in the magnitude of the GSR to various stimuli (Bagshaw, Kimble, and Pribram, 1965).

The facts cited above suggest to us that the GSR might also be useful as a base line for determining the effects of known and potential anxiolytic drugs.

GSR RESPONSE TO SHOCK IN THE RHESUS MONKEY

After acclimatization, each monkey was placed in a restraining chair 24 hr before a test. Immediately before the test, two chrome-plated recording electrodes were taped to the feet. Test sessions lasted approximately 5 hr during which a brief electric shock was delivered once every 2 min. One shock electrode was a stainless steel collar around the monkey's neck and the second electrode consisted of the metal seat and foot rests of the re-

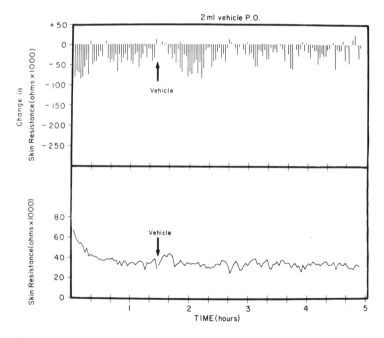

FIG. 1. Effect of oral administration of the drug vehicle (water) on skin resistance level **(lower)** and on the magnitude of changes in skin resistance after brief applications of electric shocks **(upper).** The difference in skin resistance, as measured 1 sec before and 3 sec after the shock, was used as the magnitude of the response.

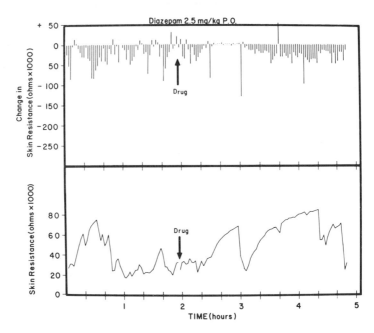

FIG. 2. Effect of diazepam, 2.5 mg/kg p.o., on skin resistance and on magnitude of response to electric shock.

straint chair. Skin resistance was measured with a digital multimeter and recorded by a digital printer 1 sec before, 3 sec after, and midway between successive shocks. The algebraic difference, if any, between the resistance readings 1 sec before and 3 sec after each shock was used to indicate the magnitude and direction of the response to the shock. The skin resistance recorded midway between shocks was used as a measure of background skin resistance. After 1.5 hr, the session was briefly interrupted and the monkey was dosed by oral gavage with either diazepam or water; the session was then continued for an additional $3\frac{1}{2}$ hr.

Figure 1 represents the basal measurements of skin resistance in a monkey and the magnitude and direction of changes in skin resistance after brief shocks for a session in which the effects of the administration of the vehicle (water) were determined. The basal skin resistance was stable and showed no change after administration of water. The response to electric shock consisted of a highly reliable brief decrease in skin resistance; this response was not affected by the administration of water.

Figures 2 and 3 show the effect of diazepam administered orally at 2.5 and 5 mg/kg, respectively. Approximately 30 min after the 2.5 mg/kg dose, there occurred a period of approximately 30 min in which shocks failed to elicit the typical drop in skin resistance. After a 5-mg/kg dose, a similar effect was elicited after approximately 30 min, but was prolonged to the end

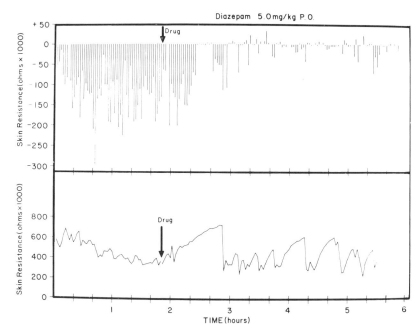

FIG. 3. Effect of diazepam, 5.0 mg/kg p.o., on skin resistance and on magnitude of response to electric shock.

of the session. The background skin resistance in these drug sessions were not stable, and no conclusions concerning this measure can be drawn. However, the data do suggest the development of slow increases in skin resistance, followed by abrupt decreases. The diminution in magnitude of the decreases in skin resistance after the administration of diazepam cannot be attributed to elevations in skin resistance, since high skin resistance could be associated with large-magnitude responses, as shown by the records for the last 2 hr of the session in Fig. 2.

HUMAN GSR IN EXPERIMENTAL SITUATIONAL ANXIETY

Three normal male volunteers, aged 28, 40, and 41, weighing 170 to 195 pounds, were used as experimental subjects. They were instructed to remain as still as possible while they were confronted with a panel containing two light sources. A green stimulus light presented for 2 min was alternated with a red light that was lit for 3 min. During exposure to the red light, the subject received two brief (0.25 sec) electric shocks to the left forearm, 1 min apart. The threshold intensity of the electric shock had been determined in an earlier session in which the shocks were presented every 15 sec, starting at 0.20 mA, and increased every third shock by an increment of 0.10 mA until the subject reported that each of two successive shocks was "aversive." This final shock intensity was then used for the duration of the experiment; the actual range of intensities employed was 1.0 to 1.50 mA. Each daily session consisted of six consecutive exposures to both red and green stimuli and was, therefore, 30 min in duration. The electrical skin resistance was measured via electrodes placed on the second and fourth fingers of the right hand. A reading was taken directly from a digital multimeter every 10 sec. Additionally, a reading was taken after each shock which represented the largest drop in resistance within 10 sec following that shock. After a number of daily sessions in which the GSR base line was relatively stable, diazepam was administered orally 1 hr before the next session. Figure 4 shows the results for one subject. The base line or nondrug sessions show a relatively stable overall resistance and a consistent drop in mean resistance after shocks. The overall resistance was approximately constant regardless of the stimulus presented. Before the seventh session, 4 mg of diazepam was given. There was no significant change seen in the basal resistance, but the change in resistance in response to shock was greatly attenuated. The next two daily sessions after diazepam showed dose-related increases in basal resistance, and the GSR response to the shock was almost obliterated. During the 10th session, when diazepam was not administered, the basal resistance stayed high, but the response to the shock remained at predrug levels. The next four drug-free sessions showed a return of basal resistance to previous nondrug

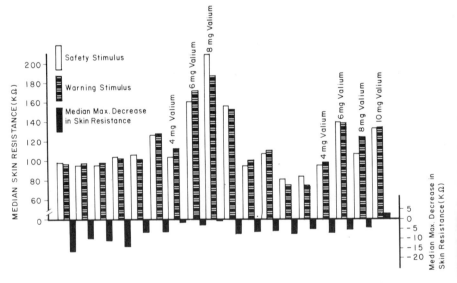

FIG. 4. Median skin resistance of subject LGL during the safe stimulus (green light), the warning stimulus (red light), and to shock presented only during the warning stimulus. The maximum decrease in skin resistance after each shock was taken as the largest drop in resistance within 5 sec after delivery of the shock.

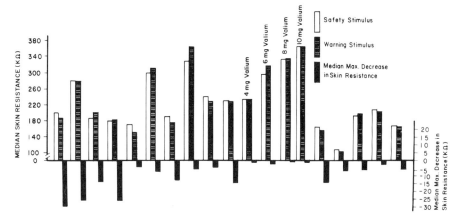

FIG. 5. Median skin resistance of subject BMM during the safe stimulus (green light), the warning stimulus (red light), and to shock presented only during the warning stimulus. The maximum decrease in skin resistance after each shock was taken as the largest drop in resistance within 5 sec after delivery of the shock.

base lines. During the last four sessions, diazepam was administered in 2-mg increments daily starting at 4 mg. Here again, there was a dose-dependent increase in basal resistance, and a decrease in responsiveness to the shock.

Figure 5 shows the data for a second subject. The first 10 sessions for this subject were without drug since he showed a great deal of session-to-session variability. However, for sessions 11, 12, 13, and 14 he received 4, 6, 8, and 10 mg of diazepam, respectively. This subject also showed dose-related increases in basal resistance as well as considerable decreases in shock responsiveness. His final five sessions, without drug, indicated a return of GSR to nondrug base line.

Figure 6 shows the data for a third subject. For sessions 8, 9, and 10, he received 5, 10, and 15 mg of diazepam, respectively. Again, there was evidence of a dose-dependent increase in basal GSR and a decrease in the GSR responsiveness to shock. The last two sessions, without drug, show a return of GSR to nondrug levels.

Diazepam, at least for the three subjects tested, produced a predictable increase in overall skin resistance and, as was seen in the experiment with monkeys, the GSR response to the shock was also reduced after small doses and completely obliterated after the largest dose tested.

BEHAVIORAL INDICES OF ANXIETY IN ANIMALS

Anxiety has been described in behavioral terms (Skinner, 1938; Millenson, 1967; 1973) as a motivational state involving an acute disruption of

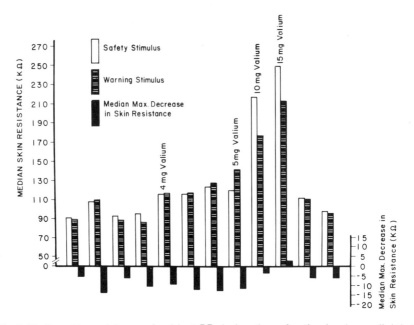

FIG. 6. Median skin resistance of subject BB during the safe stimulus (green light), the warning stimulus (red light), and to shock presented only during the warning stimulus. The maximum decrease in skin resistance after each shock was taken as the largest drop in resistance within 5 sec after delivery of the shock.

positive reinforcers associated with the presentation of a conditioned aversive stimulus. The prototypic behavioral anxiety situation in rats was first described by Estes and Skinner (1941). This "conditional anxiety" state was accomplished by pairing a tone with foot shock. After a series of such pairings, the tone alone was able to disrupt ongoing lever pressing behavior for food. Associated with the suppressed responding in the presence of the conditioned emotional stimulus (CER) were various autonomic responses, e.g., urination, defecation, and piloerection. In the main, many studies have shown that antianxiety agents restore the responding that had previously been suppressed by the conditioning paradigm (see Millenson, 1973, for an excellent review of the CER as a base line for the study of tranquilizing drugs).

Although the CER seems to be a good analogue of anxiety, the effects of antianxiety drugs on this behavior have been variable (Millenson, 1973). Recognizing this problem, Geller and Seifter (1960) designed a behavioral procedure using rats that had high validity for demonstrating the effects of antianxiety agents. Table 1 shows an extremely high correlation between the potency of antianxiety agents in a rat conflict test and their relative potencies in the clinic.

In the Geller conflict procedure, rats were trained in an approach-avoid-

TABLE 1. Comparison of clinical potency with results in the conflict test in rats

	Rat conflict			Clinical psychoneurotics		
	MED (mg/kg, p.o.)	Relative potency	Rank order	Avg. daily dose (mg) oral	Compar. studies, relative potency	Rank order
Diazepam	0.63	3.5	1	20	2	1
Chlordiazepoxide	2.2	1.0	3	40	1	2
Oxazepam	1.25	1.8	2	49	0.8	3
Phenobarbital	4.5	0.5	4	115	0.3	4
Amobarbital	5.0	0.4	5	175	0.17	5
Meprobamate	62.5	0.04	6	1410	0.03	6

MED indicates smallest dose tested that significantly ($p < 0.05$) attenuated the effects of punishment. Average daily dose (clinical) obtained from 74 published clinical reports. Complete list of references can be obtained from the authors (Cook and Davidson). Relative potency (clinical) is based on studies in which drugs were compared directly with chlordiazepoxide.
(From Cook and Davidson, 1973).

ance conflict procedure to respond on an intermittent schedule for food. Superimposed on this base line was the presentation of a tone during which each response was reinforced with food, but also accompanied by a foot shock. The intensity of the foot shock was gradually increased until all or almost all responding during the tone was suppressed. Drugs that specifically released the suppressed behavior were the benzodiazepines (diazepam, oxazepam, and chlordiazepoxide), meprobamate, and various barbiturates.

Other conflict procedures sensitive to the administration of antianxiety agents have also been reported. Leaf and Muller (1965) used a procedure in rats that required no previous training. They reported that doses of morphine increased water licking in rats that had been punished with foot shock; however, they did not test any standard antianxiety agents. Vogel, Beer, and Clody (1971), in a test similar to the one used by Leaf and Muller (except that shock was delivered between the drinking tube and the grid floor every 20th lick) found that chlordiazepoxide, diazepam, oxazepam, meprobamate, and pentobarbital all significantly increased drinking, in spite of the punishing shocks. Drugs such as d-amphetamine, magnesium pemoline, methylphenidate, scopolamine, and imipramine, did not affect the suppressed licking. However, small doses of chlorpromazine, fluphenazine, thioridazine, and amitriptyline had small but significant effects in preventing the effects of punishment in this procedure (Beer, Chasin, Clody, Vogel, and Horovitz, 1972). All the latter drugs have been reported to have some utility in clinical anxiety when given in small doses.

Recently, Migler (*in preparation*) described a procedure used with squirrel monkeys which illustrates the effects of diazepam on food-reinforced behavior that has been suppressed by punishment. A description of this procedure and the effects of diazepam administration are described below.

SQUIRREL MONKEY CONFLICT TEST

During the first 4 hr of a 5-hr session, a light was illuminated over a lever on the right side of the test panel. Each time the monkey held the lever down for 5 sec, a food pellet and a brief electric shock would be delivered. If the monkey pressed the lever, but released it before 5 sec had elapsed, there were no consequences. After 4 hr, the first light was extinguished and a light was illuminated over a lever on the left side of the test panel for 1 hr. During this period, each time the monkey held the left lever down for 5 sec, a food pellet would be delivered without an accompanying shock. Diazepam was administered by gavage 30 min after a session had started.

The typical behavior of a well-trained monkey is indicated in Fig. 7. When the monkey pressed the appropriate lever, the recording pen stepped upward at a rate of 10 steps/sec. The delivery of a food pellet is indicated by an oblique mark in the record. The 4-hr punishment period is indicated by the lower pen remaining undeflected and the 1-hr unpunished period is indicated by the deflection of the pen. During the punishment period, few responses occurred, and all but one were abortive; that is, the monkey re-

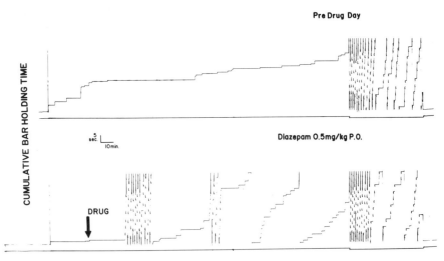

FIG. 7. Performance of a squirrel monkey (subject AL) in a conflict test (see text for details of test). **Upper:** Performance on the day prior to drug administration. During the punishment period (event pen up), only a few responses were emitted and these were almost all abortive. Responding during the unpunished period (event pen down) was not suppressed and the animal earned many pellets. **Lower:** Effect of a 0.5 mg/kg dose of diazepam administered orally on the next day. After the administration of diazepam, 5 mg/kg p.o., responding during the punishment period was greatly increased.

leased the lever before 5 sec had elapsed. During the unpunished period, many responses were made and almost all were of sufficient duration to produce reinforcement. The effect of a 0.5-mg/kg dose of diazepam, administered orally to this monkey on the next day, is also shown in Fig. 7. Approximately 30 min after drug administration, there was an abrupt onset of responding; many food pellets were delivered with accompanying shocks. The effect is typical of that seen in a number of other subjects.

BEHAVIORAL CONFLICT IN HUMANS

We first tried to develop a procedure for use with humans that was similar to the test first used in rats by Geller and Seifter (1960). It soon became evident that this procedure had some small shortcomings for use with human subjects. Our subjects showed rapid behavioral tolerance to the aversiveness of electric shocks applied to their forearms when the shocks occurred on a continuous reinforcement schedule (shock and reward following every response). When the subject could predict the occurrence of each shock, he would not be dissuaded from responding even if the shock levels were increased to the maximum, 10.0 mA. Lever pressing could not be suppressed unless the subject was unable to predict the occurrence of the shocks. In addition, it was very difficult to suppress lever pressing unless the shocks were reasonably spaced during the experimental session. We were able to use lower intensity shocks (2.0 to 4.0 mA) to suppress responding by decreasing the frequency of electric shocks and by making the shock occurrence difficult for the subject to predict. Except for the modifications mentioned above, the procedure we used was in most other respects quite similar to the Geller conflict procedure.

Three males and one female, ages 24 to 38, served as subjects. Each subject sat in front of a console having red and green stimulus lights, a telegraph response key, and counters which were used to designate the amount of money that had been earned.

Each daily session consisted of four 32-min sessions, each separated by 1 hr. Each 32-min session consisted of the presentation of a green light for 2 min during which time the subject was instructed that 1% of his responses (lever presses) would earn nickels. After the 2 min, the green light was extinguished and a red light was presented for 2 min, during which 5% of the subjects' responses earned quarters. During the red stimulus condition, every presentation of a 25-cent reward on the counter was accompanied by an electric shock delivered to the forearm. Each 32-min session included eight alternate presentations of green and red lights, 2 min each.

The results for all four subjects are presented in Fig. 8. The sessions labeled Control 1 are those in which the intensity of shock was adjusted for each subject until a reliable suppression of responding occurred. One hr later, with the shock intensity maintained at the final level of Control 1, a

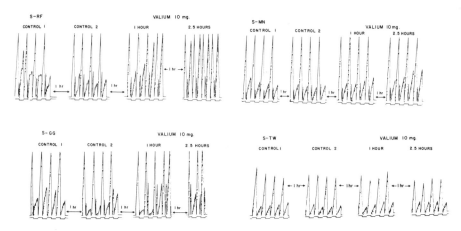

FIG. 8. Cumulative records for human subjects RF, MN, GG, and TW, indicating alternating trials of 2-min nonpunishment and punishment conditions described in text. Each session was 16 min in duration and separated from the next session by a rest period of approximately 1 hr. Diazepam was given p.o. immediately after the second control session. Each slash on the record indicates a reinforcement.

second control session (Control 2) was conducted. In all subjects, the suppression of responding in each of the red conditions was maintained at a relatively stable level. Subjects received three to seven punishing shocks during each 2-min red-light trial. At the end of the second control session, each subject was given 10 mg of diazepam orally, and was tested 1 and $2\frac{1}{2}$ hr later. Subjects RF and GG began to show greater response rates during the conflict stimulus, but not until halfway through the first drug session. The peak drug effect for subjects RF, GG, and MN occurred approximately 2.5 hr after diazepam had been administered. Subject TW showed no effects of diazepam. His base-line rate for the safe condition was low and different from those of the other subjects. Unfortunately, we were unable to try higher doses of diazepam with this subject. All four subjects reported that the shock felt as painful after administration of the drug as before.

DISCUSSION

We have demonstrated that diazepam has qualitatively similar activities across species, including humans, in two highly valid procedures used to measure the predictiveness of antianxiety agents.

Even after years of clinical experience with anxiolytic drugs, it has become apparent that the effects of these psychotropic agents are difficult to elucidate in the clinic by traditional methods. Attempts at early clinical evaluation using objective psychophysical means have indirectly relied on the emotional and intellectual background of the anxiety-neurotic patient

(Lapierre, 1974). This led Lapierre (1974) to lament recently, "A simple culture-free, IQ-free, dynamic-free method of psychophysiological assessment of anxiolytic drug effect has yet to be developed." We feel that the GSR response to anticipated danger and the conflict-punishment procedure are two reliable and valid procedures free of the constraints mentioned by Lapierre.

There are myriad advantages for standardized objective tests that can be used in normal volunteers to evaluate or predict the potential efficacy of new psychotropic drugs. These advantages include feedback to the animal laboratory that will help determine the reliability of research findings in animals. In addition, it is desirable to get an early indication of efficacy while one is still investigating the toxicologic effects of a new drug, in order to prevent the waste of normal volunteers who are now used mainly for the assessment of the adverse effects of the drug under investigation (see Fink, *this volume,* for a discussion of this problem). This early examination of the main pharmacologic effects of these new agents may be accomplished in early single-dose studies since the pharmacological activities seen in animals usually occur after single doses. Early human pharmacologic findings can also have great bearing on the selection of doses for studies in patients.

Our findings can be best described as preliminary and might be strengthened by additional studies involving placebo controls and having subjects receive other anxiolytic drugs as well as drugs from other psychotropic classes to estimate the specificity of these procedures. The effects of diazepam in our study of conflict-punishment behavior did not appear for approximately 1 hr after the drug's administration, and we did not see a peak effect until approximately 2.5 hr after drug, a finding coincident with the temporal effects of diazepam seen in the clinic. This strongly indicates that the punishment attenuation activity we report is not due to any suggestive affects but attributable to the direct pharmacologic action of diazepam. It is also worth noting that although studies with drugs from other psychotropic classes are important to study in these tests, one must also be fully aware that drugs from other classes, such as some phenothiazines and some tricyclic antidepressives, notably fluphenazine and amitriptyline, respectively, have been reported to have clinical antianxiety effects and also punishment attenuating effects in rats at some doses (Beer et al., 1972).

The utility of these procedures in humans depends mainly on whether or not subjects can tolerate them. The electric shock that was used in our studies was tolerated well by our subjects even though they were slightly apprehensive at first. Of course, the major dependent variables in these studies were physiological and behavioral measures of "apprehension" in response to aversive stimuli. Only one subject asked to be removed from the study (in an earlier version of the experiment when the shocks were given more frequently and at higher current settings than were eventually used).

We intended to provide experimental conditions for use in humans which were similar to animal procedures often reported in the literature. Although more research is needed before these procedures are acceptable for predicting clinical effects in anxious patients, this beginning indicates an optimism for that approach.

ACKNOWLEDGMENTS

We thank Dr. Lane Lenard and Mr. Rick Zinna for technical assistance. We also thank Joan Wisniewski for her skillful typing and proofreading of the manuscript and Drs. David Frost and Morton E. Goldberg for their critical editing of the manuscript.

REFERENCES

Bagshaw, M. H., Kimble, D. P., and Pribram, K. (1965): The GSR of monkeys during orienting and habituation and after ablation of the amygdala, hippocampus and inferotemporal cortex. *Neuropsychopharmacologia,* 3:111–199.

Beer, B., Chasin, M., Clody, D. E., Vogel, J. R., and Horovitz, Z. P. (1972): Cyclic adenosine monophosphate phosphodiesterase in brain: Effect on anxiety. *Science* 176:428–430.

Cook, L. and Davidson, A. B. (1973): Effects of Behaviorally Active Drugs in a Conflict-Punishment Procedure in Rats. In: *Benzodiazepines,* edited by S. Garattini, E. Mussini, and L. O. Randall. Raven Press, New York.

Darrow, C., and Gullickson, G. R. (1970): The peripheral mechanism of the GSR. *Psychophysiology,* 6:597–600.

Estes, W. K., and Skinner, B. F. (1941): Some quantitative properties of anxiety. *J. Exp. Psychol.,* 29:390–400.

Eysenck, H. J. (1969): Psychological Aspects of Anxiety. In: *Studies of Anxiety,* edited by M. H. Lader, pp. 7–20. Royal Medico-Psychological Association, London.

Geller, I., and Seifter, J. (1960): The effects of meprobamate, barbiturates, *d*-amphetamine, and promazine on experimentally induced conflict in the rat. *Psychopharmacologia,* 1:482–492.

Gullickson, G. R. (Ed.) (1973): *The Psychophysiology of Darrow.* Academic Press, New York and London.

Kaplan, R. (1963): Rat basal resistance level under stress and nonstress conditions. *J. Comp. Physiol. Psychol.,* 56:775–777.

Klüver, H., and Bucy, P. L. (1938): An analysis of certain effects of bilateral temporal lobectomy in the rhesus monkey with special reference to "psychic blindness." *J. Psychol.,* 5: 33–54.

Kugelmass, S. (1968): Experimental evaluation of galvanic skin response and blood pressure change indices during criminal interrogation. *J. Crim. Law Criminol. Pol. Sci.,* 59:632–635.

Lader, M., and Marks, I. (1971): *Clinical Anxiety.* Grune and Stratton, New York.

Lader, M. H., and Wing, L. (1966): *Physiological Measures, Sedative Drugs and Morbid Anxiety.* Maudsley Monograph No. 14, London.

Lapierre, Y. D. (1974): Galvanic skin responses (GSR) and plethysmographic changes induced by chlorimipramine, imipramine, and placebo. *Curr. Ther. Res. Clin. Exp.,* 16: No. 5, 461–469.

Leaf, R. C., and Muller, S. A. (1965): Effects of shock intensity, deprivation, and morphine in a simple approach-avoidance conflict situation. *Psychol. Rep.,* 17:819–823.

Lobb, H. (1968): Trace GSR conditioning with benzedrine in mentally defective and normal adults. *Am. J. Ment. Defic.,* 73:239–246.

Lobb, H., and Kaplun, J. (1970): Protection of GSR conditioning by dextroamphetamine. *Can. J. Psychol.,* 24:15–26.

McGonnell, P. C., and Beach, H. (1968): The effects of ethanol on the acquisition of a conditioned GSR. *Q. J. Stud. Alcohol,* 29:845–855.

Millenson, J. R. (1967): *Principles of Behavioral Analysis.* Macmillan, New York.

Millenson, J. R. (1973): The Conditioned Emotional Response (CER) as a Baseline for the Study of Tranquilizing Drugs. Presented at the First Latin American Congress of Psychobiology. Sao Paulo, Brazil, December.

Pirkko, N. (1969): Electrodermal responses as a function of quantified threat. *Scand. J. Psychol.,* 10:49–56.

Richter-Heinrich, E., and Lauter, J. (1969): A psychophysiological test as a diagnostic test with essential hypertensives. *Psychother. Psychosom.,* 17:153–168.

Skinner, B. F. (1938): *The Behavior of Organisms.* Appleton-Century, New York.

Vogel, J. R., Beer, B., and Clody, D. E. (1971): A simple and reliable conflict procedure for testing anti-anxiety agents. *Psychopharmacologia,* 21:1–7.

Wolpe, J., Lazarus, A. A., and Fried, R. (1968): Psychophysiological correlates of systematic desensitization of phobias: Preliminary findings. *Cond. Reflex,* 3:139.

Zahn, T. P., Rosenthal, D., and Lawlor, W. G. (1968): Electrodermal and heart rate orienting reactions in chronic schizophrenia. *J. Psychiatr. Res.,* 6:117–134.

Predictability in Psychopharmacology: Preclinical and Clinical Correlations, edited by A. Sudilovsky, S. Gershon and B. Beer. Raven Press, New York, © 1975.

Relationships Between Preclinical Testing and Therapeutic Evaluation of Antidepressive Drugs: The Importance of New Animal Models for Theory and Practice

Gerald L. Klerman

Department of Psychiatry, Massachusetts General Hospital, 2 Fruit Street, Boston, Massachusetts 02114

This chapter explores the theoretical and practical significance of recent research on animal models of depression. The research, although less than a decade old, offers considerable promise of contributing both to our understanding of the etiology and pathogenesis of depression and to the development of practical techniques for preclinical prediction of new types of antidepressive drugs.

There is, of course, an alternative theoretical viewpoint to the gospel (which I believe is heresy) which says that depression is uniquely human because the *sine qua non* of it is the verbal expression of either some self-depreciation or feeling of guilt; since no animal other than human can say such things, *ipso facto* any animal model is inapplicable to a theory of depression. Part of the resistance to animal models has been based on this view of the uniqueness of certain human clinical phenomena, with which I disagree. The evidence from the animal models indicates that there are major behavioral continuities within all mammalian species and that if one looks at depression and other affective states from an evolutionary standpoint as part of the adaptive apparatus of human and other species, there should be continuities across species; we humans may be adding some verbal, symbolic, and social components to it.

For example, Fig. 1 identifies some nonverbal aspects of sadness, depression, or disappointment that are easily recognizable. On the other hand, there are also certain verbal and nonverbal aspects that make depression a family affair. In exploring the more modern concepts of depression, we can detect certain signals using the example of a woman who is depressed. We can see the depression in her facial expression, in her clothing color (black, for example), in her drooping mouth and her downcast eyes; in addition, if she is also middle-aged and of pyknic build (features statistically associated with depression), we have a typical profile of a depressed woman. (The postural features she may show are similar to those that occur in depressed

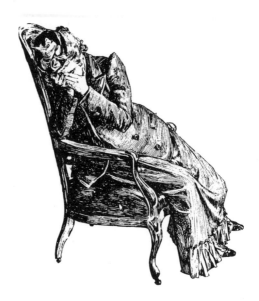

FIG. 1. Some features of the depressed state. Note that from the individual's posture, hand positioning, and other nonverbal clues we can easily recognize her sad mood and empathize with her.

monkeys and dogs, which I discuss later.) However, the husband of such a woman may have no deficiency of assertive behavior. We can imagine a sequence of events that have taken place in such a family — the wife has been depressed since an anniversary, and even though the husband has attempted to reassure her that she is still as beautiful, charming, lovely, and sexually attractive as the day they married, she doesn't believe him. He might point out: "I do like you. *You* don't like you."

This aspect of the syndrome may be uniquely human in two ways. One is the issue of self-esteem. We can imagine the conversations that have gone on in such a social diad — his attempts to reassure her as to her beauty, worth, intelligence, and other measures of self-esteem; they seem to be failing as a psychotherapeutic technique. The other aspect is that he becomes hostile, irritable, and frustrated. One of the theories of the uniqueness of human depression postulates hostility turned against oneself. Our psychoanalytic colleagues would say that he expresses his unconscious hostility and is assertive. This illustration, although reinforcing my point about the distinctiveness of the verbal and, perhaps, social components of the syndrome (which may be uniquely human) also serves to point out some of the vegetative and postural effects that seem to be common to all species, at least to all mammals.

In other fields of medicine, the availability of an animal model greatly accelerated the development of rational pharmacotherapy. Animal models provide the opportunity to understand modes of action, as distinct from descriptions of effects. When we have information about the effects of drugs on some pharmacologic response system, such as EEG or symptoms, we do not have a theory of mode of drug action—we have a description of drug effects. To understand mode of action, a theory is required that relates the manifest drug effects to one or more intervening variables. Among the possible important intervening variables are some characteristic of the subject (e.g., heredity and early development), some CNS changes (as in neurotransmitters), or some change in the environmental context in which the animal is being observed such as the schedule of reinforcement in the subject's social field (i.e., the presence or absence of significant social stimuli). Ideally, we would like to have a theory that relates drug effects to a large number of characteristics of the individual subject and brain action; for these purposes, the development of an animal model greatly facilitates research, since it allows experimental manipulations of brain, contextual, and subject variables that are not ethically or feasibly possible in human clinical research.

In 1969, McKinney and Bunney reviewed the evidence for animal models of depression and concluded that none of the existing models met the criterion of direct behavioral correlation. However, they suggested that new animal models might be likely to emerge. In less than 5 years, two new behavioral models did emerge—the separation model (Scott and Senay, 1973) and the learned-helplessness model (Seligman, 1972), in addition to a pharmacologic one, the amine-depleted animal (Klerman, 1973). It is now possible to identify experiments in both humans and animals that can test the relevance of these models to clinical psychopathology, neurochemistry, and drug evaluation. These three new animal models of depression provide fascinating possibilities for theory and practice. Of great theoretical importance, these research approaches involve not only basic neuropharmacologic (the amine-depleted animal is used for screening new drugs) and neurochemical (the role of neurotransmitters) investigations, but also behavioral models of animal depression that offer promise that experimentally produced behavioral changes, such as loss or helplessness, will induce changes in brain chemistry. Thus we can anticipate experimental verification of psychosomatic hypotheses involving two-way interactions between brain and behavior in the pathogenesis of experimental states of depression in animals.

Moreover, I believe that this research on animal models highlights important relationships among basic research, drug development, and clinical investigations. Although this general relationship is well established throughout most of medicine, it has not yet been developed fully in clinical psychiatry. Until the advent of psychopharmacology and related research in the neurosciences, clinical psychiatry had been, for the most part, both a highly pragmatic art and a highly theoretical and abstract philosophic school, with relatively little integral relationship among laboratory research, theory, and clinical practice.

GENERAL CONCEPTS IN THE PRECLINICAL DEVELOPMENT OF NEW ANTIDEPRESSIVE DRUGS

Ideally, in the scientific development of new therapeutic agents, new treatments (especially drugs) will be developed "rationally." By rationally, I mean that when a new drug is introduced for clinical study of its possible therapeutic actions, precise predictions can be made about its clinical indications, based on preclinical knowledge of the drug's mode of action. To achieve this ideal of rational pharmacotherapy, predictive knowledge is required in four areas.

1. Valid and objective clinical or laboratory criteria to identify patients with specified clinical signs or symptoms, e.g., edema, anemia, jaundice, depression, anxiety.
2. Sufficient knowledge of etiology to permit patients with given clinical manifestations to be differentially grouped, i.e., classified.
3. Understanding of the pathogenesis or pathogenic physiology, i.e., the sequence of events leading to the formulation of symptoms characteristic of the disease state.
4. Knowledge of the pharmacologic actions of classes of drugs to describe how the drug treatment interrupts the pathogenic sequence that results in symptom formation or alters the pathologic physiology characteristic of the disease state.

This ideal is seldom realized in any field of medicine, psychiatry least of all. Except for the infectious diseases (e.g., CNS syphilis), certain endocrine disorders, and the nutritional deficiency diseases (e.g., pellagra) we rarely possess such comprehensive understanding. For most mental illnesses, we have only partial information in any of the four areas. In the treatment of depression, we possess partial understanding. We do have good general diagnostic screens and a variety of effective agents (Table 1). Particularly important for clinical trials of antidepressants is the lack of agreement on the etiologic classification of patients with depression. More significant for prediction of modes of action is our dearth of knowledge about the altered physiology of the disease state, let alone its etiology.

It is important to remember that, during the brief history of treating depressed patients with effective drugs, i.e., since 1936, therapeutic efficacy has almost always been discovered in the clinical situation, usually serendipitously. In 1957, there was very little in the available animal studies of iproniazid or imipramine to suggest their possible usefulness in depressed

TABLE 1. *Drugs used in the chemotherapy of depressions*

Main group	Chemical type	Generic name	Trade name
Psychomotor stimulants	amphetamines	amphetamine	Benzedrine
		dextroamphetamine	Dexedrine
		combinations with barbiturate	Dexamyl
	others	methylphenidate	Ritalin
Monoamine oxidase inhibitors	hydrazines	isocarboxazid	Marplan
		nialamide	Niamid
		phenelzine	Nardil
	nonhydrazines	pargyline	Eutonyl
		tranylcypromine	Parnate
Tricyclic derivatives	iminodibenzyls	desipramine	Norpramin Pertofrane
		imipramine	Tofranil
		trimipramine	Unavailable commercially in United States
	dibenzocycloheptenes	amitriptyline	Elavil
		nortriptyline	Aventyl
		protriptyline	Vivactil
	dibenzoxepin	doxepin	Sinequan

patients. At that time the preclinical criterion used for predicting possible clinical antidepressive action of a drug was an increase in the gross psychomotor activity of laboratory animals, a criterion derived from experience with amphetamines and embodying the classic neuropharmacologic model of excitation-depression as a single bipolar dimension (Klerman, 1966). By this criterion, neither imipramine nor iproniazid was predicted to be antidepressive, and the unexpected demonstration of their clinical efficacy stimulated productive lines of investigation.

The Classic Model: The Stimulant-Depressant Continuum

The classic model for neuropharmacology postulated a single bipolar dimension of CNS activity, ranging from one extreme of CNS depression through an intermediate neutral state to the other extreme of CNS excitation (Table 2). This presumed state of CNS physiology is paralleled by the actions of drugs that are regarded as ordered on the stimulant-depressant dimension and by a corresponding ordering of clinical psychiatric states ranging from manic excitement through catatonic and depressed states. This theory has been applied to the actions of the amphetamines and barbiturates. Recently, it has been related to Pavlovian conditioning by Eysenck (1961) and to psychoanalytic libido theory by Ostow (1962).

TABLE 2. *Bipolar stimulant depressant continuum*

		normal	
Neurophysiology	Excitation	←————I————→	Inhibition
Mood	Elation	←————I————→	Depression
Clinical states	Mania	←————I————→	Stupor
Psychic energy	Libido plethora	←————I————→	Libido depletion
Personality	Extrovert	←————I————→	Introvert
Drugs	Stimulation	←————I————→	Depression

Metrazol	Amphetamine	Sedatives	Anesthetics
Indoklon	Caffeine	Barbiturates	Narcotics
ECT	MAO inhibitors	Bromides	
		Alcohol	

THE AMINE-DEPLETED ANIMAL MODEL

The first animal model of depression to emerge was a pharmacologic model, the amine-depleted animal. This model has been of considerable practical utility in pharmaceutical laboratories.

For many years, the possible role in depression of the sympathetic nervous system and its neurohumors, epinephrine and norepinephrine, had been the subject of intensive speculation. However, the empirical investigations of these speculations was of only limited generalizability. The crucial events in the development of the amine theory occurred from 1956 to 1958 with the suggestion that the clinical actions of reserpine and iproniazid were related to changes in brain biogenic amines. Both the animal model for chemically induced depressive psychopathology and the amine hypothesis of affective disorders are based on the clinical observation that reserpine, which depletes brain biogenic amines, produces clinical depression in 10 to 15% of hypertensive human patients, particularly when the dose is greater than 0.5 to 1.0 mg per day (Klerman, 1966). Although not universally observed in all patients treated, in those patients where depression does occur, it is severe enough to require hospitalization.

Meanwhile, clinical and pharmacologic research was elucidating the actions of MAO inhibitors. Zeller and Barsky (1962) previously noted that iproniazid and other hydrazines were inhibitors of MAO. Iproniazid, originally developed as a rocket fuel, was introduced in 1950–1951 for the treatment of tuberculosis. Adverse behavioral effects were noted in many of the tuberculosis patients treated with this compound. Isoniazid, introduced about the same time, was a more effective tuberculostatic agent, but it produced neurologic complications. In contrast, iproniazid, although less effective in the treatment of tuberculosis, produced euphoria, weight gain, increased psychomotor activity, increased social behavior, and also induced psychiatric states resembling hypomanic and schizoaffective psychoses in many patients. From 1953 to 1957, a number of astute clinicians reported these psychiatric reactions and explored the possible utility of iproniazid in the treatment of retarded schizophrenic and depressed patients (Crane, 1956a,b, 1958; Loomer, Saunders, and Kline, 1957). Simultaneous with the reports of these clinical effects, Brodie, Pletscher, and Shore (1955); Spector, Prockop, Shore, and Brodie (1958); Shore (1962); and Pletscher (1965) described the pharmacologic antagonisms between reserpine and iproniazid. A new biochemical model emerged for predicting antidepressive activities, and potential antidepressive compounds were tested for inhibition of MAO.

The introduction of imipramine in clinical therapeutics again illustrates the role of serendipity. Imipramine was developed as an iminodibenzyl derivative with potential sedative and antihistaminic properties. Because of its structural and pharmacologic similarities to chlorpromazine, the initial clinical trials in the mid-1950s were conducted in psychotic patients. These trials proved unsuccessful, but Kuhn (1958) observed significant antidepressive activity. Kuhn's observations, and the subsequent verification of his findings by other clinical investigators, initiated a new wave of clinical and laboratory investigations and introduced a new class of antidepressive drugs, the tricyclic antidepressives, imipramine, amitriptyline, nortriptyline, etc. The effectiveness of imipramine posed two problems for research. First, how could one differentiate the pharmacology of imipramine and the other tricyclic antidepressives from that of the phenothiazines, whose chemical structure and animal and human pharmacology were closely paralleled by imipramine? Second, would the clinical efficacy of imipramine, which did not inhibit MAO, serve to invalidate the attractive monoamine hypothesis of the biology of depression derived from the interactions between reserpine and iproniazid?

During the past two decades, there has been a gradual accumulation of hypotheses suggesting a probable association between the disorders of affect (depression and elation) and changes in the metabolism CNS catecholamines. The evidence for this theory is, for the most part, indirect and derives from observations that most of the agents affecting behavior and mood also have profound actions on the catecholamines and their metabolism (Bunney and Davis, 1965; Klerman and Cole, 1965; Schildkraut, 1965).

Although the view of the importance of the monoamine oxidase system in the degradation of catecholamines required considerable modification after the demonstration by Armstrong, McMillan, and Shaw (1957) and by Axelrod (1962) of the catechol O-methyl-transferase pathway, therapeutic changes caused by inhibitors of MAO are still hypothesized to be related to drug-induced changes in CNS amines either catecholamines, indoleamines, or both (Feldstein, Hoagland, Wong, Oktem, and Freeman, 1964; Feldstein, Hoagland, Oktem, and Freeman, 1965).

As was well known, reserpine profoundly reduces the psychomotor behavior of animals. Sulser and associates (Sulser, Watts, and Brodie, 1960, 1962; Sulser and Brodie, 1962; Sulser, Bickel, and Brodie, 1964) observed that imipramine and its metabolite, desmethylimipramine, reverse this effect. Previously, many investigators had demonstrated that imipramine antagonized many other actions of reserpine, especially its autonomic effects, without affecting reserpine-induced depletion of brain amines (Domenjoz and Theobald, 1959; Costa, Garattini and Valzelli, 1960; Chen and Bohner, 1961; Garattini, Giachetti, Jori, Pieri, and Valzelli, 1962). However, in animals whose brain catecholamines are selectively depleted prior to the administration of reserpine, imipramine no longer antagonizes the behavioral effects of reserpine. This finding indicates that these actions of imipramine are dependent on the presence of catecholamines in the brain (Scheckel and Boff, 1964; Sulser et al., 1962).

Since about 1960, the effects of a new compound on the reserpine-treated or amine-depleted animal were used in many laboratories as a screening test for possible antidepressive drug effects. Although there are many limitations to this model, the catecholamine-depleted animal (especially one also treated with reserpine) is currently the most widely used and valid biochemical and behavioral analogue of some, if not all, depressed states in humans.

The use of animals under the influence of drugs such as reserpine, tetrabenazine, or guanethidine, which deplete amines in the brain or peripheral tissues, has proved to be very fruitful for testing new compounds suspected to have antidepressive properties (Costa et al., 1960; Chen and Bohner, 1961; Garattini et al., 1962). From the psychiatric viewpoint, the amine-depleted animal is of considerable interest. It may provide an experimental analogue of depression, especially since the administration of reserpine and alpha-methyldopa, both depletors of amines, may produce depression in man.

Research in the amine-depleted animal has stimulated a great deal of theorizing about the role of biogenic amines in affective disorders. However, it is important to acknowledge that after almost 10 years of intensive research, the catecholamine hypothesis of affective disorders remains unverified. As Gershon and Shopsin (1973), Mendels and Frazer (1974), and others have pointed out, the theory has given insufficient attention to the indoleamines and acetylcholine neurotransmitters. Attempts to verify the theory clinically by studying various body fluids (especially CSF) in patients have yielded inconclusive and inconsistent findings.

As an animal model for predicting the relationship between preclinical and clinical actions of new drugs, the amine-depleted animal has three major deficiencies.

1. The behavior of the animal treated with such amine depletors as reserpine and benzoquinolines does not correspond completely to the behavior of clinically depressed humans. Amine-depleted animals demonstrate sedation, autonomic changes, and reduction in psychomotor activity, but these changes are not completely similar to the behavior of patients with clinical depression, and are strikingly less so than those in the other animal models to be discussed later.
2. There is a lack of correspondence of drug effects in the animal to clinical efficacy. For example, most of the studies involving the amine-depleted animal indicate that norepinephrine and related catecholamine compounds are more prone to reverse the state than are serotonin-related compounds. Thus drugs like dopa and amphetamines are often found in screening for potential new drugs. In clinical practice, however, dopa has had no beneficial effect in the treatment of depression, nor have amine-depleting substances like alpha-methyltyrosine and methyldopa produced the characteristic depressive features predicted by the amine-depleted model.
3. Perhaps the most serious criticism of the amine theory is that the new drugs detected by use of this model have had chemical and pharmacologic properties almost identical to those of marketed tricyclics. This result is, of course, not unexpected given the nature of this animal model, but only points out that all animal models are limited.

ANIMAL SEPARATION MODELS

Folklore and clinical experience have long noted that separation or loss in humans and animals is followed by behavioral symptoms suggesting depression. Almost all pet lovers are aware of the striking changes that animals, particularly dogs, exhibit when their masters go away. Human clinical studies had documented the importance of separation in child development and suggested that separation and loss might be important precipitants of adult clinical depression. Only in the past 8 or 10 years, however, have there been intensive experimental studies on the psychologic, behavioral, and neurochemical consequences of separation in animals. Research in dogs and monkeys has been most extensive.

The research in dogs by Fuller and Scott (1970) which began in the 1950s and progressed rapidly in the 1960s demonstrated that, after separation, puppies develop behavioral syndromes similar to human depression, and vocalization of distress was most characteristic. Scott and his associates (Scott and Senay, 1973) found that imipramine was the most effective of a wide variety of compounds studied in reducing the vocalization of these separated animals (Fig. 2) without producing sedation or adverse autonomic effects. In fact, dogs who had been separated and then given large doses of imipramine appeared to be no different from the controls given placebo except for a marked reduction in rate of vocalization. The effects of imipramine were in sharp contrast to the lack of effect of antianxiety drugs such as meprobamate and diazepam, barbiturates, alcohol, and phenothiazines. Interestingly, reserpine enhanced the rate of vocalization and other manifestations of the separation syndrome in dogs.

More recently, primates (particularly the rhesus monkey) have been studied as animal models of depression; this work was the topic of a recent AAAS symposium (Scott and Senay, 1973). The Wisconsin group (Harlow, Harlow, and Suomi, 1971) has done the most significant work for possible drug prediction. Early in their research, they used total social and physical isolation, sometimes coupled with use of surrogate wire monkey mothers (Harlow, 1974). This extreme set of conditions produced in young rhesus

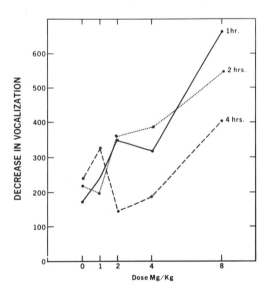

FIG. 2. Effects of imipramine on vocalizations of dogs following separation from significant others. Note the dose relationship between imipramine action in reducing vocalization, a major predictor index of separation in animals.

monkeys a very severe developmental psychopathology that has some similarities to psychoses. Separation experiments have since been modified to include separation of the infant rhesus from either the mother or peers. The sequence of changes includes a two- and, perhaps, three-stage pattern of development (Fig. 3). The protest stage (first) is followed by the stage of despair; if reunion is allowed or surrogate objects are provided, a recovery stage follows. These stages are amazingly consistent with observations from other primate laboratories and also with human research, particularly that of Spitz (1945) and Bowlby (1969).

Mother-infant separations carried out in almost all primate laboratories indicate that, after separation, the infants enter the initial protest stage, characterized by increased psychomotor activities, increased search behavior, anxiety, agitation, and increased vocalization. Shortly thereafter, the subjects enter a phase of withdrawal. Although the form and duration of the despair or withdrawal state vary, the psychomotor changes are similar to those of humans. There is a decrease in psychomotor activity, characteristic facial and motor changes, and a decrease in appetite. Furthermore, subsequent learning is impaired if separations are repeated or prolonged.

Many variables influence the complex behavioral response to loss, including the age of the animal, the degree of confinement, and the presence of peers or of mother surrogates. McKinney and Bunney (1969) have carried this research further to study the neurochemistry of the brain of separated monkeys. They recently reported preliminary findings on changes in amines

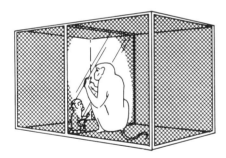

FIG. 3. Diagrammatic representation of the protest (top) and despair (bottom) stages that follow mother-infant separation.

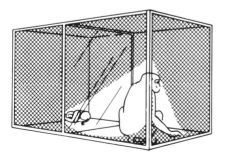

in the brains of young rhesus monkeys separated from their mothers. Catecholamines were reduced in brains of animals killed during the despair or withdrawal stage.

Unfortunately, there are very few well-designed studies of the effects of known or new antidepressive drugs on the behavior of primates separated from their mothers or peers and exhibiting these characteristic syndromes. Boelkins and Cady (1970) indicated that amitriptyline reversed some of the behavioral effects seen during the stage of withdrawal or despair.

The separation model is of particular importance for three reasons.

1. The stimuli inducing the behavioral state are similar to precipitants of human depression, i.e., loss and separation. This state seems closest to so-called reactive depression pattern after grief and bereavement.
2. The behavioral effects have amazing similarity to those in human studies of children and adults. Seeing pictures of the monkeys or dogs, one does not have to be a clinical psychiatrist to feel empathetically that these animals are experiencing a depressive state of some sort.
3. The biochemical and pharmacological studies will soon indicate whether we have a truly psychosomatic model, that is, if behavior induced by changes of the social environment of the animal, i.e., loss, will induce brain biogenic amine changes and if these behavioral and biochemical changes may, in fact, be reversible by drugs known to be antidepressive.

INDUCED BEHAVIORAL HELPLESSNESS

The newest animal model of depression derives from the work of Seligman (1972) and his associates at the University of Pennsylvania. This work is not yet widely known to clinical or pharmacologic audiences. Seligman's "learned helplessness" syndrome refers to a stable behavioral pattern characterized by the animal's failure to initiate potentially adaptive responses to escape traumatic events. Dogs who have been trained to escape shock in a shuttlebox are then subjected to repeated inescapable electric shock while they are strapped in a classic Pavlovian harness. When these dogs later receive electric shock in a shuttlebox, they fail to cross the barrier to escape, even though they have previously learned to do so. This passive behavior, learned helplessness, is in marked contrast to the previous behavior of the same dogs or to the behavior of dogs that have not been exposed to the inescapable shock in the harness. During shuttlebox training, prior to enforced helplessness and unavoidable aversive conditioning, both the matched controls and the experimental animals learn that their response (jumping the barrier) ends the shock in the shuttlebox. In the dog, learned helplessness was reversed by forcibly dragging the dog to the other side of the shuttlebox; this enforced learning seems to break the cycle.

Seligman has generalized a behavioral theory from these experiments and has predicted certain aspects of nontraumatic situations in which the subject, animal or human, fails to make use of previously learned experience. He has demonstrated to the subjects that their own responses can be instrumental in terminating noxious stimuli, enhancing their cognitive or motor performance, or gaining access to otherwise rewarding experiences.

There are many behavioral similarities between the depressive syndromes in humans (Table 3) and animals. Seligman's animals show reduced psychomotor activity, have characteristic facial and postural changes, lose weight, have decreased sexual activity, and fail to learn. He extended his search to clinical observations on the role of negative self expectations in reducing the effectiveness of the depressed individual working to change his environment. He infers that the subjective experiences of hopelessness, helplessness, and weakness that characterize depressed persons correspond to the animal's passivity and failure to make use of previous learning. He recently reported well-designed experiments showing relationships among self-perception, performance, and reinforcement in depressed humans.

There are relationships between Seligman's work and the recent theoretical, psychologic concepts of Beck (1969) who focused on negative cognitive set in depression, i.e., the relationship between perception of one's self as helpless, hopeless, and weak and engaging in depressive and suicidal be-

TABLE 3. *Frequency of depressive symptoms and behaviors in 35 hospitalized depressed women at time of admission*

Symptom or behavior	Patients manifesting (No.)	(%)
Loss of interest in work or activities	35	100
Sad or depressed feelings	34	97
Feelings of hopelessness	34	97
Feelings of helplessness	33	94
Sleep difficulty	32	91
Somatic manifestations of anxiety	32	91
Suicidal thoughts	30	86
Loss of weight	29	83
Feelings of guilt	28	80
Psychomotor agitation	28	80
Feelings of worthlessness	27	77
Anorexia	25	71
Diurnal variation	21	60
Psychomotor or cognitive retardation	19	54
Headache	17	49
Constipation	11	31
Obsessional and compulsive symptoms	11	31
Lack of insight as to being ill	10	29
Paranoid symptoms	9	26

havior. Lewinsohn (1974), a social psychologist who utilizes a Skinnerian behavioral frame of reference, commented on naturalistic observations of social factors that produce a low rate of positive reinforcement in the life situation of depressive individuals. For humans, the most powerful reinforcers are in the social field and include expressions of sympathy, reassurance, love, praise, attention, and other indicators of interpersonal or group cohesion.

The studies by Beck (1969), Seligman (1972), and Lewinsohn (1974) indicate a relationship of behavioral contingencies in the life situation of certain individuals to depressive mood. There are, however, two important research efforts that have not yet been undertaken and that would be necessary to demonstrate fully the validity of this animal model. These two stages of research are:

1. Biochemical studies of the brains of dogs or other animals exposed to enforced or learned helplessness. Do CNS changes parallel to the behavioral sequence occur, i.e., an initial agitation, a protest stage followed by a withdrawal or passive stage? I predict that the brain chemistry findings would parallel these two stages; during the stage of protest or agitation, there would be increased CNS biogenic amine activity but, during the stage of passivity or helplessness, there would be a selective decrease in brain amines (Mirsky, 1968).

2. Practically no work has been done on the use of pharmacologic agents in the treatment of the helplessness of the animal. Tricyclic antidepressives or MAO inhibitors should reverse the syndrome. Conversely, amine depletors, such as reserpine or AMPT, should potentiate the syndrome. If so, we will have a kind of pharmacologic congruency that would enhance the utility of the model.

Like the primate separation model, the helplessness model has great theoretical and practical advantages and intensive research may result in it becoming a screen for new drugs.

CONCLUSIONS

This research has implications for both practice and theory. The practical advantage is that new models for depression in animals, particularly in nonprimates, could lead to effective preclinical screens to predict new classes of antidepressive drugs. Theoretically, we now see the emergence of a number of alternative theories that offer a potent combination of practical utility and intellectual elegance.

The three models reviewed here remove some of the false dichotomy between mind and body that has plagued Western science since Descartes. If these three animal models are validated and developed into preclinical screening techniques for new drugs, they will be of theoretical importance because of their truly psychosomatic interrelationships. In one case, the amine-depleted animal, pharmacologically induced biochemical changes in the brain induce behavioral manifestations. This might best be called a somatopsychic model. It would be well within the classic tradition of biologic psychiatry. The other two models, however, are truly psychosomatic. Psychologic changes, due either to separation of the animal from other animals socially important to it or to changes in capacity to adapt to the environment, may produce brain chemical changes associated with characteristic depressive behavioral symptomatology, i.e., the protest-despair stages.

The development of these animal models contrasts with the earlier history of the discovery of antidepressive drugs — mainly the role that has been too often played by serendipity. Thus it now seems that investigators are on the verge of being able to link the results of behavioral studies in animals with pharmacotherapeutic findings. To make this linkage complete, it is necessary to study the effects of animals' separation on CNS metabolism, particularly on the catecholamines, indoleamines, and acetylcholine neurotransmitters, and also on electrolytes and hormones. Presently, since the situation remains inconclusive, one can consider two alternative theories. A unitary theory put forth recently by Akiskal and McKinney (1973) proposes that depression is a final common pathway mediated by CNS amine changes (Fig. 4). The alternative theory, which I label pluralistic, postulates multiple pathways in the pathogenesis of depression. Variable response to drug treatment offers indirect support for the hypothesis that there are multiple subgroups within the depressive state, each of which may have different etiologies (constitutional, genetic, behavioral, developmental) and each of which may have different pathophysiologic mechanisms and respond differentially to treatment with various types of antidepressive drugs, including some yet to be discovered.

In addition, clinical experience is difficult to integrate into a unitary theory, especially the inconsistent role of loss in precipitating acute depressions. Although this fact does not necessarily limit the importance of the animal studies, it may mean that the separation-loss model provides only a partial explanation of depression. To the extent that this partial explanation is true, it would support the development of a pluralistic, rather than a unitary, theory of depression. Also supporting a pluralistic theory are suggestions that some adult depressions may derive from the vulnerability of certain adults to even minimal stress, a vulnerability acquired during multiple losses suffered in childhood. This theory has been supported by clinical investigations, particularly in psychodynamics, and might explain depressive mechanisms in a subgroup whose members, as the result of childhood influences, are predisposed or vulnerable and show acute adult depression precipitated by relatively minor adaptive changes rather than by major losses or severe external stress. An alternative source of this

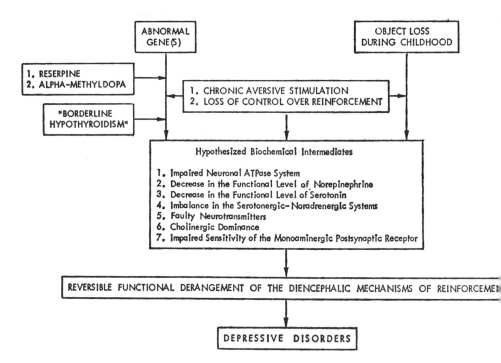

FIG. 4. A multidisciplinary model of the pathogenesis of depressive disorders.

vulnerability may be genetic variability. Winokur, Clayton, and Reich (1969) reviewed the evidence for genetic subtypes on the basis of clinical relationships and the roles of sex and age at onset of depression.

Thus the possibility exists that there are multiple pathways in the pathogenesis of depression. Various etiologic mechanisms may be operative, including early experience and immediate loss. Animal models offer an opportunity to test these theories by experimental research.

REFERENCES

Akiskal, H. S., and McKinney, W. T. (1973): Depressive disorders: Toward a unified hypothesis. *Science,* 182:20–29.

Armstrong, M. D., McMillan, A., and Shaw, K. N. F. (1957): 3-Methoxy-4-hydroxy-D-mandelic acid, a urinary metabolite of norepinephrine. *Biochem. Biophys. Acta,* 25:422.

Axelrod, J. (1962): The effect of psychoactive drugs on the metabolism of catecholamines. In: *Psychosomatic Medicine, The First Hahnemann Symposium,* edited by J. H. Nodine and J. H. Moyer, pp. 312–317. Lea and Febiger, Philadelphia.

Beck, A. (1969): *Depression: Clinical, Experimental and Theoretical Aspects.* Harper and Row, New York.

Boelkins, R. C., and Cady, P. (1970): Drug therapy in a model of infant depression. *AAAS,* Chicago, December 27.

Bowlby, J. (1969): *Attachment and Loss.* Basic Books, New York.

Brodie, B. B., Pletscher, A., and Shore, P. A. (1955): Evidence that serotonin has a role in brain function. *Science,* 122:968.
Bunney, W. E., and Davis, J. M. (1965): Norepinephrine in depressive reactions. *Arch. Gen. Psychiatry,* 13:483–494.
Chen, G., and Bohner, B. (1961): The anti-reserpine effects of certain centrally acting agents. *J. Pharm. Pharmacol.,* 131:179.
Costa, E., Garattini, S., and Valzelli, L. (1960): Interactions between reserpine, chlorpromazine, and imipramine. *Experientia,* 16:461.
Crane, G. E. (1965a): Further studies on iproniazid phosphate, isonicotinilisopropylhydrazine phosphate, Marsilid. *J. Nerv. Ment. Dis.,* 124:322.
Crane, G. E. (1956b): The psychiatric side-effects of iproniazid, *Am. J. Psychiatry,* 112:494.
Domenjoz, R., and Theobald, W. (1959): Zur Pharmakologie des Tofranil (N-(3-Dimethyl-aminopropyl)-iminodibenzyl-Hydrochlorid). *Arch. Int. Pharmacodyn. Ther.,* 120:450.
Eysenck, H. J. (1961): *Experiments with Drugs.* Pergamon Press, London.
Feldstein, A., Hoagland, H., Wong, K. K., Oktem, M. R., and Freeman, H. (1964): MAO activity in relation to depression. *Am. J. Psychiatry,* 120:1192.
Feldstein, A., Hoagland, H., Oktem, M. R., and Freeman, H. (1965): MAO inhibition and antidepressant activity, *Int. J. Neuropsychiatry,* 1:384–387.
Fuller, J. L., and Scott, J. P. (1970): Social deprivation in the dog: Genetic variation in vulnerability. *AAAS,* Chicago, December 27.
Garattini, S., Giachetti, A., Jori, A., Pieri, L., and Valzelli, L. (1962): Effect of imipramine, amitriptyline, and their monomethyl derivatives on reserpine activity. *J. Pharm. Pharmacol.,* 14:509.
Gershon, S., and Shopsin, B. (Eds.) (1973): *Lithium: Its Role in Psychiatric Research and Treatment.* Plenum Press, New York.
Harlow, H. (1974): *Learning to Love.* Jason Aronson, New York.
Harlow, H. F., Harlow, M. K., and Suomi, S. J. (1971): From thought to therapy: Lessons from a primate laboratory. *Am. Sci.,* 59:538–549.
Klerman, G. L. (1966): Modes of action of antidepressant drugs. In: *Pharmacotherapy of Depression,* edited by J. O. Cole and J. R. Wittenborn. Charles Thomas, Springfield.
Klerman, G. L. (1973): Pharmacological aspects of depression. In: *Separation and Depression.* Edited by J. P. Scott and A. C. Senay, *AAAS,* Washington, D.C., pp. 69–89.
Klerman, G. L., and Cole, J. O. (1965): Clinical pharmacology of imipramine and related antidepressant compounds. *Pharmacol. Rev.,* 17:101–141.
Kuhn, R. (1958): The treatment of depressive states with F22355 (imipramine hydrochloride), *Am. J. Psychiatry,* 115:459–464.
Lewinsohn, P. M. (1974): A behavioral approach to depression. In: *The Psychology of Depression: Contemporary Theory and Research,* edited by R. J. Friedman and M. M. Katz. Winston-Wiley, Washington, D.C.
Loomer, H. P., Saunders, J. C., and Kline, N. S. (1957): A clinical and pharmacodynamic evaluation of iproniazid as a psychic energizer. *Psychiat. Res. Rep.,* 8:129–141.
McKinney, W. T., and Bunney, W. E. (1969): Animal models of depression. *Arch. Gen. Psychiatry,* 21:240–248.
Mendels, J., and Frazer, A. (1974): Brain biogenic amine depletion and mood. *Arch. Gen. Psychiatry,* 30:447–451.
Mirsky, I. A. (1968): Some comments on psychosomatic medicine. *Exc. Med. Int. Congress Series,* 187:107–125.
Ostow, M. (1962): *Drugs in Psychoanalysis and Psychotherapy.* Basic Books, New York.
Pletscher, A. (1965): Pharmacology of antidepressants. In: *Psychopharmacology,* edited by N. S. Kline and H. E. Lehmann, p. 861. International Psychiatry Clinics, Little Brown and Co., Boston.
Scheckel, C. L., and Boff, E. (1964): Behavioral effects of interacting imipramine and other drugs with *d*-amphetamine, cocaine, and tetrabenazine, *Psychopharmacologia,* 5:198.
Schildkraut, J. J. (1965): The catecholamine hypothesis of affective disorders: A review of supporting evidence. *Am. J. Psychiatry,* 122:509–522.
Scott, J. P., and Senay, E. C. (Eds.) (1973): *Separation and Depression: Clinical and Research Aspects.* AAAS, 94, Washington, D.C.
Seligman, M. E. P. (1972): Learned helplessness. *Ann. Rev. Med.,* 23:407–412.

Shore, P. A. (1962): Release of serotonin and catecholamines by drugs. *Pharmacol. Rev.,* 14:531.

Spector, S., Prockop, B., Shore, P. A., and Brodie, B. B. (1958): Effect of iproniazid on brain levels of norepinephrine and serotonin. *Science,* 127:704.

Spitz, R. A. (1945): Hospitalism. *Psychoanal. Study Child,* 1.

Sulser, F., Bickel, M. H., and Brodie, B. B. (1964): The action of desmethyl-imipramine in counteracting sedation and cholinergic effects of reserpine-like drugs. *J. Pharmacol.,* 144: 321.

Sulser, F. and Brodie, B. B. (1962): The mechanism of action of a new type of antidepressant drug which does not block monoamine oxidase. *Chicago Med.,* 65:9.

Sulser, F., Watts, J., and Brodie, B. B. (1960): Antagonistic actions of imipramine (tofranil) and reserpine on central nervous system. *Fed. Proc.,* 19:268.

Sulser, F., Watts, J., and Brodie, B. B. (1962): On the mechanism of antidepressant action of imipramine-like drugs. *Ann. NY Acad. Sci.,* 96:279.

Winokur, G., Clayton, P., and Reich, T. (1969): *Manic Depressive Illness.* C. V. Mosby Co., St. Louis.

Zeller, E. A., and Barsky, J. (1962): *In vivo* inhibition of liver and brain monoamine oxidase by 1-isonictinyl-2-isopropylhydrazine. *Proc. Soc. Expr. Biol., Med.,* 81:459–461.

DISCUSSION

Krapcho: I wonder if people have tried the effective anticholinergic agents in the howling dog, because it is quite possible that the decrease in salivation might produce a decrease in howling.

Klerman: As far as I know, it hasn't been done.

Krapcho: Will a decrease in salivation affect howling?

Klerman: I personally don't think so, but, as I say, my experience with dogs is limited to watching my neighbor's pets.

Blackwell: There is another animal model I want to tell you about. It's kind of disappeared from sight, but it was an intriguing idea. Apparently, in a species of monkey called the African Queen, when you disrupt the hierarchy for the male, its scrotum changes from pink to blue in response to a loss of hierarchial position within the colony. John Price, a friend of mine who works in Newcastle, had a whole colony of these monkeys, and his idea was that if he could find the biochemical cause of the change in color, he'd probably have the answer to depression. That was two or three years ago, and I've heard nothing of the idea since.

Klerman: Well, one of your other English colleagues has written a similar paper on the effects of different positions in a dominant status level on susceptibility to depression — the argument being that people who have had drops in status level, and animals who've dropped in status level because of some change in age, structure, or dominance hierarchy exhibit depressive-like phenomena (at least in natural observations) and that this "depression" is a way of inhibiting their aggression, because if they express it towards the new dominant individuals they would not survive. He has taken this and elaborated a rather speculative theory about inhibition of aggression in relationship to change in dominance. It is conceivable that one can develop experimental dominance changes. No one has yet done it, but that's another model that is possible. What's intriguing is that once you begin to think about these models and get away from the bind that we clinicians have tended to be in that only humans can get depressed, all sorts of possibilities emerge. One can be quite inventive developing animal or even human models of depression. There is a human model being developed by Fisher and McNair at Boston University in which they use one-arm bandits. As students come in to the laboratory, it is advertised that they have an opportunity to participate in games of chance. The one-arm bandits are rigged so that first the students win and then they stop winning. This is analogous to various extinction schedules used with animals. The students get depressed, they report themselves "high" on mood scales, and their faces look depressed. The next step is to introduce various drugs, but I don't think they have done it yet. They are trying to develop this. This obviously has some appeal, because one can develop various theories about reward and one can get very speculative about the noradrenergic mediation of reinforcement. There is a pharmacologic literature about drugs like the tricyclics and their influence on noradrenergic mechanisms of behavior influenced by reinforcement. It is very speculative, but it's also imaginative.

Horovitz: I certainly couldn't agree with you more that these behavioral tests of reward that closely resemble human conditions should be studied pharmacologically. Does it bother you that in many of them, at least from what you describe and I think in more of them, we find that drugs like imipramine work on the first administration, rather than after a week to 10 days, as the human situation?

Klerman: I think the folklore that it takes 2 to 3 wk for tricyclics to take effect is based upon a misinterpretation of the data and the fact that earlier studies were done with too low doses. There are now a number of good studies that pick up tricyclic-placebo differences at week 1 if higher doses and more sensitive outcome measures are used. Rickels has a couple of studies; DiMascio and I have a study that we presented at the CINP in July, 1974. We have been able to pick up imipramine effects in 1 wk on higher doses, if you start at 150 mg the first week rather than doing 25 mg, 50 mg, and agonizing up with the patient. I think part of the problem was that in the first round with the tricyclics, the doses were just too low. That's my interpretation of it.

Gale: I heard Seligman talk recently in a seminar at Washington University. He mentioned that anticholinergic drugs could, in fact, reverse learned helplessness. This makes sense if you consider that what is being learned is, in fact, non-responding during extinction. The animal unable to make an escape response during the shock situation is actually being extinguished for responding. In similar situations involving extinction, anticholinergic drugs seem to prolong extinction. Thus, an anticholinergic compound administered during the learned-helplessness situation might be expected to reverse the effects of the training in this procedure.

Klerman: Did he say what drug was used, what kind of dosage, or anything like that?

Gale: I don't have that information with me, but I think it was atropine or perhaps scopolamine.

Klerman: That just confirms my feeling that the existence of these models opens up all sorts of imaginative kinds of experiments that get us out of what Sam calls "the rut" of only having the amine-depleting model.

Gale: How does that compare with the human situation in terms of trying to treat a depressed patient with atropine or scopolamine?

Gershon: Not very well.

Klerman: However, it has been argued that almost all of the antidepressant drugs have some anticholinergic components.

Gershon: But when you give atropine, you don't get it.

Minn: I wonder whether a significant number of depressed animals is not produced in a very severely overcrowded situation, and whether that might not be a decent source of depressed animals.

Klerman: I really don't know.

Weliky: There are studies that were done with mice colonies by Dr. Calhoun in which they had the overcrowded situation he calls "behavioral sink," with marked behavioral changes of this type.

Bunney: It was suggested some time ago that the dolphin might make an interesting animal behavioral model for depression, because it's supposedly the only species known in which there have actually been recorded suicides after separation, where they actually drown themselves.

Klerman: The dog models, I think, sound a little bit more practical.

Gershon: I agree with the point that Dr. Klerman made about the reserpine model contributing something, but it has also created a lot of problems. I have here about 14 slides (which I am not going to show) of drugs that have fulfilled the criteria of the animal models for catecholamine function and not one of them has thymoleptic activity. The other point is that all of the behavioral models that Dr. Klerman proposes should really be looked at carefully to get out of this treadmill activity, and that what Dr. Bunney mentioned really is not dismissable, because drug companies spend as much money, or more, on whatever they do now that I don't know if dolphins are out of the ball park on economic grounds. Finally, the other point is that you don't always have to have behavioral analogues of depression. You might get arbitrary interactions. The one we have been pushing for years is simply blood-pressure measures. It's not an analogue of the behavior, but there is a drug interaction with blood pressure that produces a change, and I am particularly delighted to show this. This was published before all the clinical data were in, so I am innocent of postdating it. This is our story of giving yohimbine to a conscious dog and getting the yohimbine response. All we are measureing is blood pressure. The dog is not down and flat; he is alert, excited, and so on. If you give him amphetamine, there is no potentiation of this response, and if you give him imipramine, the pressure goes up about 40 to 50 mm Hg. TRH at 50 to 100 mg/kg i.v. does not produce potentiation, and those people who heard the reports at the ECDEU meeting in Miami recently, including the report by Dr. Sugarman, know from the current data on TRH that this agent is not a thymoleptic.

Predictability in Psychopharmacology: Preclinical and Clinical Correlations,
edited by A. Sudilovsky, S. Gershon and B. Beer. Raven Press, New York,
© 1975.

Problems in Predicting New Psychotropic Agents Through Studies in Animals

Zola P. Horovitz

The Squibb Institute for Medical Research, Princeton, New Jersey 08540

It is well established that most major breakthroughs in the continuing search for new agents with psychotropic activity in man have resulted from astute clinical observations. The phenothiazines and the antidepressives, important psychotropic agents, were introduced to clinical investigation for reasons other than their eventual prime usefulness in the psychotropic area. It seems clear, however, that in the future the ideal way to discover new therapeutic agents will be to utilize selective animal screens with good scientific rationale that are soundly linked to disease in man, and then to study as many as possible of the new compounds that proved active in these screens in well-designed trials in the human. Both the preclinical and clinical studies are necessary, and scientists on both ends of this spectrum must be innovative and communicative.

Although our basic scientific knowledge and expertise have increased rapidly in the last decade, many forces have inhibited progress in drug development in both the preclinical and clinical areas. Three factors have interfered with clinical experimentation.

First, regulatory agencies throughout the world have been demanding an ever-increasing number of preclinical requirements that have limited the number of compounds that could be prepared for testing in man. Second, much tighter moral and ethical controls have been imposed on clinical investigation itself. Although few can argue against the need for adequate regulatory, moral, and ethical restrictions, it is quite clear that they have not only made the cost of early, unique clinical investigations quite high, but they have probably prevented the less tenacious clinician from doing many studies that might have been useful in discovering new psychotropic drugs.

The third limiting factor is the relative absence of astute, well-trained clinical psychopharmacologists who are willing to become involved in the search for new drugs. It is quite apparent that, with few exceptions, there has been an almost complete lack of development of clinical models of psychiatric diseases in which new compounds could be tested. The factors cited above have obviously slowed the development of such models. A few of the chapters in this volume indicate some new efforts in this area, but more are definitely needed.

On the other hand, two main problems in the preclinical sciences seem to have prevented progress in discovering new psychotropic agents. The first relates to the clinical area. Because of the deficient clinical feedback relating to the assessment of new and unique chemical agents and test procedures, the validity of these procedures and of new theories of mechanisms of action has not been confirmed in the ultimate proving ground. Second, most of our animal screens have been developed on the basis of the activity of presently available compounds and, therefore, too many preclinical scientists have become mired in the quicksand of convenient procedures that will detect only compounds similar to those already available.

Despite all these problems, I remain confident that new and useful psychotropic agents can be discovered. In the following pages, I will attempt to describe the procedures presently used for developing new agents in each of the three major psychotropic areas, their main drawbacks, and the potential for newer tests in both animals and man.

ANTIPSYCHOTIC AGENTS

Inhibition of the conditioned avoidance response (CAR) has been the prime test procedure in animals for evaluating the potential of new antipsychotic agents ever since the early work with the first phenothiazine, chlorpromazine. There are many variations of this procedure, but they all measure the disruption in the avoidance of an aversive stimulus by a trained animal after the administration of a test compound at a dose that does not produce severe motor debilitation. Although the rat is most commonly employed, this procedure has been used with almost every mammalian species. Figure 1 shows the dose response effects of chlorpromazine on the CAR (Cook and Weidley, 1957). (See also Courvoisier, Fournel, Ducrot, Kolsky, and Koetschet, 1953; Irwin, 1961; Izquierdo, 1962; Mercier, Dessaigne, and Etzensperger, 1962; and Niemegeers and Janssen, 1960, for descriptions of these various tests.)

Excellent correlations exist between the potencies of the two chemical types of antipsychotic agents the phenothiazines and butyrophenones in blocking avoidance behavior in animals and their potencies in affecting psychotic behavior in patients. Cook (1964) demonstrated that avoidance procedures can also be used in human volunteers, and that chlorpromazine produces the same decrease in avoidance behavior in humans as it does in various animals (Fig. 2).

Although both of these major chemical types of antipsychotic agents (phenothiazines and butyrophenones) work very well in the CAR procedure they also have another common denominator (Ayd, 1961)—their ability to produce extrapyramidal side effects (EPS) (Fig. 3). One might conclude that the CAR, the most widely used animal procedure, is merely measuring

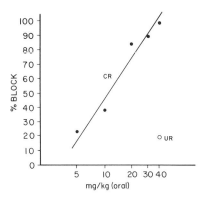

FIG. 1. Block of conditioned response by chlorpromazine. Percentage block represents the proportion of a group of 10 rats at each dose level that failed to respond to the CS (tone) within 30 sec. The points represent the maximum block in each treatment group that occurred over a period of 5 hr after drug administration. The point designated UR indicates that proportion of the 40 mg/kg treatment group which failed to respond to the shock. (From Cook and Weidley, 1957, with permission.)

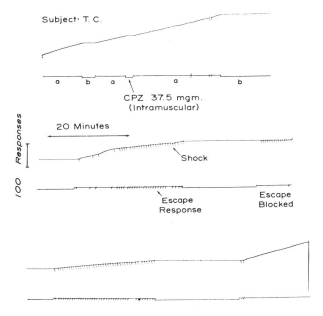

FIG. 2. Effect of chlorpromazine on continuous (Sideman) conditioned avoidance behavior. Periods designated (a) represent avoidance. Shock-shock intervals and response-shock intervals were both 30 sec. Shock duration was 10 sec, or until escape occurred. Pips on cumulative record indicate delivered shocks; pips on baseline represent escape responses. Onset of avoidance block occurred 1 hr postdrug administration. (From Cook, 1964, with permission.)

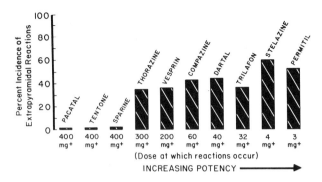

FIG. 3. Relationship between potency of various phenothiazine neuroleptics and incidence of extrapyramidal reactions in patients. (From Ayd, 1961, with permission.)

the ability of compounds to produce side effects. Data from the use of such compounds as thioridazine and clozapine (which have a low propensity to produce EPS) support the view that the CAR procedure is more predictive of antipsychotic activity, but the validity of its predictive value will remain in doubt until a potent blocker of the CAR response has been proved in man to be a potent antipsychotic agent that does not produce EPS.

In the last few years studies of the relationship between the known antipsychotic activity of agents and their actions on dopaminergic receptors and dopamine-containing neurons have led to the use of such measurements as antiapomorphine activity as predictors of antipsychotic activity (Janssen, 1961; Janssen, Niemegeers, and Schellekens, 1965). Once again, it could be that the EPS caused by the antipsychotic agents are also related to their action on the dopamine system. It is possible that antagonism of the actions of dopamine in selected regions of the brain may account for both the therapeutic and adverse effects of the antipsychotic agents. If this is so, perhaps agents can be developed that possess a selective affinity for one part of the brain over another. Appropriate pharmacologic studies using this approach may be very productive in identifying antipsychotic agents with fewer side effects than are caused by agents presently available.

ANTIANXIETY AGENTS

The antipunishment effects of the classic antianxiety agents such as chlordiazepoxide, as described in the Geller conflict procedure (Geller and Seifter, 1960) and modifications of it, appear to be the prime measurements of the antianxiety effects of these compounds. The description of this procedure and data to support its validity are described in detail by Beer and Migler in this volume. All antianxiety agents are effective as antipunishment compounds; potency in the rat conflict procedure is closely correlated with clinical activity; and the former is a good prediction of the latter. Most antianxiety agents also, however, are somewhat sedative and cause muscle relaxation. How much these sedative effects contribute to side effects or prime therapeutic activity is unknown, as is the relationship of sedative and muscle-relaxant effects to the antipunishment response. Gluckman (1965) and others have speculated about the use of inhibition by these agents of pentylenetetrazole-induced convulsions as a procedure for detecting new antianxiety agents.

Once again, it appears to this author that the anticonvulsant effects of the known antianxiety agents might be related to their depressive and muscle relaxant effects. Since most anticonvulsants are not anxiolytic in man anticonvulsant activity is not likely to predict new types of antianxiety agents. It will take an antianxiety agent without either sedative properties or anticonvulsive effects to answer the important questions of what are the prime animal predictive tests in this area. A recent paper (Sokalis, Sathananthan, Collins, and Gershon, 1974) describes a new type of antianxiety agent that is not depressant or anticonvulsant and may be the first lead to answering the questions raised above. The compound discussed therein is one of a series of cyclic AMP phosphodiesterase inhibitors that Beer, Chasin, Clody, Vogel, and Horovitz (1972) described. They speculate that there is a correlation between antianxiety activity in the human, antipunishment effects in animals, and depression of the phosphodiesterase enzyme.

The antiaggressive effects of the benzodiazepines in animals have been examined extensively to determine their value in predicting utility both as antianxiety agents and as antiaggressive compounds in humans. Valzelli (1973) described experiments in animals that separate the muscle-relaxing properties of benzodiazepines from their antiaggressive effects (Fig. 4). DiMascio (1973) points out, however, that in many cases the benzodiazepines are not only ineffective against human aggression and hostility but may exacerbate these conditions. He postulates that the benzodiazepines may release aggressiveness that can be of therapeutic benefit to the patient and was only being suppressed by an overlying anxiety. If true, this postulation supports the importance of the most commonly measured behavioral

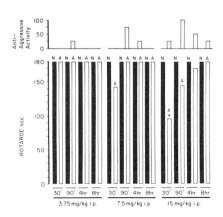

FIG. 4. Effect of chlordiazepoxide at different dosages and time of intraperitoneal administration on rotarod performance in normal (N) and aggressive (A) mice, and on aggressive behavior of mice. ($P < 0.01$ with respect to N at the same time and dosage.) (From Valzelli, 1973.)

effect of these agents—the release of suppressed behavior as determined in the antipunishment tests.

The importance of antipunishment procedures in predicting new anti-anxiety agents and the development of antianxiety measures in normal human volunteers are well described in the chapters in this volume by Beer and Migler, Blackwell and Whitehead, and Ulenhuth, Stern, Schuster, and Domizi.

ANTIDEPRESSIVE AGENTS

Antidepressive agents are probably the poorest of the three major psycho-tropic drug classes for predictability of preclinical tests for clinical activity. Based on the effects of the imipramine-like agents, application of the theory of blockade of norepinephrine reuptake has led, in the last 15 years, to the use of various reserpine-treated animals in the search for antagonists of norepinephrine reuptake (Schildkraut, Davis, and Klerman, 1968). The biggest problem with this theory is that the effects of the antidepressives appear immediately after administration in animals but take 7 to 14 days to appear in man. In addition, many reports, exemplified by a series of papers by Gershon (Hekimian, Gershon, and Floyd, 1970), have shown that there is not a good correlation between the activities of compounds that block the effects of reserpine-like agents in animals and their clinical antidepressive activities. What amazes this author is why no one has tested the acute anti-reserpine activity of some of these compounds in the human to answer the question of whether these agents that failed as antidepressives in humans actually had antireserpine activity in humans.

Another theory about antidepressive activity developed in our labora-tories at The Squibb Institute for Medical Research postulates a selective action of these agents on the amygdala (Horovitz, 1967). Procedures such as mouse-killing (muricide) (Horovitz, Piala, High, Burke, and Leaf, 1966) and low intensity brain stimulation sensitization (Babington and Wedeking, 1973) have been used to detect selective effects of the antidepressives on this area of the brain and, more recently, to relate the effects of electro-convulsive shock to an action of the amygdala (Babington, in press). Al-though the use of biochemical and neurophysiologic rationales for de-veloping new compounds in this area remains valid, it appears that new procedures, such as the development of behavioral measures that simulate the symptoms of depressive disease in man as advocated by Klerman (this volume) and by McKinney (1974), should also be pursued.

DISCUSSION

It seems quite obvious to anyone working on the development of new psychotropic agents that two things are needed. First, new structural types of agents that work on the central nervous system must be explored. There are many analogues of available agents that provide gains in safety or slightly different types of activity, but what are needed are new types of structures in the major classes of psychotropic activity that might provide broader spectra of therapeutic activity, while hopefully improving also on the therapeutic ratio. Second, new models in the preclinical area must be found that more closely resemble the disease state in man. Of course, these new models have to be confirmed in man and the only way this can be done is by finding an agent that works on these models and determining whether it has clinical activity in the human. Chapters by Blackwell and Whitehead, Beer and Migler, Fink, Uhlenhuth et al., and others in this book speak to the problem of developing clinical pharmacologic tests that are similar to procedures in animals. Such tests could be used to determine quickly whether a new pharmacologic agent has the same action in the human as it does in a procedure in an animal. There also would be a very fast evaluation of the approximate active dose of this new agent and a quick response to see if this agent has any pharmacologic activities in the human. These pharmacologic procedures in normal volunteers could be used with minimally acceptable risks and costs to pick out the best compound from a series of agents active in animals. It should be pointed out that these early clinical pharmacologic tests do not necessarily assure the eventual usefulness of these agents; only large-scale testing in patients and evaluation of side effects can establish clinical utility. Finally, the most important advantage of these clinical pharmacologic tests which mimic animal tests is that their use would minimize the exposure of human beings to a drug at a very early stage of development (a fact of both moral and ethical importance), would reduce the costs of developing a drug, and might speed up the progress of finding new and better agents to treat psychiatric patients.

Irwin (1968) has argued for many years that comparisons between animals and humans are used inadequately in the search for new psychotropic agents. He states, "A major problem in animal-human comparisons is the fact that drug effects on human behavior are all too rarely determined using the techniques or measures employed with animals . . . The problem, essentially is to focus on animals most nearly like humans in their patterns of response, qualitatively and quantitatively, and to employ measures and procedures applicable and relevant across species, e.g., observational or conditioning techniques. Often overlooked is that drugs affect behavior through mechanisms essentially similar for humans and other animal species. I submit that regardless of the quantitative differences that have evolved in capacity, patterns, and complexity of organization and possibilities for psychiatric disorder, the essential primitive physiologic and behavioral functions making such differences possible are in the main shared by all mammalian species." Irwin, who has been a proponent of the use of observational, neurological examination procedures in animals, has pointed out that profiles of activity similar to those developed for various psychotropic agents in animals can be obtained in man, and that new chemical structures that show interesting activity in observational procedures in animals should be tested the same way in normal volunteers. Use of such a procedure poses many problems in interpretation and evaluation, but it certainly has some merit if it can be done consistently by the same laboratory.

The electroencephalogram (EEG) is widely used to evaluate drugs in animals and man. Although one may have serious reservations about the relationship of EEG changes to actual therapeutic effects rather than to the side effects of psychotropic agents, the quantification procedures developed and described by Fink and colleagues in this volume are certainly worth considering as tools for predicting the early efficacy of new drugs.

Although at times in this chapter I have been quite pessimistic about both the preclinical and clinical environment for finding new and useful psychotropic agents, I believe that by the continuation of both original research by old and new investigators and of dialogue between preclinical and clinical investigators in such forums as the meetings of the American College of Neuropsychopharmacology and the symposium that stimulated this volume, obstacles can be overcome and new and useful CNS drugs will appear.

ACKNOWLEDGMENTS

The author would like to thank Drs. B. Beer, D. Frost, M. E. Goldberg, and A. Sudilovsky for their constructive editorial and scientific comments on this manuscript.

REFERENCES

Ayd, F. J., Jr. (1961): Neuroleptics and extrapyramidal reactions in psychiatric patients. In: *Extrapyramidal System and Neuroleptics,* edited by J. Bordeleau, Montreal. pp. 355–363. Editions Psychiatriques.

Babington, R. G. Antidepressives and the kindling effect. In: *Antidepressants,* edited by S. Fielding and H. Lal. Futura Publishing, Mt. Kisco, New York. (*in press*).

Babington, R. G., and Wedeking, P. W. (1973): The pharmacology of seizures induced by sensitization with low intensity brain stimulation. *Pharmacol. Biochem. Behav.,* 1:461–467.

Beer, B., Chasin, M., Clody, D. E., Vogel, J. R., and Horovitz, Z. P. (1972): Cyclic adenosine monophosphate in brain: Effect on anxiety. *Science,* 176:428–430.

Cook, L. (1964): Effects of drugs on operant conditioning. In: *Ciba Symposium on Animal Behavior and Drug Action,* pp. 23–43. Little, Brown & Co., Boston.

Cook, L., and Weidley E. (1957): Behavioral effects of some psychopharmacological agents. *Ann. NY Acad. Sci.,* 66:740–752.

Courvoisier, S., Fournel, J., Ducrot, R., Kolsky, M., and Koetschet, P. (1953): Proprietes pharmacodynamiques du chlorhydrate de chloro-3 (dimethylamino-3′ propyl)-10 pheno-thiazine (4.560 R.P.) Etude expérimentale d'un nouveau corps utilisé dans l'anésthésie potentialisée et dans l'Libérnation artificielle. *Arch. Int. Pharmacodyn. Ther.,* 92:305–361.

DiMascio, A. (1973): The effects of benzodiazepines on aggression: Reduced or increased? In: *Benzodiazepines,* edited by S. Garrattini, E. Mussini, and L. O. Randell, pp. 433–440. Raven Press, New York.

Geller, I., and Seifter, J. (1960): The effects of meprobamate, barbiturates, *d*-amphetamine and promazine on experimentally induced conflict in the rat. *Psychopharmacologia,* 1:482–492.

Gluckman, M. I. (1965): Pharmacology of axazepam (Serax), a new antianxiety agent. *Curr. Ther. Res. Clin. Exp.,* 7:721–740.

Hekimian, L. J., Gershon, S., and Floyd, A. (1970): The clinical evaluation of four proposed antidepressants: Relationship to their animal pharmacology. *Int. Pharmacopsychiatry,* 3:65–76.

Horovitz, Z. P. (1967): The amygdala and depression. In: *Excerpta Medica. Proc. First Int. Sym. Antidepressant Drugs, Milan, April 1966* edited by S. Garattini and M. N. G. Dukes, pp. 121–129.

Horovitz, Z. P., Piala, J. J., High, J. P., Burke, J. C., and Leaf, R. C. (1966): Effects of drugs on the mouse killing (muricide) test and its relationship to amygdaloid function. *Int. J. Neuropharmacol.,* 5:405–411.

Irwin, S. (1961): Correlation in rats between the locomotor and avoidance suppressant potencies of eight phenothiazine tranquilizers. *Arch. Int. Pharmacodyn. Ther.,* 132:279–286.

Irwin, S. (1968): A rational framework for the development, evaluation, and use of psychoactive drugs. *Am. J. Psychiatry (Suppl.),* 124:1–19.

Izquierdo, I. (1962): Observations on conditioned and unconditioned on- and off-behavioural responses to a buzzer. (Letter to the Editor.) *J. Pharm. Pharmacol.,* 14:316–318.

Janssen, P. A. J. (1961): Vergleichende pharmakologische Daten uber sechs neue basische 4'-Fluorobutyrophenon-Derivate. *Arzneim. Forsch.,* 11:819–824.

Janssen, P. A. J., Niemegeers, C. J. E., and Schellekens, K. H. L. (1965): Is it possible to predict the clinical effects of neuroleptic drugs (major tranquillizers) from animal data? *Arzneim. Forsch.,* 15:1196–1206.

McKinney, W. T., Jr. (1974): Animal models in psychiatry. *Perspect. Biol. Med.,* 17:529–542.

Mercier, J., Dessaigne, S., and Etzensperger, P. (1962): Détermination de l'accoutumance expérimentale par une méthode psychophysiologique. V. Etude de quelques drogues neuroplégiques, tranquillisantes et hypnotiques. *Ann. Pharm. Fr.,* 20:131–149.

Niemegeers, C. J. E., and Janssen, P. A. J. (1960): Influence of haloperidol (R 1625) and of haloperidide (R 3201) on avoidance and escape behaviour of trained dogs in a "jumping box." *J. Pharm. Pharmacol.,* 12:744–753.

Schildkraut, J. J., Davis, J. M., and Klerman, G. L. (1968): Biochemistry of depressions. In: *Psychopharmacology. A review of Progress 1957–1967,* edited by D. H. Effron, pp. 625–648.

Sokalis, G., Sathananthan, G., Collins, P., and Gershon, S. (1974): SQ 65,396: A non-sedative anxiolytic. *Curr. Ther. Res.,* 16:861–863.

Valzelli, L. (1973): Activity of benzodiazepines on aggressive behavior in rats and mice. In: *Benzodiazepines,* edited by S. Garrattini, E. Mussini, and L. O. Randell, pp. 405–417. Raven Press, New York.

Predictability in Psychopharmacology: Preclinical and Clinical Correlations, edited by A. Sudilovsky, S. Gershon, and B. Beer. Raven Press, New York © 1975.

Evaluation of the Duke University Behavioral Rating Inventory for Drug-Generated Effects (BRIDGE)

A. Sudilovsky, E. H. Ellinwood,* F. Dorsey,* and L. Nelson*

*The Squibb Institute for Medical Research, Princeton, New Jersey 08540; and *Duke University Medical Center, Durham, North Carolina 27710*

A major condition concerning the value of animal experimentation for predicting psychotropic drug effects in man is the selection of therapeutically relevant measures of drug activity. This condition is centrally linked to the possibility of establishing, in both animals and humans, levels of detectable phenomena that permit profitable comparisons. Motor activity might be one such productive framework, since it constitutes, among all attributes of behavior, the most basic observable property of animal life and remains a primary source of information on adjustment of the individual to his circumstances (King, 1954). In fact, there is sufficient experimental evidence that alterations in motor activity reflect disordered mental states in humans; excellent reviews of the extensive literature on the evaluation of specific measures of psychomotility in psychiatric populations have been made by Yates (1961), King (1965, 1969), and Holzman (1972).

From a more general standpoint, however, it has been documented for more than a century that certain characterizations of physical movement in man relate to specific psychopathologies (Kraepelin, 1889; Bleuler, 1950; Kraüpl-Taylor, 1966). Reich (1949) developed the concept that at the base of many psychiatric problems there is a core of motor dysfunctions and Schilder (1951) speculated on the relationship between psychopathology, as manifested by the motility in schizophrenic patients and reflex activities in experimental animals. Furthermore, the presence of psychomotor peculiarities has been empirically utilized for the diagnostic appraisal of patients. Nathan, Zare, Simpson, and Andberg (1969) have shown, for example, that diagnoses of psychotic states most often result from observation of increased psychomotor behavior. Conversely, an important component of the "neuroleptic syndrome" in humans, as defined by Delay and Deniker (1961), is the "slowing-down of psychomotor functions." Quantitation of general motor activity in psychiatric patients by means of various devices (Heusler, Ulett, and Blasques, 1959; Kast, 1964), as well as the analysis of the behavior of schizophrenics in terms of motor pattern (Itil, 1969), have been proposed as indexes of psychotropic drug action and of intensity of psychopathology. Recently, Drtil and colleagues (Drtil, Vinar, and Tosovsky, 1973; Drtil and Tosovsky, 1974) found significant correlations in psychotic patients between spontaneous psychomotor activity and several symptoms of psychopathology, quantified by use of the Brief Psychiatric Rating Scale.

Since psychomotor behavior and response to drug action are not exclusive features of man, motor function in animals attains, from such a perspective, a psychopathologically meaningful dimension. Smythies (1970) pointed out that a model is a strategy that lays down the challenge to see and to make comparisons of the basic phenomenology in clinical disorders. In this connection, there is a need to approach animal behavior from a direct clinical standpoint. Physical activities observed in experimental situations have frequently been suggested as correlates of human symptomatology. For example, striking similarities in facial and motor changes in primates with those observed in human depression are obtained in mother-infant separation experiments (Harlow, 1974). Florio, Fuentes, Ziegler, and Longo (1972) refer to shaking movements of the head, aimless paw movements, bizarre postures, staring gaze, and hissing as elements of "hallucinatory" pattern of response to the administration of four amphetamine derivatives in cats. Utena (1966) qualified as autistic (i.e., analogous to the autistic behavior of schizophrenic patients) the withdrawal tendency, monotonous sluggishness, and disorganized excitement observed in mice and cats after the long-term administration of amphetamine. More specifically, repetitious side-to-side looking movements in treated cats, monkeys, and chimpanzees have been related to the looking movements associated with fear and suspiciousness that often occur in amphetamine addicts preceding or during a psychotic reaction (Ellinwood and Sudilovsky, 1973). Measurement of drug-induced cataleptic manifestations, as well as of stereotyped motor responses to amphetamine or apomorphine are currently used in the screening of new agents with potential antipsychotic activity (Fielding and Lal, 1974).

The importance attached to studying the effects of psychotropic drugs on animal models of psychopathology rather than merely on normal animals is reflected in the many efforts made during the past 25 years to pharmacologically alter either human or animal behavior in the direction of psychosis. Of all drugs known to be amenable to use in the production of a model psychosis, amphetamine is thus far the most valuable (Bell, 1973; Snyder, 1973). Because the paranoid-like psychotic episode induced by amphetamine evolves with time, it provides a unique opportunity to study the consecutive stages that precede the developing psychosis. In previously reported studies (Ellinwood, Sudilovsky, and Nelson, 1973b), we explored the relationship of chronic amphetamine intoxication in experimental animals to amphetamine psychosis, particularly the common phenomenologic progression that may be involved. We found that an accurate behavior-rating system was needed for an evaluation of the similarity of behavioral phenomena among cats, monkeys, and men and for understanding underlying mechanisms in a complex syndrome. Reliability of the behavioral rating is doubly important in chronic drug studies in which end-stage behaviors become the anchor to which other measures are related, since control of time, absolute drug dose, tolerance, and the interactions of these factors are very difficult. One of the main problems in such studies is the impossibility of measuring the multivariate, overlapped, and patterned phenomena in this behavioral motor syndrome with currently available univariate tools. We found it necessary to develop a multidimensional behavior-rating system that would reflect variations in the quality and intensity of motor activity and detect subtle changes in the formation and disintegration of behavioral complexes at different phases of the period of chronic intoxication. Such a rating system should have four specific features.

1. *Completeness:* All of the behaviors observed and considered relevant should be codable in one of the established categories. Very few should be recorded in a miscellaneous category.
2. *Level of detail:* The scale must be able to reflect subtle changes in the animal's behavior, since a syndrome may develop gradually in chronic abusers of the drug.
3. *Conciseness and communicability:* The items of a rating scheme should employ well-defined entries and simple abbreviations, so that ratings can be remembered, recorded quickly, and communicated easily to others.
4. *Reliability:* Having learned the scale, two raters should be able to agree reliably on the correct rating of a sample of behavior. A single rater should be able to reliably reproduce his own ratings of a given sample of behavior.

This chapter reports the development and refinement, along these guidelines, of the Duke University Behavioral Rating Inventory for Drug-Generated Effects (BRIDGE).

METHODS

Experimental Conditions

Female cats, 2 to 4 kg, were surgically implanted with electrodes and fitted with a permanent connector to allow repeated and chronic electrophysiologic (EEG) recording from various subcortical nuclei. All animals were housed singly and fed *ad libitum* throughout the experiment. At least 2 weeks were allowed for recovery after surgery. Thereafter, each cat underwent an acclimation period (2 hr each day during 5 days) in the experimental environment, which consisted of a commercially available metal cage, 17.5″ × 24″ × 19.5″ high with a wooden floor and Plexiglas front and side that was placed in a closed room separated from the recording room by a one-way mirror. The animal was observed both through the mirror and via a remote-controlled video camera. The only constraint on the animal within the cage was an EEG recording cable attached to the connector on the top of the head. This cable passed through the top of the cage, through the junction box, to the recording polygraph. The cable attached to the cat was arranged with enough slack to allow the head to reach all points within the cage.

The *standard recording session* consisted of a 20- to 30-min acclimation period, followed by a 3-min period during which video and EEG recordings were taken. Either saline or methamphetamine hydrochloride was then injected intraperitoneally and recordings were made for 3-min intervals beginning at 20 sec and 10, 20, 30, and 90 min after injection.

STUDY _____ SUBJECT _____ DAY _____ CONDITION _____ DATES _____ ____

| | | | | | | | | | | | | | | recorded | | rated | |
INTERVAL	1	2	3	4	5	6	7	8	9	10	11	12	13	14	15	16	17	18
PLACE																		
ORIENTATION																		
ATTITUDE																		
AROUSAL																		
MOVEMENT SPEED																		
HEAD POSITION																		
HEAD MOVEMENT																		
LOOKING CHARACTER																		
LOOKING LOCATION																		
SNIFFING INVOLVEMENT																		
BODY POSITION																		
BODY MOVEMENT																		
FORELEG POSITION																		
FORELEG MOVEMENT																		
HINDLEG POSITION																		
HINDLEG MOVEMENT																		
TAIL POST TAIL MVT.																		
GROOMING CHARACTER																		
GROOMING LOCATION																		
S.MODAL S.RELAT.																		
DYSTONIA																		
DISJUNCTION																		
ATAXIA																		
AUTONOMIC RESP.																		
MISCELLANEA																		

FIG. 1. Rating form used to encode one 3-min segment of behavior.

During the initial 5-day acclimation period, saline (1 ml) was administered daily and actual recordings were taken on the third and fifth days to produce baseline data for the evaluation of drug-induced behavior and changes in EEG.

For the next 11 days the animal was injected twice each day with progressively larger doses of methamphetamine. Recording sessions in the environment took place immediately after the first injection on the 1st, 3rd, 8th, and 11th days.

In developing the rating scale, we used a large number of animals over a period of 2 years to assess their behavioral repertoire in the experimental setting before and after drug administration. Observable elementary motor, postural, and autonomic phenomena were recorded in an open-end catalogue, defined operationally, and coded for scoring on a rating chart designed to record any selected item within the categories indicated. Figure 1 is the sheet on which the 18 segments (each 10 sec long) that comprise one 3-min record are rated. In use, ratings are made for each 10-sec segment of the video tape, which is linked with EEG records by synchronous signals. For each 10-sec segment, entries are made on the rating sheet for each of the 27 categories of the inventory, which include position and orientation in the cage, attitude, arousal and movement speed, position and movement of the various body segments (head, trunk, forelegs, hindlegs, and tail), orientation and quality of the animal's gaze, presence of any grooming, sniffing, autonomic reactions, ataxia, dystonia, disjunction, as well as notation of the modality and relatedness of any head stereotypy to that of other regions of the body.

The Inventory

In the following Catalogue of Definitions for the BRIDGE system, all categories have been grouped in three main areas of interest (Animal-Environment Relationship, Motor Profile, and Autonomic and Reflex Responses), and Miscellanea, which comprise the less frequently observed behaviors.

I. Animal-Environment Relationship

A. Physical relationship

1. *Place* (2)[1]

Refers to the actual location of the animal within the cage, as determined by the relation of his trunk to several theoretically separate zones of the floor of the cage; may be designated as *Front* (*F*), *Back* (*B*), *Right* (*R*), or *Left* (*L*) half of the cage.

---

[1] To convert the ratings to computer-readable format, it was necessary to limit the number of behaviors coded in each category for each 10-sec interval. The number in parentheses indicates the entries allowed.

When appropriate, the more specific designation of *Front-right* (*Fr*), *Back-right* (*Br*), *Front-left* (*Fl*), or *Back-left* (*Bl*) should be used. If the animal occupies two diagonally opposite quadrants or the boundary zone between two halves, the ratings are *Diagonal* (*D*) or *Midline* (*M*) location, respectively. Ratings reflect the order of occurrence of location and are made on the basis of time spent by the animal at specific cage locations. If possible, two entries should be made indicating the two locations that account for the largest part of the 10-sec interval. If the animal uses the major part of the 10-sec interval for translative movements, so that no specific location is occupied, the appropriate score is *Changing* (*Ch*).

2. *Orientation* (2)

Describes the orientation of the animal's body within the cage, as determined by the direction of his longitudinal axis (represented by the spine); may be rated as *Front* (*F*), *Back* (*B*), *Right* (*R*), *Left* (*L*), or as *Front-right* (*Fr*), *Front-left* (*Fl*), *Back-right* (*Br*), and *Back-left* (*Bl*). Alternatively, if the animal is moving, the corresponding score will be *Changing* (*Ch*). Rating of this category follows the rules indicated for the previous one (*Place*) with respect to number and order of entries.

B. Psychomotor relationship

1. *Arousal* (1)

Refers to the degree of readiness or alertness of the animal, as indicated by his static and kinetic configurations and the conjunction of several features contributing to these. Such features are useful in defining the five levels of arousal described below, but should be regarded merely as indicators for the recognition of each ratable level. Arousal, as we consider it, conceptualizes the intensity of the relationship between the animal and his environment. Thus, knowledge of his habitual behavior in the experimental setting is necessary to discriminate the various possible states. *Level 1* represents the sleeping state, generally characterized by closed eyes, dropped head, muscular relaxation, and relative unresponsiveness. *Level 2* corresponds to a somnolent state usually manifested by slow, progressive, and nonsustained closing of the eyes, decreased muscle tone (head nodding), slow postural readjustments, and decreased sensorial availability (receptivity and responsiveness) to environmental stimuli. *Level 3* indicates the syntonic state (baseline behavior of a normal awake animal), characterized by adequate but selective sensory-motor availability to environmental stimuli in the absence of muscular tension greater than the minimum necessary to maintain posture. *Level 4* is equivalent to the aroused state, characterized by increased muscular tension indicative of readiness to move, moderate apprehension or curiosity toward the environment, and restricted distractibility. *Level 5* represents the hyperaroused state, usually manifested by marked apprehensiveness, hypersensitivity to external stimuli, and exaggerated muscular tension with disproportionate reactions and/or restlessness.

2. *Attitude* (1)

Defined by the attentional mode and involvement of the animal, as manifested by his postural appearance and motor activity in relation to his surroundings and his own body (environment). Whereas posture represents the endpoint of a movement or action, attitude reflects the quality of the animal-environment relationship. Classifications are *Asleep* (*A*): Self-explanatory; *Indifferent* (*I*): Lack of manifest attentional involvement with the environment; *Interested* (*IN*): Directed attentional contact with the environment or a part of it as selected stimulus, but without definite physical approach; *Investigative* (*IV*): Selected attentional contact and active reaching out or approaching and examining of one or more parts of the environment. In the *IN* attitude, the animal may single out aspects of the environment, but in the *IV* attitude an active interaction with those aspects is achieved through a selected response; *Reactive (R)*: An abnormal attitude characterized by shifting attentional contact manifested in increased peering about the environment, frequent postural readjustments, and sudden inadequate or apparently unmotivated movements with a tense and jumpy quality; *Unaware (U)*: An abnormal attitude in which detachment from the environment is detected through a lack of sensorial availability (analogous to that seen in stuporous states).

The *IN* and *IV* attitudes may present a nervous, tense, or apprehensive quality after administration of a psychostimulant drug in relatively large doses. In that case, they are termed *Interested Abnormal (INA)* or *Investigative Abnormal (IVA)*, respectively. On occasion, a given attentional mode (directed, selected, or shifting) can persist even as the animal changes his posture or level of activity. In that case, a focused quality is indicated by scoring either *Interested Focused (INF)*, *Investigative Focused (IVF)*, or *Reactive Focused (RF)*.

3. *Looking Activity* (2 for each aspect)

Two aspects are rated. The first is the Character of the animal's looking activity. *Vacant (V)*: Eyes open, with no specific or appreciable visual placing. *Casual (C)*: Transient glancing or visual placing on the environment in general. *Observant (O)*: Attentive visual contact and/or looking movements in relation to one or a few specific aspects of the environment. *Staring (S)*: Intense and/or relatively sustained observant looking activity. *Frozen-staring (F)*: Persistent staring with no head movement or during a "pure" stereotypy of the head (see II A 3, *Head Movements*).

The second aspect is the Location of the animal's gaze. *Close (Cl)*: Localized in the immediate surrounding, that is, within the space limited by the cage walls. *Image (I)*: Visual placing on the animal's own reflection on any of the cage walls. *Ceiling (C)*: Visual placing on or through the roof of the cage. *Distant (D)*: Visual placing in either the immediate or distant area outside the Plexiglas sides of the cage.

If the animal's eyes are closed, the corresponding score for both aspects of this category is *None (N)*.

4. *Sniffing Activity* (1)

Discrete (D) or *Throughout (T)*, depending on its duration within the 10-sec interval.

5. *Grooming Activity* (2 for each aspect)

Two aspects are rated. The Character of any grooming is indicated as *Paw-wiping (P)*, *Licking (L)*, *Biting (B)*, or *Scratching (S)*. An *Abortive (A)* character is scored if one of the motor components of a grooming pattern occurs without consummation of the grooming activity. This phenomenon frequently appears as a tonic leg posturing, with the leg either flexed or extended and occasionally showing sudden phasic flexor or extensor movements.

The bodily location of the grooming is designated as *Face (F)*, *Ear (E)*, *Back (B)*, *Chest (Ch)*, *Abdomen (A)*, *Groin (G)*, *Foreleg (Fo)*, *Hindleg (H)*, or *Tail (T)*.

II. Motor Profile

A. Motor output

1. *Movement Speed* (1)

A five-point scale is used to evaluate speed of movement. *Level 1* is complete immobility, that is, no movement in any region of the body. *Level 2* is a state of slow mobility, as in a drowsy, relaxed, or stuporous condition. *Level 3* is the usual moving speed of an awake and normally aroused animal. *Level 4* is a state of fast mobility, but with maintenance of the flowing harmony of the movements. *Level 5* is a state of nonharmonic, fast mobility in which reactive movements are predominant. Thus, levels 2, 3, and 4 represent the range of movement speed under normal conditions with levels 2 and 4 being extremes of that range.

Familiarity with the animal's range of movement speed in the experimental setting will facilitate accuracy. Occasionally, in order to decide on the score for a given 10-sec interval, it may be helpful to observe the ongoing movements for a longer period.

2. *Head Position* (2)

Head position is determined by the angle formed by the intersection of the cervico-occipital region of the head with the spine. *Upright (U)*: Whenever the angle so formed is less than 180 degrees. *Lowered (L)*: Whenever the angle so formed is equal to or larger than 180°. If either *U* or *L* is accompanied by definite neck extension, the corresponding scores will be *Upright-extended (Ue)* and *Lowered-extended (Le)*. In any case, if the head is turned relative to the animal's body, this is specified by scoring, in addition, either *Facing-side (s)* or *Facing-back (b)*, depending on the extent of the turn. *Dropped (D)*: A position in which the head is not completely supported by the neck. *Changing (Ch)*: Scored if no clear position is adopted.

3. *Head Movements* (2)

Transient (T): Transitory movements without sequential relationship to those preceding or following. It may be a single displacement (horizontal or vertical) or a composed one (bobbing, dipping, casual scanning, etc.). *Tremor (Tm)*: Small rhythmic oscillatory movement. *Stagger (Sg)*: Coarse and nonrhythmic movements of the head-neck ensemble suggestive of lack of stability. If this movement appears in more than a few consecutive 10-sec intervals, it can be taken as indicative of ataxia. *Shake (Sh)*: Sudden and more or less violent consecutive movements. *Recoil (R)*: Sudden retreating movement usually associated with unexpected stimuli and occasionally incorporated into a stereotypy pattern (see below). *Look (L)*: A head movement clearly directed for visual placing on a specific object or in a specific direction.

Stereotyped (S): Any movement repeated sequentially and describing a path of displacements recognizable as a kinetic configuration is rated as stereotyped by placing an *S* before the symbol. The most frequently observed stereotypy configurations have been given specific names. These are *Minutia-search (M)*: pecking-like movements executed by rotation of the head around the interauricular axis; *Side-to-side (Si)*: horizontal head-neck movement around the base of the neck or rotational movement of the head around the occipito-atlantoid articulation; *Up-and-down (U)*: vertical head-neck movement (smooth or jerky) around the base of the neck or rotational movement of the head around the occipito-atlantoid articulation; *Balinese (B)*: circumduction head-neck movement around the base of the neck by which the tip of the animal's nose describes a more or less irregular ovoid or circular path.

The stereotypy may be "pure" or "impure," if contaminated by other nonsequential movements. Thus, scoring of two codes is indicative of interrupted ("impure") stereotypy. The stereotypy configurations may also, in the course of their evolution, incorporate a transitory movement or pause, thereby acquiring a distinctive characteristic. This incorporation is represented by adding to the stereotypy code a symbol for the incorporated element [*look (l)*, *pause (p)*, *dip (d)*, or *recoil (r)*], using the lower case to differentiate it from nonincorporated interruptive occurrences of the same behavior. Finally, if no movement occurs during the 10-sec interval, this will be indicated by scoring *None* (*N*).

4. *Body Posture* (2)

Lying (*L*): Either side of the animal is supported on the floor of the cage. No signs of active body support or of an effort to maintain such posture should be detectable. *Sphinxing* (*Sp*): Support is provided by the animal's abdomen on the floor with hindlegs completely flexed and forelegs either flexed or extended forward. *Crouching* (*Cr*): The animal is supported on all four flexed legs while the abdomen is close to, but not in contact with, the floor of the cage. This posture is similar to that of an animal preparing to spring or shrinking with fear, but not necessarily as tense. *Sitting* (*Si*): Support is shared by extended or partially flexed forelegs and completely flexed hindlegs, with the hindquarters in contact with the floor. *Standing* (*S*): Support is given by all four extended or slightly flexed legs. *Standing-on-hindlegs* (*Sh*): Forelegs are off the ground, body is vertical and rests on the hindquarters; it is similar to the rearing posture in the rat. *Pushed-up front quarter* (*Pf*): Front quarter is off the floor and actively supported by the forelegs, while the hindquarters are in a lying or sphinx-like position. *Pushed-up hindquarters* (*Ph*): Forelegs are flexed or extended forward, abdomen is off the ground, and hindlegs are relatively extended, elevating the hindquarters; it may look similar to an estrous-crouch. *Camelback* (*c*): The back is arched at the dorsal-lumbar level and looks like a hump. In a sitting cat, this is seen as an exaggeration of the normal curvature of the back.

5. *Body Movements* (2)

Tremor (*Tm*), *Staggering* (*Sg*): Coarse, irregular, vacillating body movements, usually indicative of ataxia. *Swaying* (*Sw*): Relatively large oscillatory movements to the sides, most easily detectable when the animal is standing quietly. *Stretching* (*Sx*): Slow, deliberate elongation of the forelegs, hindlegs, or trunk with a tensing of the muscles in the elongated region of the body. *Twitching* (*Tw*): Sudden and instantaneous contraction of a muscle or of a restricted group of muscles. *Jerking* (*Je*): Similar to twitching, but resulting in sudden displacement of a body region. *Hunching* (*H*): Transitory elevation of the back forming a momentary camelback or exaggerating an existing one. If dependent on the execution of an ongoing stereotyped motor response at the head-neck region, this should be indicated by scoring *Hunching-associated* (*Ha*). *Falling* (*F*): Loss of any body posture resulting from absence of gravitational equilibrium. *Jumping* (*J*): Rapid upward displacement, leaving no part of the body in contact with the floor. *Standing on hindlegs* (*Sh*): Moving from a quadrupedal to a bipedal stance. *Push-up forequarters* (*Pf*): Change from flexion to extension of the forelegs with maintenance of the hindquarters posture. *Push-up hindquarters* (*Ph*): The same movement as push-up forequarters but occurring in the hindquarters and having a slight Repositioning quality (see II A 7, *Leg Movements*). *Pumping* (*P*): Up and down displacement due to successive flexion and extension of all four legs simultaneously, without their being lifted from the floor. *Advancing* (*A*): Moving forward or in a forward direction. *Retreating* (*R*): Moving backwards. These last two movements imply displacement of the body (change of place and/or orientation) and may involve stepping with all four legs or with only the forelegs or hindlegs if a large enough single step is taken. *Pivoting* (*Pi*): Oscillating movement around a fixed point, usually the hindquarters. Most frequently, the forelegs step alternately to the right and left of the relatively fixed hindlegs. *Turning* (*T*): Changing direction while moving. *Circling-cage* (*Cc*): Locomotor displacement that almost uninterruptedly follows a path around the perimeter of the cage. *Circling-self* (*Cs*): Continuous or almost continuous turning in a single direction, bringing the animal to his original orientation. *Spinning* (*Sn*): Fast circling-self.

In the case of turning, circling, and spinning movements, direction should be indicated by adding the codes (*r*) for *right* or (*l*) for *left* after the symbol. Some of the body movements described above may become stereotyped; *P, Pi,* and the combination of *A* and *R* are usually apparent stereotypy configurations. In any case, an *S* should be placed before the corresponding mnemonic symbol.

6. *Leg Posture* (2)

Flexed (*F*) and *Extended* (*E*) have the accepted anatomical definitions based on the angle of the leg joints. The *rabbit* attribute, indicated by following the symbol with an *r* refers to a peculiar leg posture in which support is maintained by the paws and also by placing the first segment of the leg in contact with the floor. *Wide-base* (*W*): Greater than normal separation between fore- or hindlimbs while supporting the body.

7. *Leg Movements* (2)

Twitching (*T*) and *Jerking* (*J*) are defined as in Body Movement above, but are here confined to the legs. *Claw-extending* (*C*): Spreading of the toes to expose the claws. *Sliding* (*Sl*): Movement of the legs while maintaining continuous contact with the floor. Sliding usually occurs while the animal is leaning against a wall of the cage or is in a wide-based stance; it is indicative of dystonia. *Shaking* (*Sh*): Rapid movement of the leg, as if trying to get rid of something sticky and, especially in the hindlimbs, having a fast, clonic quality. *Raising* (*Ra*): A pulling-up movement, usually differentiated from Repositioning by its slowness of execution and by maintenance of the raised position for a short period. *Reaching-out* (*Re*): A foreleg movement directed toward a specific point in the environment, although the foreleg does not necessarily make contact with that point. *Treading* (*Tr*): Alternating pushing movements of forelegs or hindlegs. *Pushing* (*Pu*): As in the Push-up or Pumping body movements or pushing against the walls of the cage when the animal is in a lying position. *Repositioning* (*R*): Placement and removal of one or more legs on the cage floor, with or without shifting the body weight and without modifying place and orientation. *Stepping* (*St*): Placement of one or more legs on the cage floor with shift in body weight and modification of place and/or orientation. *Walking* (*W*): Sequential stepping with displacement of the animal in the cage.

If any of these leg movements becomes stereotyped, an *S* should be placed before the corresponding mnemonic symbol.

8. *Tail Posture and Tail Movements* (2 for each item)

Raised (*R*): Forming an angle greater than 45° with the hindlimbs. *Lowered* (*L*): Forming an angle equal to or less than 45° with the hindlimbs. *Dropped* (*D*): Hanging and apparently not being included in the animal's behavioral state, or resting entirely on the floor.

Transient (*T*): Any movement of the tail aside from *Squirrel* (*Sq*): A fast, repetitive, flowing twitch.

Waxy (*w*): A plastic quality to any tail posture or movement.

9. *Stereotyped Activity* (1 for each aspect)

Two aspects of the stereotyped activity displayed by the animals are rated. The first is the nature of Modality of the head stereotypy, which includes *Sniffing* (*Sn*), *Looking* (*L*), and the combination of *Sniffing and Looking* (*Snl*). Execution of the head stereotypies always involves groups of muscles normally subserving either orientation (*L*) or exploration (*Sn*) activities. The identification of the stereotypies as being of the *Sn* and/or *L* modalities implies only an activation of the motor components of those behaviors.

The second aspect is the Relatedness, by virtue of alternation, simultaneity, or opposition, of concomitant regional stereotypies. Such relatedness is indicated by listing the body regions seen to be related: *Head-Body (Hb), Head-Legs (Hl), Body-Legs (Bl),* or *Head-Body-Legs (Hbl).*

B. Motor function

1. *Dystonia* (1)

Recognizable in either abnormal *postures (P)* or abnormal *movements (M)*. If both are present, *PM* is scored. Dystonia is characterized by hyperflexion or hyperextension of body regions with awkward appearance.

2. *Disjunction* (1)

Identified by lack of proper relationship among *postures (P)* or *movements (M)* in two or more body regions, resulting in a fragmentation of the static or kinetic configuration of the body. *PM* indicates disjunction of both the postural and movement types.

3. *Ataxia* (1)

Characterized by inadequate control of the range and precision of movements and/or by quivering of flexed and/or extended regions of the body; it refers to kinetic or static manifestations, or both. Thus, if an animal keeps a certain posture, staggering or swaying movements are indicative of this motor alteration. *Level 1* indicates a moderate degree of ataxia. If marked incoordination is present, so that the animal tends to fall or is grossly unable to coordinate all four legs in order to walk or to maintain a standing posture, *Level 2* should be scored. Absence of ataxia is indicated by scoring *None (N)*.

III. Autonomic and Reflex Responses (3)

Pupil dilation: Equal bilateral dilation *(Pe)* is differentiated from *unequal or unilateral dilation (Pl)* if left is larger or *(Pr)* if right is larger. *Eyes-wide (E):* Increased palpebral opening. *Sneeze (Sn), Salivation (Sa), Panting (P), Yawning (Y), Gagging (G), Vomiting (V), Pilorection (Pi),* and *Defecation (D)* can also be indicated. If none of these responses is present, *None (N)* is entered.

IV. *Miscellanea* (3)

Response to stimulus: Clear and sudden postural shifting or movement activity corresponding to a *visual (Rv), auditory (Ra),* or *undetermined (Ru)* source or event. If a normally stimulating event does not provoke a response, a *failure to respond (Rf)* is scored. *Claw Sharpening (Cl), Meowing (M), Hissing (H), Face-twitch (Tw),* and *Ear-twitch (E)* are self-explanatory. *Licking (L):* Actual licking of an object in the environment (Plexiglas, cage floor, etc.) not related to a grooming activity. *Biting (B):* Actual biting (not related to grooming) of an object in the environment (EEG cable, cage wires, etc.). *Chewing (Ch):* Suggested masticatory movement not associated with eating. *Tongue protrusion (T):* Tongue hanging out or moving in and out of the mouth. *Fly-catching (F):* A fast sudden turning or swinging head movement with opening and closing of the mouth and, on occasion, protrusion of the tongue. It may be accompanied by other body movements, such as pawing, headshaking, etc. *Nose-wiping (Nw):* Slow swinging head movement, usually describing an arc tangential to the floor and almost rubbing the nose against it. *Wet lips (W):* Wetting of the lips with the tongue. This often precedes gagging and vomiting. It may be associated with increased salivation. *Hallucinating (H):* Rated by analogy with the human phenomenon on the basis of hissing, motor reactions (such as striking at nonexistent objects in the air, sudden retreating movements, or eluding jumps apparently related to "internal" cues), character of looking activity (most frequently staring gaze), and facial expression. *Akathisia (A):* Restlessness and/or repeated weight-shifting movements of the legs (generally repositioning or stepping movements), with or without changing of place or orientation. *Obstinate progression (O):* Persistent, propulsive pushing against an immovable obstacle.

Evaluation

Table 1 is a synopsis of the sequential steps in evaluating the BRIDGE scale. To assess the rating system, three raters were used — one "expert" and two "students." The expert (A.S.) was the primary developer of the scale, and was also the sole rater for four large research projects (step 1). The students were laboratory technicians who had no previous experience in rating animals' behavior. They were trained in the system over a period of 3 weeks, the training consisting of sessions for discussion of all the items in the catalogue followed by several practice rating sessions in which expert and students compared ratings (step 2). Training was terminated when general agreement on the definitions and ratings assigned on practice segments was reached between both expert and students.

Test ratings were then done by each rater on eight previously unviewed subjects. The first 15 (3-min) segments evaluated by the expert were rated blindly (step 3), having been chosen from the entire set of unviewed tapes and projected by a fourth party, so that the rater was unaware of the day or

TABLE 1. *Synopsis of sequential steps in evaluating the BRIDGE rating system*

1. First rating by "expert" of subjects for delayed re-rating comparison (ED1) (a totally different set of subjects from those in steps 3–6 below).
2. Communication of BRIDGE system to "students."
3. Blind rating by "expert" of 15 3-min segments from recordings of the eight *test* (previously unviewed by either "expert" or "students") subjects (B1). Ten of these segments are from day 11.
4. Non-blind ratings of day 11 recording session in the eight *test* subjects by the "expert" (N1) and by the "students" (*N2* and *N3*).
5. Second non-blind rating by the "expert" of recordings used in step 4 (*NN1*).
6. Reconciliation by the "expert" of any discrepancies between *N1* and *NN1* ("consensus").
7. Second rating (non-blind) by the "expert" of subjects for delayed re-rating comparison (*ED2*).

Data Comparisons

Delayed re-rating	(ED1	: ED2)	student 1 : student 2	(N2 : N3)
Proximal re-rating	(N1	: NN1)	student 1 : "consensus"	(N2 : "consensus")
Blind evaluation	(B1	: N1)	student 2 : "consensus"	(N3 : "consensus")

time since injection shown in each segment. Unknown to the rater, 10 ot these segments were actually chosen from data recorded on day 11 of the intoxication cycle and were thus the same as records to be rated later. The purpose of this blind rating was to determine whether there were any effects associated with knowledge of the duration of intoxication or of the interval after a specific injection ("drug state"). In acute experiments the autonomic effects of amphetamine usually serve to distinguish treated animals from untreated controls; in contrast autonomic effects are seen during recording sessions at all stages of chronic intoxication.

All video tape segments were then rated by both expert and students throughout the entire recording session on the 11th day of drug administration (step 4). This day was chosen for test rating because it showed the most varied as well as the most bizarre behaviors. In order to produce the best rating against which to test the students, the expert rated the day 11 behavior a second time (step 5). He then reconciled all disagreements between his first and second ratings (step 6), producing a "consensus" rating against which the students were tested.

The double rating by the expert also allowed evaluation of the intrarater agreement in an expert rater. This comparison will be called the *proximal* rerating, since these two ratings were accomplished within 4 to 6 weeks of each other, and during a time when the rater was continuously using the rating system and was intimately familiar with it.

A second rating of several subjects (step 7), different from those included in the proximal rerating and therefore from those in the consensus determination, was made 1 year after the last experience of the expert rater with the rating scale, which was also 18 months after the original rating of these subjects (step 1). This *delayed* rerating provides a "worst condition" that allows assessment of the need for continuous practice in the system. In addition, the delayed comparison provides a means of measuring the deterioration of rating consistency over an extended period.

The delayed and proximal intrarater comparisons assess the time factor in rater reliability. The comparison of the expert's blind rating with his first nonblind rating of the same subjects (i.e., the first of the two proximal ratings) was made to assess the effect of any bias due to knowledge of the drug state.

To determine the intra- and interrater agreement rates, the percent agreement was calculated in the following way: (a) Two relevant sets of ratings (e.g., "student 1" versus "consensus" or "blind" versus "first nonblind") were compared interval by interval and category by category, and the total number of disagreements in each category was tabulated across all 10-sec intervals. (b) The percent disagreement was calculated as:

$$\frac{\text{number of disagreements}}{\text{number of possible disagreements}} \times 100$$

The number of possible disagreements was determined by the total number of entries per interval allowed for a given category (see footnote, page 0). If two entries per interval were allowed[1] in a given category, and 25 intervals were compared to determine the agreement rate, there would be 50 possible disagreements. If there were five actual disagreements recorded, the percent disagreement for that category would be $(5/50) \times 100$, or 10%. (c) Percent agreement, which is reported here, is 100% minus percent disagreement.

RESULTS AND DISCUSSION

A representative subset of the behavioral categories was analyzed according to the methods outlined above. In this subset we tried to include those categories most relevant to the use of the animal amphetamine intoxication as a model of amphetamine psychosis. Table 2 is a precis of these categories with their relevant behaviors and mnemonic codes. The following is a discussion of how the original scale fared when tested against each of our four original criteria.

TABLE 2. *Precis of behaviors included in the selected representative subset of categories from the original rating system*

Attitude	Arousal	Sniffing involvement
Asleep (A)	Asleep (1)	*Discrete (D)
Indifferent (I)	Somnolent (2)	*Throughout (T)
Interested, normal (INN)	Normal (3)	
Interested, abnormal (INA)	Aroused (4)	Dystonia and disjunction
*Interested, focused (INF)	Hyperaroused (5)	
Investigative, normal (IVN)		*Postural (P)
Investigative, abnormal (IVA)		*Motor (M)
*Investigative, focused (IVF)	Movement speed	None (N)
Reactive (R)		
*Reactive, focused (RF)	No movement (1)	Ataxia
Unaware (U)	Slow (2)	
	Normal (3)	Level 1 (1)
	Fast (4)	Level 2 (2)
	Sudden, reactive (5)	None (N)

Unstereotyped	Stereotyped	Incorporated into stereotypy
*Tremor (Tm)		*Look (1)
*Stagger (St)	Minutia search (M)	*Pause (p)
*Shake (Sh)	Balinese (B)	*Dip (d)
*Recoil (R)	Up-and-down (U)	*Recoil (r)
*Look (L)	Side-to-side (Si)	
Transient (T)		

[a] Items consolidated with other behaviors or dropped from the system.

Completeness

Our first criterion, completeness, was well met. In the rating of 13,917 10-sec intervals by the expert rater, 392,099 behaviors were entered. Only 4.9% were contained in the miscellanea category. Thus, of those behaviors displayed that were relevant to the model, very few were not defined.

Level of Detail

To arrive at an adequate level of detail presents a problem in that, if distinctions between behaviors within a category are too fine, there will frequently be apparent errors in judgment made by the raters. On the other hand, if the code is so general as to produce no disagreements between raters, it is too crude and many significant features will not be rated. The problem has been discussed previously (Altmann, 1965, Hutt and Hutt, 1970), and Altmann's rule of thumb, "to split (categories) when in doubt," has been applied here. If, on analysis, the distinctions made are not significant, the categories can be combined. If what are, in fact, distinct patterns are combined during observation, nothing can be done to recover the lost data. In our original system, we attempted to specify maximum detail within the limits of what we felt could be distinguished. On subsequent evaluation, we employed progressively coarser versions of the scale until a satisfactory agreement level had been reached. Specific behaviors not found to be significant or relevant were also dropped. Specific changes made to date in our scale as a result of such procedures are discussed in the section on Reliability, below. Table 3 is a precis of the system as it has been modified by these iterative procedures. It reflects what is currently a realizable level of detail in our experience. Other researchers might, through this process, develop more or less specific scales in other contexts.

Conciseness and Communicability

By definition, the mnemonic code for the behaviors is concise since each symbol consists, at most, of three characters; however, the real test of conciseness is the rating speed. Using the BRIDGE system, trained observers rate video tapes in less than 10 times real time, which indicates that 10% of the samples of ongoing "real" behavior could be rated by use of this system. With videotaped data, rating 10% of the samples taped would take only as long as the original experimental session. The final testing of the communicability of the system lies in the measures of reliability discussed below.

Reliability

The measures of reliability used in this discussion are rates of agreement, as discussed above. In defining minimal acceptable level of agreement, two different situations must be recognized.

TABLE 3. *Precis of behaviors in the analyzed subset after consecutive reductions of detail made to maximize percent agreement among the raters*

Attitude	Movement speed
Asleep (A)	No movement (1)
Indifferent (I)	Slow (2)
Interested, normal (INN)	Normal (3)
[a]Interested, abnormal (INA)	Fast (4)
Investigative, normal (IVN)	Sudden, reactive (5)
[a]Investigative, abnormal (IVA)	
[a]Reactive (R)	**Sniffing involvement**
Unaware (U)	
	Absent (N)
Arousal	[c]Present (1)
Asleep (1)	
Somnolent (2)	**Dystonia and disjunction**
Normal (3)	
Aroused (4)	Absent (N)
Hyperaroused (5)	[d]Present (1)
Head movement	**Ataxia**
[b]Transient (T)	Level 1 (1)
Minutia search (M)	Level 2 (2)
Balinese (B)	None (N)
Up and down (U)	
Side to side (Si)	

[a] Includes corresponding focused attitude.
[b] Includes stagger, shake, recoil, look, tremor, incorporated transitory movements.
[c] Includes discrete and throughout.
[d] Includes motor and postural.

1. The expert's intrarater agreement and the students' interrater agreement; and
2. The students' agreement with consensus—the measure that we have assumed, in this analysis, to be the correct rating.

Table 4 lists the interrater agreement between students and consensus, and between student and student. In addition, the intrarater agreement rate on proximal rerating and on blind rating by the expert is shown for the selected categories.

Although the percentages presented in columns 1, 2, and 5 of Table 4 for expert intrarater and students' interrater agreement are measures of consistency, but not necessarily measures of correctness, columns 3 and 4, which compare the students with consensus, represent percent agreement with "correct" ratings. We feel, perhaps arbitrarily, that these latter percentages, since they are probabilities of making a correct rating, should exceed 70%.

TABLE 4. *Percent agreement for several comparisons of selected categories in the original rating system*

Category	Intrarater		Interrater		
	Proximal (N1:NN1)[a] 648[b]	Blind (B1:N1)[a] 180[b]	Student 1: consensus (N2:consensus)[a] 216[b]	Student 2: consensus (N3:consensus)[a] 216[b]	Student 1: student 2 (N2:N3)[a] 216[b]
Attitude	94.3	84.4	51.8	35.6	56.9
Arousal	98.6	98.9	40.7	48.6	83.8
Movement Speed	92.7	89.4	49.5	63.9	77.8
Head Movement	95.2	85.7	78.9	56.9	57.4
Head stereotypy[c]					
Presence	98.8	96.4	87.7	83.8	85.9
Type	98.8	96.4	87.3	83.8	76.6
Sniffing Involvement	94.3	98.9	82.9	83.8	89.3
Dystonia	90.2	63.9	36.6	30.1	40.7
Disjunction	83.8	87.8	39.8	54.6	47.7
Ataxia	97.4	99.4	63.0	70.4	92.6

[a] Mnemonic (see Table 1).
[b] Number of intervals.
[c] Derived from head movement category. *Presence:* Agreement on the presence of head stereotypy, regardless of type. *Type:* Agreement on both the presence and type of head stereotypy.

Our reasoning is that with this as a minimum, the probability that two independent ratings of the same interval would agree on the correct behavior is $0.7 \times 0.7 = 0.49$, i.e., less than 50% of the time, an unacceptable occurrence. The expert self-consistency and the student interrater columns, since they do not represent agreement with a standard, may include agreements on erroneous ratings and are, therefore, unrelated to probabilities of correct ratings. Because of this, minimal acceptable agreement levels cannot be defined in terms of probabilities, but "high" consistency seems desirable and, indeed, was often attained.

Upon immediate rerating, the expert agreed well with his original determinations, indicating that there are conditions under which consistent results can be obtained with the system. In the delayed rerating situation, agreement rates were much lower, ranging from 79.86% for Presence of Head Stereotypy (derived from the Head Movements category), to 54.29% for the Head Movements category. These results demonstrate the well-known, highly detrimental effect of time lag and absence of practice on the consistency of the rater. Twelve months had elapsed since the rater had had any practice in using the scale. Although a short briefing session had been conducted before the delayed rerating, it certainly was not extensive enough to constitute retraining in the system. The time between ratings of the same subjects in the delayed situation was at least 18 months, whereas in the proximal rerating, the time between ratings of the same subjects was, at most, 6 weeks. It is possible that the original rating, in the case of proximal rerating, was remembered by the rater. The time lag and the interpolated rating of other samples in the delayed rerating would allow the rater to forget more fully the general impression of the animal's behavior that had been gained from his original rating. An additional factor unique to our situation lies in the fact that there was interpolated between the first and second ratings, in the delayed rerating set, the communication of the rating system to the students. During these communication sessions, the scale may have become more precise, due to feedback from the students, and may even have undergone subtle changes. Such results underlie the need for very close control and monitoring of current rating status in order to keep the system consistent, or to make one aware of any evolution in the system. Measures that might be used to implement such a monitoring are discussed later.

The expert's blind rating, done to determine if knowledge of the experimental situation influenced ratings, demonstrates a lack of such influence. Self-consistency from blind to nonblind (Table 2, column 2) is of the same order as that of the proximal rerating. Had there been major differences, blind ratings or correction factors applied to nonblind ratings would be mandated for all situations, to assure comparability of data.

In comparing the student raters with the consensus (Table 4), we find that, in the original system, they have high agreement in a few categories. An appreciable portion of the disagreement is eliminated as the scale becomes less specific (Table 5). We feel that factors such as previous experience and training of the raters in the areas being rated play a role both in the disagreements generated by the original scale and in the lack of agreement remaining as the scale is modified. The expert was not only involved in developing the scale, but also had extensive previous experience in observing clinical neurological and psychiatric disorders, whereas the student raters had no such experience. The importance of this experience factor is underlined by the agreement rates of the students with each other. Table 4 shows that this mutual consistency was higher than the agreement rate of either student with the expert and was, in general, acceptable. The students' poor agreement with consensus, coupled with their acceptable level of interrater agreement, indicates that the latter includes agreements in error perhaps reflecting their common lack of experience.

In an attempt to produce a system less vulnerable to the detrimental effects of time lag, communication, and degree of previous experience, consecutive reductions were made in the level of detail within some categories. Table 5 shows the effects of these reductions in specificity on the agreement rates.

We found in the Attitude category that the evaluations most affected by the time lag (delayed rerating) were different from those affected by communication or experience (students to consensus). Confusion between the qualifiers Abnormal and Focused within the Interested and Investigative at-

TABLE 5. *Percent agreement for several comparisons of selected categories in the modified BRIDGE rating system*

	Intrarater		Interrater		
			Student 1: consensus	Student 2: consensus	Student 1: student 2
Category	Proximal (N1:NN1)[a] 648[b]	Blind (B1:N1)[a] 180[b]	(N2:consensus)[a] 216[b]	(N3:consensus)[a] 216[b]	(N2:N3)[a] 216[b]
Attitude	94.6	86.1	63.0	53.2	65.3
Arousal	98.9	98.9	83.8	100.0	91.7
Movement Speed	92.7	89.4	40.7	48.6	83.8
Head Movement	95.8	99.2	83.1	63.0	69.2
Head stereotypy[c]					
Presence	98.8	96.7	89.8	83.8	89.6
Type	98.8	96.7	89.1	83.8	85.2
Sniffing Involvement	94.6	98.9	82.9	84.7	90.7
Dystonia	99.8	98.9	89.4	63.0	56.9
Disjunction	93.5	87.8	60.7	54.6	60.7
Ataxia	97.4	99.4	63.0	70.4	92.6

[a] Mnemonic (see Table 1).
[b] Number of intervals.
[c] Derived from head movement category. Presence: Agreement on the presence of head stereotypy, regardless of type. Type: Agreement on both the presence and type of head stereotypy.

titudes accounted for 60% of the disagreements in the delayed comparison, and a shift from rating of Reactive attitude to Focused Reactive attitude on second rating accounted for another 11%. Thus, by eliminating the indication of Focused, and subsumming this designation under the corresponding Abnormal qualifier, we decreased our error rate by 71% in the delayed comparison. The effect of this consolidation on the communication and experience factors, reflected by the student to consensus agreement rates, was not as dramatic. Further analysis indicated the consolidation to be favorable to the student:consensus comparison only within the categories of Interested and Investigative attitudes.[2] In the case of the Focused Reactive attitude, however, the students did not confuse this with the basic Reactive attitude, but rather with the Abnormal Interested attitude.[3] At no time, in either the delayed or proximal comparisons, did the expert change an interval originally designated Focused Reactive. The distinction between the Focused Reactive and the Abnormal Interested attitudes thus seems to be a subtle one, not subject to decay over time, and either dif-

[2] All of the intervals identified as either INF or IVF by the expert were misrated by the students. Student 1 rated 85% of these with the corresponding Abnormal attribute. Student 2 rated 100% with the corresponding Abnormal attribute.
[3] All intervals identified as Focused Reactive in the consensus were misrated by the students. Student 1 rated 87% to be Abnormal Interested. Student 2 rated 100% to be Abnormal Interested.

ficult to communicate or difficult to comprehend without the tuned appreciation of the expert. We have maintained this distinction in our modified scale
as one that is highly relevant to the model psychosis and all raters must be
trained to recognize.

The Attitude category presented the most dramatic example of behaviors
differentially affected by time delay and experience or communication. In
all other categories the difference was small. The modifications below are
based entirely on the delayed comparison.

In Arousal, the elimination of the distinction between the aroused and
the hyperaroused states (levels 4 and 5) has a profound effect on the student
consensus agreements (compare Tables 4 and 5), as well as on the delayed
rerating comparison (increased from 66.16 to 90.91%). The rating of these
levels of arousal seems to stand out in our analysis as a difficult distinction
to agree upon. The ability of the expert to distinguish these states when using
the scale continuously (proximal rerating) argues for the maintenance of
the distinction. Also, the need for the sensitivity such a distinction would
allow within the range of arousal associated with the amphetamine effect
justifies use of the full 5-point scale — with the reservation that the rater
must be sensitive to this distinction and must constantly re-evaluate this
sensitivity against known standards to maintain his consistency.

In the category of Head Movements, we applied two transformations.
We found that the small unstereotyped reactive-type movements (Look,
Recoil, Shake, Stagger, and unstereotyped Dip) were frequently confused.
We included these movements under the Transient designation. In the case
of Stereotyped movements, the concept of incorporation (see Head Movements in Catalogue of Definitions) proved very difficult to handle. We thus
treated incorporated movements as transient unstereotyped movements.
The combined application of these two transformations reduced our error
rate in this category by 20% in the delayed rerating situation. The Head
Stereotypy determination was also affected by the inclusion of incorporated
movements under Transient. However, the effect was slight, as can be
seen by comparison of Tables 4 and 5.

The categories of Dystonia and Disjunction were both modified by eliminating the distinction between the postural and motor manifestations, leading
to scales that indicated only the presence or absence of these disorders.
Although the modification dramatically increased the agreement rate in the
Dystonia category, the Disjunction category remains at a lower than acceptable agreement level for both students and for the delayed comparison.
Disjunctive behavior, like the Focused Reactive attitude, is of sufficient
importance to the whole picture of the amphetamine psychosis to warrant
further definition of this phenomenon in order to bring its reliability to
acceptable levels.

In several categories we concluded that there was either no reasonable
reduction in level of detail to be applied, or that whatever reduction was

possible did not materially increase the reliability of the system. In the Movement Speed category, the students tended to rate lower than the expert, a situation that can be remedied only by more intensive training. In Sniffing Involvement, the agreement was sufficiently high initially. Reduction of the Ataxia category to a present or absent basis resulted in no appreciable increase in the agreement rates. However, the scores in this category in four of the five comparisons reach acceptable levels. We feel that with further training of the raters all scores could be brought to an acceptable level.

A precis of selected behaviors for a rating system that has the qualities for which BRIDGE was designed, namely, completeness, adequate level of detail, conciseness and communicability, and reliability is presented in Table 3. Some precautions are required in its use. One consideration is the previous experience and adequacy of the raters' training, since the students' disagreements with the expert indicate that their scales were not uniformly identical. However, the agreement rates between the student raters indicate that a consistent rating system was, in fact, communicated to them. A second consideration is the matter of proximity of the rating sessions. If the system is to be reliable in use, either the rater should do all ratings within a relatively short period or there should be some standard retraining device. One aid to such retraining, which we are currently developing, is a video-tape catalogue with voice description containing numerous examples of each behavior. A rater could then run through this catalogue to refresh his memory as to the fine points involved. Such a catalogue would also be used for quality control to prevent unintentional evolution of the scale. Another test tape, consisting of many randomized examples of the behaviors, as well as several examples of frequently misidentified segments, will be developed. Portions of this tape could then be rerated periodically as a test, to insure that the integrity of the rating system is being maintained. Periodic cross-ratings, when several raters are available, would also enhance reliability. If the data were sufficiently few, or the time sufficiently great, ratings of the same sample of data by two trained raters could be made. The raters could then resolve any disagreements together. Such a course would have two distinct benefits. It would homogenize the learned rating scale of the two raters and it would record the most nearly correct result for each category.

The present results demonstrate the feasibility of a rating system for chronic amphetamine intoxication that can represent the various postural, motor, and attitudinal aspects in such a way that they are amenable to analysis and evaluation. The behavioral rating system can, of course, be extended for use with other compounds that have a reasonably similar postural motor expression; definitions derived from descriptions in our studies have been applied by Cools (1973) in cannulation studies of the extrapyramidal system in cats.

In our own use of the scale, we are interested primarily in assessing the behavioral syndrome that follows chronic amphetamine intoxication as it evolves over time. Some of the results we obtained after treatment of experimental animals, as well as the relevance of individual items in this rating system, and their relationship to the analogous signs and symptoms in the amphetamine psychosis, have been reported elsewhere (Ellinwood, Sudilovsky, and Nelson, 1972; Ellinwood and Sudilovsky, 1973; Sudilovsky, Nelson, and Ellinwood, 1974). Additionally, differential behavioral changes in the process of chronic amphetamine intoxication, as affected by disulfiram pretreatment, were evaluated by means of the scale (A. Sudilovsky, *unpublished observations*), but the extensiveness of these observations precludes their discussion here. By using selected specific behavioral categories, we have defined a "hallucinatory psychotic state" in the cat and correlated it with changes in EEG spindle activity from the amygdala and olfactory bulb (Ellinwood, Sudilovsky, and Nelson, 1974). We have also explored the correlation between various behaviors referred to in this chapter and concomitant electrophysiologic recordings from subcortical nuclei after the administration of disulfiram (Sudilovsky and Ellinwood, 1973), amphetamine, or a combination of both (Ellinwood, Sudilovsky, and Gabrowy, 1973a; Ellinwood and Sudilovsky, 1974). A comprehensive presentation of our work in this area has been made by Ellinwood (1974). Currently, we are using various aspects of the scale to measure behavioral changes in studies involving intraventricular cannulation in cats.

Appropriate derivations of the BRIDGE rating scale can also be used with other animal species in which different types of biochemical or physiologic correlations are more economical. For example, a succinct rating scale for use in rats (Ellinwood and Balster, 1974), capable of describing the array of amphetamine-induced behaviors as well as of providing accurate dose-response measures for neuroleptic drugs, e.g., pimozide, has been derived from the system described in this chapter.

ACKNOWLEDGMENTS

Supported by NIMH Grant MH15907 and NIDA Grant DA00057. We appreciate the expert technical assistance of Nancy Wagoner and An LaBarre. Thanks are also due to Dr. David Frost for editing this manuscript.

REFERENCES

Altmann, S. A. (1965): Sociobiology of rhesus. II. Stochastics of social communication. *J. Theor. Biol.,* 8:490–522.
Bell, D. S. (1973): The experimental reproduction of amphetamine psychosis. *Arch. Gen. Psychiatry,* 29:35–40.

Bleuler, E. (1950): *Dementia Praecox or the Group of Schizophrenias.* International Universities Press Inc., New York.

Cools, A. R. (1973): Serotonin, a behaviorally active compound in the caudate nucleus of cats. *Isr. J. Med. Sci.,* 9:5–16.

Delay, J., and Deniker, P. (1961): *Méthodes Chimiothérapiques en Psychiatrie. Les Nouveaux Médicaments Psychotropes.* Masson, Paris.

Drtil, J., and Tosovsky, J. (1974): Comparison of psychopathology scores determined by a psychiatric rating scale and computed on the basis of spontaneous psychomotor activity. *Act. Nerv. Super. (Praha),* 16:206–208.

Drtil, J., Vinar, O., and Tosovsky, J. (1973): An attempt to correlate some experimental measures of psychomotor activity with the psychotic symptomatology. *Act. Nerv. Super. (Praha),* 15:78.

Ellinwood, E. H., Jr. (1974): Behavioral and EEG Changes in the Amphetamine Model of Psychosis. In: *Neuropsychopharmacology of Monoamines and Their Regulatory Enzymes,* edited by B. Usdin, pp. 281–297. Raven Press, New York.

Ellinwood, E. H., Jr., and Balster, R. L. (1974): Rating the behavioral effects of amphetamine. *Eur. J. Pharmacol.* 28:35–41.

Ellinwood, E. H., Jr., and Sudilovsky, A. (1973): Chronic Amphetamine Intoxication: Behavioral Model of Psychoses. In: *Psychopathology and Psychopharmacology,* edited by J. O. Cole, A. M. Freedman, and A. J. Friedhoff, pp. 51–70. The Johns Hopkins University Press, Baltimore.

Ellinwood, E. H., Jr., and Sudilovsky, A. (1974): Arousal and EEG. Changes in the amphetamine model of psychosis. *J. Pharm. Belg.,* 5:27.

Ellinwood, E. H., Jr., Sudilovsky, A., and Nelson, L. (1972): Behavioral analysis of chronic amphetamine intoxication. *Biol. Psychiatry,* 4:3, 215–230.

Ellinwood, E. H., Jr., Sudilovsky, A., and Grabowy, R. (1973a): Olfactory forebrain seizures induced by methamphetamine and disulfiram. *Biol. Psychiatry,* 7:2, 89–99.

Ellinwood, E. H., Jr., Sudilovsky, A., and Nelson, L. (1973b): Evolving behavior in the clinical and experimental amphetamine (model) psychosis. *Am. J. Psychiatry,* 130:1088–1093.

Ellinwood, E. H., Jr., Sudilovsky, A., and Nelson, L. (1974): Behavior and EEG analysis of chronic amphetamine effect. *Biol. Psychiatry,* 8:2, 169–176.

Fielding, S., and Lal, H. (1974): Pre-Clinical Neuropsychopharmacology of Neuroleptics. 3: Screening Tests Using Higher Animals. In: *Industrial Pharmacology, Vol. 1, Neuroleptics,* edited by S. Fielding and H. Lal, pp. 64–75. Futura Publishing Co., New York.

Florio, V., Fuentes, J. A., Ziegler, H., and Longo, V. G. (1972): EEG and behavioral effects in animals of some amphetamine derivatives with hallucinogenic properties. *Behav. Biol.,* 7:401–414.

Harlow, H. (1974): *Learning to Love.* Jason Aronson, New York.

Heusler, A., Ulett, G., and Blasques, J. (1959): Noise-Level Index (an objective measurement of the effect of drugs on the psychomotor activity of patients). *J. Neuropsychiatry,* 1:23–25.

Holzman, Ph. S. (1972): Assessment of perceptual functioning in schizophrenia. *Psychopharmacologia,* 24:29–41.

Hutt, S. J., and Hutt, C. (1970): *Direct Observation and Measurement of Behavior,* pp. 34–37. Charles C Thomas, Springfield.

Itil, T. M. (1969): Quantitative analysis of "motor pattern" in schizophrenia. In: *Schizophrenia, Current Concepts and Research,* edited by D. V. S. Va Sankar, pp. 210–219. PJD Publications, New York.

Kast, E. C. (1964): Observations of psychomotor behavior as an index of psychopharmacologic action. *J. Neuropsychiatry,* 5:577–584.

King, H. E. (1954): *Psychomotor Aspects of Mental Disease, An Experimental Study,* p. 3. Harvard University Press, Cambridge.

King, H. E. (1965): Psychomotor changes with age, psychopathology, and brain damage. In: *Behavior, Aging and the Nervous System,* edited by A. T. Welford and J. E. Birren, Chapter 25. Charles C Thomas, Springfield.

King, H. E. (1969): Psychomotility: A Dimension of Behavior Disorder. In: *Neurobiological Aspects of Psychopathology,* edited by J. Zubin and C. Shagass, pp. 99–128. Grune & Stratton, New York.

Kraepelin, E. (1889): *Psychiatrie. Ein Kurzes Lehrbuch fuer Studierende & Aertze,* Third edition. Abel, Leipzig.

Kraüpl-Taylor, F. (1966): *Psychopathology, Its Causes and Symptoms,* pp. 191–200. Butterworth Inc., Washington.

Nathan, P. E., Zare, N., Simpson, H. F., and Andberg, M. M. (1969): A systems analytic model of diagnosis. I. The diagnostic validity of abnormal psychomotor behavior. *J. Clin. Psychol.,* 25:3–9.

Reich, W. (1949): *Character-Analysis.* Orgone Institute Press, New York.

Schilder, P. (1951): *Brain and Personality.* International Universities Press Inc., New York.

Smythies, J. R. (1970): A Model for Schizophrenia? Discussion. In: *The Mode of Action of Psychotomimetic Drugs,* edited by J. R. Smythies, pp. 7–15. N.R.P. Bulletin, 8:1.

Snyder, S. H. (1973): Biochemical Models of Psychosis, Focus on Amphetamines. In: *Pharmacology and the Future of Man, Vol. 1: Drug Abuse and Contraception,* edited by J. Cochin, pp. 106–124. Karger, Basel.

Sudilovsky, A., and Ellinwood, E. H., Jr. (1973): EEG changes and motor impairment after disulfiram administration to cats. *Fed. Proc.,* 32:791.

Sudilovsky, A., Nelson, L., and Ellinwood, E. H., Jr. (1974): Amphetamine Dyskinesia: A Direct Observational Study in Cats. In: *Drug Addiction, Vol. 4: New Aspects of Analytical and Clinical Toxicology,* edited by J. M. Singh and H. Lal, pp. 17–37. Stratton Int. Med. Book Corp., New York.

Utena, H. (1966): Behavioral Aberrations in Methamphetamine-Intoxicated Animals and Chemical Correlates in the Brain. In: *Progress in Brain Research, Vol. 21B, Correlative Neurosciences, Part B: Clinical Studies,* edited by T. Tokizane and J. P. Schade, pp. 192–207. Elsevier Publishing Co., Amsterdam.

Yates, A. J. (1961): Abnormalities of Psychomotor Functions. In: *Handbook of Abnormal Psychology, an Experimental Approach,* edited by H. J. Eysenk, Chapter 2. Basic Books, New York.

Predictability in Psychopharmacology: Preclinical
and Clinical Correlations, edited by A. Sudilovsky,
S. Gershon, and B. Beer. Raven Press, New York © 1975.

Conditioned Avoidance: A Predictor of Efficacy and Duration of Action for Long-Acting Neuroleptic Agents

Donald E. Clody and Bernard Beer

The Squibb Institute for Medical Research, Princeton, New Jersey 08540

One of the most recent advances in the treatment of schizophrenia is the introduction of the long-acting neuroleptic. Long-acting pharmacologic agents may have widespread use, especially for patient populations that are notorious for their failure to adhere to therapeutic regimens.

A major problem in the treatment of schizophrenia is the failure of the patient in remission to maintain adequate levels of the prescribed neuroleptic, which usually precipitates rehospitalization. Whether this failure is another symptom of the disease or a function of the aversiveness of the neuroleptic is not completely clear. These problems, however, are obviated by the use of a drug with prolonged activity. The long-acting neuroleptic gives the physician control of the amount of drug administered and provides the patient with a more stable, active level of drug for a long period than can be attained with repeated doses of a conventional short-acting neuroleptic.

The first long-acting neuroleptics, fluphenazine enanthate and fluphenazine decanoate, have been shown to produce antipsychotic effects lasting 2 to 4 weeks. These long-duration effects appear to be due to a slow, but sustained, release of fluphenazine from tissue depots.

We have been involved in delineating some of the behavioral and biochemical effects of the long-acting neuroleptics in rats. The first question we asked was, "How does one decide which of the many animal tests available is the best predictor of neuroleptic activity?" Neuroleptics, like all drugs, have multiple biologic activities, any one of which, at one time or another, has been touted as having the best correlation with antipsychotic activity. Some criteria can be applied to animal procedures that are purportedly predictive of clinical efficacy.

First, all agents that are effective in the clinic should be effective in the test procedure. Further, the relative potencies and time courses of the agents in the clinic should be correlated with their relative potencies and time courses in the test procedure. The duration of or tolerance to both the clinical effect of the drug and the effect of the drug in the test procedure should be similar. Finally, in cases in which the test procedure can be adapted to patient populations, or at least to normal human subjects, these subjects should respond in a predictable fashion to doses of the drug that are efficacious for the patients' disease state.

Let us apply these criteria to the various behavioral or biochemical test procedures that are commonly used *in vivo* to identify neuroleptic activity. When administered to rats, neuroleptic agents, among other effects, produce catalepsy, antagonize the behavioral effects of apomorphine (stereotyped behavior in rats; emesis in dogs), affect the dopamine system in the brain, and produce a profound inhibition of conditioned avoidance responding.

CATALEPSY

Catalepsy is usually measured by the length of time an animal remains fixed in any position in which it has been placed. Treatment with most neuroleptics will result in a marked prolongation in that time. This procedure, however, does not identify all effective antischizophrenic agents. Clozapine, for example, is devoid of cataleptic effects (Stille et al., 1971). Furthermore, animals develop tolerance to the cataleptic effects of neuroleptics within 3 to 7 days after repeated administration of short-acting neuroleptics (Asper, Baggiolini, Burki, Lauener, Richaud, and Stille, 1973) or a single injection of a long-acting neuroleptic (Nymark, Franck, Pedersen, Boeck, and Møller-Nielsen, 1973).

STEREOTYPED BEHAVIOR

Compulsive gnawing and grooming or licking movements are elicited in rats by treatment with apomorphine, amphetamine, or methylphenidate. This stereotyped behavior is rather specifically antagonized by pretreatment with a neuroleptic agent. The blockade of stereotypy procedure seems to have more face validity than the catalepsy test for predicting neuroleptic activity in that it entails normalizing behavior that has been altered by treatment of an animal with amphetamine or apomorphine. As was the case for the catalepsy test, drug-induced stereotypy is not antagonized by clozapine (Stille et al., 1971); animals develop tolerance to the inhibition of stereotyped behavior by neuroleptics after repeated administration of various short-acting neuroleptics (Asper et al., 1973; Møller-Nielsen, Fjalland, Pedersen, and Nymark, 1974) or a single injection of a long-acting neuroleptic (Bossier, Simon, and Linoff, 1966; Christensen and Møller-Nielsen, 1974).

ANTIEMETIC BEHAVIOR

Another procedure that has been used to predict neuroleptic activity is the prevention of apomorphine-induced emesis in dogs. Although this procedure lacks face validity, it does seem to identify antipsychotic agents, except for clozapine. The antiemetic test is also apparently more sensitive to neuroleptics than are other procedures, e.g., emesis is blocked at doses smaller than those producing avoidance deficits in dogs (Laffan, High, and Burke, 1965). Dreyfuss, Ross, Shaw, Miller, and Schreiber (*in preparation*) reported that the duration of action of fluphenazine decanoate relative to that of fluphenazine enanthate in blocking emesis gave the same ratio (2:1) as that reported for antipsychotic activity. The absolute duration of action of these compounds in the antiemesis test (approximately 120 days for fluphenazine decanoate and 60 days for fluphenazine enanthate), however, is far greater than the duration of activity found in other test procedures and in patient populations.

BRAIN DOPAMINE ACTIVITY

Looking for changes in the dopaminergic system of the brain as predictors of neuroleptic activity is based on a rationale similar to that for the antagonism of apomorphine-induced emesis. Since apomorphine, and possibly amphetamine, produces profound behavioral alterations in animals as a result of stimulation (either direct or indirect) of dopaminergic receptors, psychotic behavior may be related to overstimulation of dopaminergic receptors. Therefore, antipsychotic activity should be predictable from test procedures that measure the effects of blockade of dopaminergic receptors.

Treatment with a neuroleptic agent produces a blockade of dopaminergic receptors in the brain and results in an increased mobilization of dopamine that leads to an increase in levels of homovanillic acid (HVA), the major metabolite of dopamine. This finding is observed only after the acute administration of a neuroleptic; tolerance to the effect develops after 3 to 7 days of administration of the drug (Asper et al., 1973; Burki, Ruch, Asper, Baggiolini, and Stille, 1974). Clozapine again appears to differ from other neuroleptic drugs in that the increase in the concentration of HVA after one injection of clozapine does not differ from that achieved after seven injections of the drug (Burki et al., 1974). Tolerance to the decrease in dopamine level seen after a single injection of almost any neuroleptic agent develops after seven daily injections. Clozapine again differs from the other neuroleptic agents; a single injection of a large dose of clozapine causes a slight increase in striatal-dopamine level that is maintained even after seven daily injections of either a small or large dose of clozapine (Burki et al., 1974). It appears, therefore, that the effects of antipsychotic agents on the metabolism of brain dopamine are independent of the clinical effectiveness of these agents; one antipsychotic agent, clozapine, appears to have effects on the dopaminergic system opposite to those produced by other neuroleptic agents, yet all these drugs are clinically efficacious in the treatment of schizophrenia. If one wanted to correlate the dopamine effects of the neuroleptic agents with a single aspect of their clinical profile, the extrapyramidal effects (EPS) produced by these agents would be a good candidate. Clozapine, which is virtually without extrapyramidal effects (Simpson and Varga, 1974), has effects on dopamine metabolism opposite to those of neuroleptics that produce relatively strong EPS effects.

CONDITIONED AVOIDANCE BEHAVIOR

One procedure that seems to fulfill the criteria mentioned above is the conditioned avoidance paradigm. Little or no tolerance, as measured by a decrease in conditioned avoidance behavior, develops after the repeated administration to rats of a conventional neuroleptic such as haloperidol (Møller-Nielsen et al., 1974) or after a single injection of a long-acting agent, such as fluphenazine enanthate (Bossier et al., 1966) or flupenthixol decanoate (Nymark et al., 1973).

All clinically effective antipsychotic agents produce qualitatively similar decreases in avoidance behavior, and the relative potencies of the various neuroleptics in avoidance procedures are very well correlated with their relative clinical potencies (Cook and Catania, 1964). Cook and Catania (1964) have also shown that chlorpromazine produces very selective decreases in avoidance behavior in normal human subjects. However, it has not yet been demonstrated that antipsychotic agents produce deficits in the avoidance behavior of schizophrenic subjects when given at dose levels that are effective in controlling the subjects' schizophrenia.

The conditioned avoidance procedure may be seen as having some face validity for predicting antipsychotic activity. One can view the primary symptom of schizophrenia as being the inability to inhibit responsivity to stimuli, and the other symptoms, thought disorder, hallucinations, and delusions, as secondary to or a result of this primary deficit. In this analysis, the delusional and hallucinatory symptoms become a means of handling the mass of stimuli flooding the schizophrenic's sensorium. The disorderly thinking in schizophrenic patients can also be viewed as a failure to inhibit the intrusion of extraneous stimuli into consciousness.

Chapman (1966), in a report on the early symptoms of schizophrenia, suggested that ". . . one of the schizophrenic patient's main difficulties seems to be in regulating and organizing sensory intake so that it is kept at the optimum required for assimilation at a given time." This is most clearly demonstrated by the verbal report of one of Chapman's patients (Case 10).

> ". . . It has to do with what is going on around me – taking in too much of my surroundings – vital not to miss anything. I can't shut things out of my mind and everything closes in on me. It stops me thinking and then the mind goes a blank and everything gets switched off. I can't pick things up to memorize because I am absorbing everything around me and take in too much so that I can't retain anything for any length of time. . . ."

The major function of the antipyschotic agent, then, is to reduce or suppress stimulus input. The conditioned avoidance procedure provides a simple method for analyzing the effect of drugs on the effectiveness of stimuli. Neuroleptic agents would be expected to cause a relatively specific suppression of responsivity to the conditioned avoidance stimulus, and they do.

We have recently reported some behavioral and biochemical effects of several long-acting neuroleptics in rats (Clody, Haubrich, Herman, and Beer, 1974). At the outset of these studies, we predicted that the behavioral and biochemical effects of long-acting neuroleptics would parallel the effects produced by chronic administration of relatively short-acting or conventional neuroleptics.

We have used a conditioned avoidance procedure (shelf-jump avoidance, Tenen, 1966) to measure the relative durations of activity of several long-acting neuroleptics. The test chamber utilizes a motorized wall that moves back and forth, making a shelf accessible to the rat. A trial starts with the rat on a grid floor; after 10 sec, the wall retracts, exposing the shelf. The conditioned stimuli (CS) available to the animal consists of the sound and other stimuli accompanying the movement of the wall. If the animal does not jump onto the shelf (avoidance) within 10 sec after the onset of the CS, electric shocks are delivered through the grid floor, at a rate of 1 per sec. Escape responses are those occurring during the shock. After a response (either avoidance or escape), the animal is allowed to remain on the shelf for 10 sec. The wall then moves back into the box, gently pushing the rat back onto the grid floor. After an additional 10 sec, the CS is again presented, initiating the next trial.

In the first experiment, we were interested in determining the relative durations of action of four clinically effective long-acting antipsychotic agents.

In all experiments in which an avoidance base line is used to test duration of action, we are testing for performance effects, i.e., the rats are trained to a 90 to 100% avoidance criterion (which takes approximately 3 to 5 sessions) before any drug is administered.

The four long-acting neuroleptics studied in the first experiment were fluphenazine enanthate, fluphenazine decanoate, flupenthixol decanoate, and fluspirilene. The doses were injected based on the recommended total milligram dosage for patients, but were administered to the rats on the basis of body weight (mg/kg). Control animals were injected intramuscularly with an equivalent volume of sesame oil. All animals were tested for avoidance effects one day after injection and approximately two or three times per week until avoidance levels were again within normal limits. The results of this experiment are shown in Table 1, which also shows the recommended doses for patient populations and their reported durations of action. The duration of action in the avoidance procedure was based on significant differences from control values ($p < 0.05$, Mann-Whitney U Test). The

TABLE 1. *Effects of long-acting neuroleptics and fluphenazine HCl, clinically and in animals*

Drug	Intramuscular initial dose (mg)	Reported duration	Intramuscular dose (mg/kg)	Duration (days)	Maximum effect observed (percent decrease in avoidance behavior)
Fluphenazine enanthate	12.5–25.0	2 weeks	12.5	24–34	69 (day 3)
			25.0	48–52	64 (day 3)
Fluphenazine decanoate	12.5–25.0	4 weeks	12.5	24–34	60 (day 3)
			25.0	48–52	63 (day 6)
Flupenthixol decanoate	20	2 weeks	20	10–13	62 (day 3)
Fluspirilene	2	5–7 days	2	6–10	20 (day 3)
Fluphenazine HCl			25	6–7	83 (day 1)

last column at the right shows the maximum percent decrease in avoidance behavior that was observed over the course of the experiment, as well as the day on which this deficit occurred.

As may be seen from Table 1, all four long-acting drugs showed a fairly good correlation between duration of action in patients and duration of action in rats (avoidance procedure). Second, the duration of action of both fluphenazine enanthate and fluphenazine decanoate in the avoidance procedure is dose related, i.e., halving the dose results in a halving of the duration of action. Anomalously, however, fluphenazine enanthate and fluphenazine decanoate have the same duration of action in the avoidance test at equal doses, in contrast to the durations of activity for these agents in psychotic patients, and to the relative durations of antiemetic activity.

It may also be seen in Table 1 and Figs. 1, 2, and 3 that the maximum effect on avoidance of a long-acting neuroleptic usually occurred one or more days after injection (usually on day 3), whereas fluphenazine hydrochloride (Table 1; Fig. 3), injected intramuscularly as an emulsion in oil, had its maximal effect during the first day after injection. This difference may indicate a slower onset of action by the long-acting agents or may be related to some other biochemical or behavioral variable.

Figures 1, 2, and 3 illustrate the effects of these long-acting neuroleptics on conditioned avoidance and on escape behavior (mean number of shocks/trial) during the experiment. Figure 1 compares the effects of single intramuscular injections of flupenthixol decanoate and fluspirilene (24 hr before the test on day 1 and again on day 27). Fluspirilene, 2 mg/kg, produced approximately the same magnitude (20 to 25% decrease) and duration (5 to 7 days) of effect after each injection. After the injection of fluspirilene, the maximum decrease in avoidance behavior was observed on the second test session, whether the second test session occurred 3 or 7 days after injection.

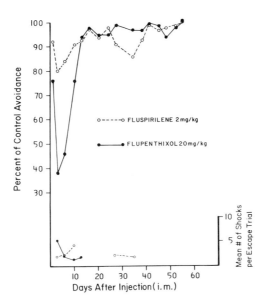

FIG. 1. The effects of single intramuscular injections of either fluspirilene (2 mg/kg) or flupenthixol decanoate (20 mg/kg) on avoidance and on escape behavior of rats. The avoidance effects are plotted as percent of avoidance levels from control (oil injected) rats. Also shown are the effects of these neuroleptics on escape behavior, as indicated by the number of shocks taken per escape trial. Flupenthixol decanoate was injected 24 hr before the first test session; fluspirilene was injected 24 hr before the test on days 1 and 27.

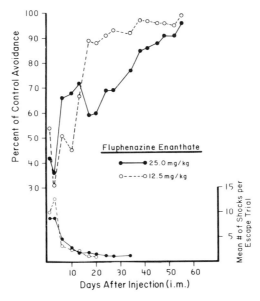

FIG. 2. The effects of single intramuscular injections of two dose levels of fluphenazine enanthate on the avoidance and escape behavior of rats.

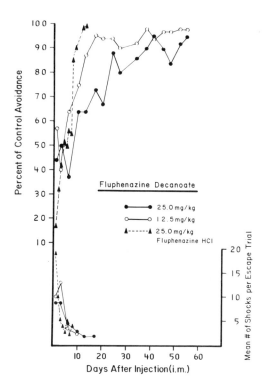

FIG. 3. The effects of single intramuscular injections of two dose levels of fluphenazine decanoate and one dose level of fluphenazine hydrochloride on the avoidance and escape behavior of rats.

Flupenthixol, 20 mg/kg, produced its maximum avoidance effect in the second test session and had a duration of effect of 10 to 13 days. In most cases, the decrease in avoidance behavior was accompanied by a deficit in escape behavior, i.e., the rats tended to take slightly (but significantly) more shocks before an escape response than did control animals.

Figure 2 shows the effects of single injections of fluphenazine enanthate. Both groups of rats treated with fluphenazine enanthate (12.5 and 25.0 mg/kg) showed approximately the same maximum decrease in avoidance behavior in the second test session; the group given the smaller dose showed a duration of activity approximately half that observed after the larger dose. After 10 days, the mean number of shocks per escape trial was only slightly greater than control values. Thus, 10 or more days after injection, fluphenazine enanthate affected avoidance behavior without causing any substantial deficit in escape behavior. Figure 3 shows the effects of single injections of fluphenazine decanoate (12.5 and 25.0 mg/kg), which were very similar to the pattern of effects observed with fluphenazine enanthate. Figure 3 also shows the effects of a single injection of fluphenazine hydrochloride (25 mg/kg). Fluphenazine hydrochloride had its maximum avoidance effect one day after injection, and the effect lasted seven or eight days. This agent also produced a significant effect on escape behavior (increase in number of shocks per escape trial) for seven to eight days; thus, fluphenazine hydrochloride did not show any differential effects on avoidance and escape behavior. These data suggest that the duration of activity of a short-acting neuroleptic, such as fluphenazine hydrochloride, can be prolonged by injecting it intramuscularly as an emulsion in oil.

In separate groups of animals, we studied the effects of single injections of these neuroleptics (injected intramuscularly in oil and at the same doses used in the avoidance study) on the brain (striatum) dopamine system. Measurements at various times after treatment with a neuroleptic showed that levels of HVA increased to a maximum at 24 hr, declined over the next few days, and returned to normal after 6 days. Fluphenazine enanthate, fluphenazine decanoate, and fluphenazine hydrochloride all raised levels of HVA by four to five times during the first 24 hr. These levels were only slightly elevated 3 days after injection and had returned to control values by day 6. Fluspirilene and flupenthixol showed substantially the same time course, except that the level of HVA was approximately twice normal on day 1 and had returned to control values by day 6. The effects of these long-acting neuroleptics on HVA levels correlate well with the time course for the effects of repeated injections of short-acting neuroleptics on the metabolism of dopamine (Asper et al., 1973). The effects of neuroleptics on avoidance behavior appear to outlast their effects on the system of brain dopamine. Although these two effects of the neuroleptics appear to be dissociable, proof of this separateness would require a demonstration of both effects in the same animals, i.e., that tolerance to the effect of the neuroleptic on dopamine metabolism develops in animals that show a deficit in avoidance behavior.

As mentioned above, animals treated with long-acting neuroleptics do not show a maximum decrease in avoidance behavior until some time after the first test session. This lag could be due simply to the fact that the drug does not attain maximal tissue concentrations within the first 24 hr after administration. Another possible explanation is that the effects of the neuroleptics on dopamine metabolism antagonize their behavioral effects. The neuroleptic blockade of dopaminergic receptors results in an initial increased output of dopamine which, in turn, competes with the neuroleptic for the receptor site, thus resulting in a submaximal neuroleptic blockade. As this feedback-inspired increase in dopamine activity wanes, there is decreased competition for receptor sites, resulting in an enhancement of the effect of the neuroleptic on behavior. This explanation does not seem likely, since clozapine, which has neuroleptic-like effects on avoidance behavior (Stille et al., 1971; Clody, *unpublished data*), has effects on dopamine levels opposite to those of other neuroleptics. This difference again suggests that the effects of antipsychotic agents on avoidance behavior and on brain dopamine activity are independent of one another.

The apparent increase with time in the effectiveness of neuroleptics on avoidance behavior may be related to a learning or training variable. If the duration of action of the long-acting neuroleptics were due simply to the sustained release of active drug, one would expect that animals tested at the same time after injection, regardless of whether they had been tested previously, would show the same deficit in the performance of the avoidance task. If, however, a learning variable is involved in these avoidance effects, then one would expect that animals that had not been tested for a long period of time after injection would differ from animals that had been tested. A second behavioral experiment was designed to test these possibilities. In this study, the duration of action of fluphenazine decanoate was assessed in six separate groups of animals; the groups were tested as long as 70 days after injection. The groups differed only in the number of days that elapsed between injection and the first test session.

Forty-six rats were first trained to perform the avoidance task to a 90 to 100% avoidance criterion and were then injected with fluphenazine decanoate, 25 mg/kg, i.m. Initial tests for avoidance were made either 1, 7, 14, 21, 28, or 35 days after injection (see Table 2); a partial replication study was made for days 7, 14, and 21. It would appear from Table 2 that the duration of effect of fluphenazine decanoate on avoidance behavior is approximately 21 to 28 days. When the groups were tested repeatedly for avoidance, however, a different profile of effects emerged. Table 3 shows the percent avoidance responses for the six groups when they were tested for as long as 70 days after injection. Groups 1 and 2 showed no significant differences in avoidance performance throughout the course of testing, and were therefore combined for subsequent statistical analysis. Group 3 did not significantly differ from groups 1 and 2, although the avoidance performance of these animals tended to be higher in their first two test sessions (days 14 and 19) than those of groups 1 and 2. Animals that were first tested for

TABLE 2. Effects of fluphenazine decanoate on the avoidance behavior of different groups of rats tested at various times after injection

Day of test					
1	7	14	21	28	35
Mean percent avoidance					
49	50	66	89	91	92
	57"	69"	88"		

" Replicate value.

TABLE 3. *The interaction of effects of fluphenazine decanoate (25 mg/kg, i.m.) and time of testing on the avoidance behavior of rats*

		Day of test													
Group	n	1	3	7	12	14	19	21	23	28	33	35	40	51	61	70
		Mean percent avoidance													
1	8	49	56	60	45	56	47	55	52	66	69	61	65	69	83	80
2	8	–	–	50	47	43	62	60	57	59	69	79	77	74	79	90
3	8	–	–	–	–	66	63	61	58	67	66	70	70	73	76	89
4	8	–	–	–	–	–	–	89[a]	88[a]	81[a]	83	75	81	86	91	95
5	8	–	–	–	–	–	–	–	–	91[a]	92[a]	87	86	89	92	95
6	6	–	–	–	–	–	–	–	–	–	–	92[a]	81	77	84	91

[a] Different from groups 1 and 2 ($p < 0.05$).

avoidance effects 21 days after injection (group 4) differed significantly from groups 1 and 2 ($p < 0.05$, 2-tailed Mann-Whitney U Test) during the first three test sessions (days 21, 23, and 28).

Similarly, animals tested initially at 28 days (group 5) differed significantly in mean percent avoidance from groups 1 and 2 on days 28 and 33. The animals in group 6, tested initially at 35 days, differed significantly from groups 1 and 2 only on their first test session (day 35). The animals in groups 4 and 5 showed a significant decline ($p < 0.05$, Wilcoxon Matched-Pairs Signed-Ranks Test, Siegel, 1956) in avoidance behavior in the course of testing. Group 6 also showed this same trend, but the decline in avoidance was not statistically significant. These results demonstrate that if animals are treated with fluphenazine decanoate and are not tested in the avoidance situation for at least 21 days, no substantial avoidance deficit occurs in the first few test sessions. In contrast, animals that are tested for the first time 14 days after injection or sooner show a sustained effect of fluphenazine decanoate on avoidance behavior. Furthermore, the animals in groups 4, 5, and 6 also showed a decline in avoidance performance with repeated testing, which suggests that fluphenazine decanoate was still showing activity at these times and that the avoidance behavior of these animals was altered under the influence of the drug. The data demonstrate clearly that the duration and magnitude of avoidance deficits produced by neuroleptics depend not only on dosage and injection parameters but also on the time between injection and the first test and on the frequency of test sessions.

Do these findings, then, invalidate the utility of the avoidance procedure either as a predictor of neuroleptic activity or for measuring the duration of action of neuroleptics? We think not. First, the predictive reliability of the avoidance procedure, as discussed earlier, is not affected by our findings. However, our data do suggest the need for caution in using an avoidance procedure to predict the duration of action of a long-acting neuroleptic agent. In our study, one would have come to quite different judgments about the duration of action of fluphenazine decanoate if only group 1 had been tested or if the various groups had been tested at only one time. Although these findings do not negate the utility of the avoidance procedure for predicting the duration of neuroleptic activity, they do raise some methodologic questions about the design of such experiments. There are also clinical implications to our data. It is possible that clinical assessments of duration of action of long-acting neuroleptics are influenced by the same variables that were identified in the studies in animals. Do long-acting neuroleptics show different durations of action depending on whether the patients are rated (tested) daily, weekly, or monthly? It is suggested that the variables that were shown to interact with the behavioral effects of neuroleptic agents in animals may also be present in the clinical setting and can therefore affect the determination of the efficacy and duration of activity of these agents in the treatment of schizophrenia.

REFERENCES

Asper, H., Baggiolini, M., Burki, H. R., Lauener, H., Richaud, W., and Stille, G. (1973): Tolerance phenomena with neuroleptics catalepsy, apomorphine stereotypies, and striatal dopamine metabolism in the rat after single and repeated administration of doxepin and haloperidol. *Eur. J. Pharmacol.*, 22:287–294.

Bossier, J. R., Simon, P., and Linoff, J. M. (1966): Pharmacologic study of a long-acting neuroleptic: Fluphenazine enanthate. *Med. Pharmacol. Exp.*, 14:435–442.

Burki, H. R., Ruch, W., Asper, H., Baggiolini, M., and Stille, G. (1974): Effect of single and repeated administration of clozapine on the metabolism of dopamine and noradrenaline in the brain of the rat. *Eur. J. Pharmacol.*, 27:180–190.

Chapman, J. (1966): The early symptoms of schizophrenia. *Br. J. Psychiatry*, 112:225–251.

Christensen, A. V., and Møller-Nielsen, I. (1974): Influence of flupenthixol and flupenthixol-decanoate on methylphenidate and apomorphine-induced compulsive gnawing in mice. *Psychopharmacologia*, 34:119–126.

Clody, D. E., Haubrich, D. R., Herman, R. L., and Beer, B. (1974): Effects of long-acting neuroleptics on avoidance behavior and striatal HVA and 5-HIAA levels in rats. Abstracts of the IX Congress of CINP. *J. Pharmacol. (Paris)*, 5:19.

Cook, L., and Catania, C. (1964): Effects of drugs on avoidance and escape behavior. *Fed. Proc.*, 23:818–825.

Laffan, R. J., High, J. P., and Burke, J. C. (1965): The prolonged action of fluphenazine enanthate in oil after depot injection. *Int. J. Neuropsychiatry*, 1:300–306.

Møller-Nielsen, I., Fjalland, B., Pedersen, V., and Nymark, M. (1974): Pharmacology of neuroleptics upon repeated administration. *Psychopharmacologia*, 34:95–104.

Nymark, M., Franck, K. F., Pedersen, V., Boeck, V., and Møller-Nielsen, I. (1973): Prolonged neuroleptic effect of α-flupenthixol decanoate in rats. *Acta Pharmacol. Toxicol.*, 33:363–376.

Siegel, S. (1956): *Nonparametric Statistics for the Behavioral Sciences*. McGraw-Hill, New York.

Simpson, G., and Varga, E. (1974): Clozapine – A new antipsychotic agent. *Curr. Ther. Res.*, 16:679–686.

Stille, G., Lauener, H., and Eichenberger, E. (1971): The Pharmacology of 8-chloro-11-(4-methyl-l-piperazinyl)-5H-dibenzo[b,e][1,4]diazepine (Clozapine). II. *Farmaco.* 26:603–625.

Tenen, S. S. (1966): An automated one-way avoidance box for the rat. *Psychonomic Sci. Sect. Anim. Physiol. Psychol.*, 6:407–408.

Predictability in Psychopharmacology: Preclinical and Clinical Correlations, edited by A. Sudilovsky, S. Gershon, and B. Beer. Raven Press, New York © 1975.

Antipsychotic Drugs and Central Dopaminergic Neurons: A Model for Predicting Therapeutic Efficacy and Incidence of Extrapyramidal Side Effects

B. S. Bunney and G. K. Aghajanian

Departments of Psychiatry and Pharmacology, Yale University School of Medicine and the Connecticut Mental Health Center, 34 Park Street, New Haven, Connecticut 06508

In 1952, acting upon the suggestions of Laborit, Delay demonstrated that chlorpromazine was therapeutically effective in the treatment of psychosis (Caldwell, 1970). Since then hundreds of drugs have been studied in the hopes of finding better antipsychotic (neuroleptic) agents. From these studies only a handful of new drugs have emerged as being good neuroleptics. All but two have a moderate to high incidence of extrapyramidal side effects. Numerous animal behavioral tests have been devised to help predict which of the myriads of potential neuroleptics may actually have antipsychotic properties, and possess a low enough incidence of side effects to make them worth testing in man. No single test or group of tests has proved to be 100% accurate in predicting antipsychotic efficacy. In addition, we are unaware of any current tests that accurately predict incidence of extrapyramidal side effects. We have recently begun to develop an animal model which preliminary studies suggest may accurately predict both the antipsychotic efficacy and incidence of extrapyramidal side effects of putative neuroleptics. This is a model which is not based on drug-induced changes in animal behavior but rather on drug-induced changes in the activity of a particular neuronal system in the brain—the dopamine system.

NEUROANATOMY OF THE DOPAMINE SYSTEM

This system was first identified in mammalian brain by Andén, Carlsson, Dahlström, Fuxe, Hillarp, and Larsson (1964*a*) and Dahlström and Fuxe (1964) using fluorescence histochemical techniques. By combining lesioning techniques with fluorescence histochemistry, Ungerstedt (1971) mapped the monoamine systems of the rat brain in even greater detail. These investigators found that the great majority of dopamine cells are located in the zona compacta (ZC) of the substantia nigra and the adjacent midbrain ventral tegmental (VT) area (Fig. 1). The ZC dopamine cells project to the caudate

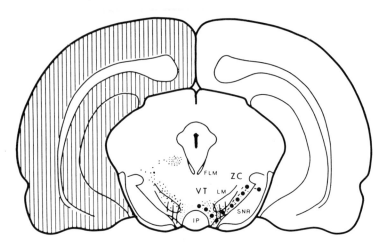

FIG. 1. Representative transverse section of the rat midbrain at the level of the interpeduncular nucleus, showing location of dopamine-containing cell bodies. Black dots represent dopamine cells in the ZC of the substantia nigra and in the VT area. FLM, fasciculus longitudinalis medialis; IP, nucleus interpeduncularis; LM, lemniscus medialis; SNR, substantia nigra, zona reticulata. (Modified from Ungerstedt, 1971.)

nucleus whereas the VT dopamine cells have terminals mainly in the olfactory tubercles and accumbens nucleus. It is important to note that although these two groups of cells are immediately adjacent to each other they project to entirely different areas of the brain. Although extensive mapping of these systems has been carried out (mainly in the rat brain), two recent reports—one by Nobin and Björklund (1973) using human fetuses and another by Olson, Nystrom, and Seiger (1963) using adult autopsy material—have demonstrated that the human dopamine system is almost identical to that of the rat. In general, the precise identification of a neuronal system both anatomically and biochemically makes it useful as a model in investigating the central action of drugs. Why do we choose this particular system around which to build a model for predicting putative neuroleptic antipsychotic efficacy and extrapyramidal side effects?

REASONS FOR CHOOSING DOPAMINE SYSTEM FOR PREDICTIVE MODEL

During the last 20 years the antipsychotic drugs have been shown to have a wide variety of effects on the biologic system of animals and man: they are good electron donors; they inhibit oxidative phosphorylation; they stabilize membranes; and they even change the pecking order of pigeons (Matthysse, 1973). However, there is only one biochemical effect which correlates with the antipsychotic action of these drugs and that is their effect on the catecholamine system of the brain, particularly the dopamine system. In 1963, a group in Sweden headed by Arvid Carlsson showed that small doses of chlorpromazine and haloperidol enhanced the accumulation of O-methylated catecholamine metabolites (3 methoxytyramine and normetanephrine) induced by the inhibition of monoamine oxidase (Carlsson and Lindqvist, 1963). Promethazine, a phenothiazine lacking antipsychotic efficacy and extrapyramidal side effects, was found to have no effect on catecholamine metabolism. Based on this evidence, Carlsson suggested that antipsychotic drugs might increase dopamine turnover secondary to a blockade of dopamine receptors. He further hypothesized that this blockade would then lead to an increase in the activity of dopamine-containing cells mediated through an as yet unidentified neuronal feedback pathway. The increase in neuronal activity would thus explain the increase in turnover of the neurotransmitter. Numerous studies using more sophisticated biochemical techniques confirmed Carlsson's original findings that many antipsychotic drugs increase dopamine turnover (Glowinski, Axelrod, and Iversen, 1966; Nybäck, Borzecki, and Sedvall, 1968; Andén, Corrodi, and Fuxe, 1972). In support of Carlsson's feedback hypothesis, both Andén, Corrodi, Fuxe, and Ungerstedt (1971) and Nybäck and Sedvall (1971) demonstrated that an anatomically intact dopaminergic system is essential for the phenothiazines to cause changes in dopamine metabolism. Using X-ray crystallography techniques, Horn and Snyder (1971) have shown that part of the three-dimensional configuration of the chlorpromazine molecule is directly superimposable on the dopamine molecule, lending some credence to Carlsson's hypothesis that dopamine receptors can react with antipsychotic drugs and may be blocked by them. Thus there is extensive evidence that the antipsychotic drugs produce marked changes in dopamine metabolism.

There is evidence suggesting that at least some of the parkinson-like side effects of the antipsychotic drugs are attributable to their effect on the dopamine system. The dopamine-containing cells in the ZC of the substantia nigra are degenerated in Parkinson's disease (Hassler, 1953). From the pioneering work of Hornykiewicz (1963), we know that this degeneration leads to a depletion of dopamine in the neostriatum which in turn is thought to be responsible for at least some of the symptoms of Parkinson's disease (Hornykiewicz, 1963). Many antipsychotic drugs produce very similar symptoms. This is not so surprising if we accept Carlsson's hypothesis that antipsychotic drugs block dopamine receptors. Such a blockade would lead to a functional "depletion" of dopamine in the striatum. Whether there is a drug-induced functional depletion or an actual one as is seen in Parkinson's disease, it is reasonable to believe that the end result would be a common clinical syndrome. It is this kind of reasoning that has led people to suggest that the extrapyramidal side effects of antipsychotic drugs may be mediated through the nigrostriatal dopamine system.

The antipsychotic properties of neuroleptics have also been linked to a part of the dopamine system. In particular it has been suggested that they

may be mediated through their effect on limbic areas innervated by VT dopaminergic neurons (Snyder, 1972; Matthysse, 1973; Stevens, 1973). However, here the evidence is much less conclusive than that for the extrapyramidal site of action of the neuroleptics. The evidence that is available includes
the following:

(1) It has been shown biochemically that two drugs with good antipsychotic properties and little extrapyramidal side effect increase dopamine
metabolite levels to a greater extent in the limbic system than in the striatum
(clozapine, Andén and Stock, 1973; thioridazine, Roth, *personal communication*).

(2) Many amphetamine addicts who develop psychosis display stereotyped compulsive behavior (Ellinwood, 1967). Both the psychosis and
stereotyped behavior are readily reversed by antipsychotic drugs. Known
dopamine-receptor stimulators (amphetamine, apomorphine, L-DOPA)
produce stereotyped behavior in animals (Andén, Rubenson, Fuxe, and
Hökfelt, 1967; Ernst, 1967; Butcher and Engel, 1969; Randrup and Munkvad, 1972) which is thought by some to be the animal concomitant of psychosis in man (Snyder, 1972). Dopamine-receptor blockers (i.e., the antipsychotic drugs) block and reverse stereotyped behavior. McKenzie (1972)
reported that destruction of the nucleus accumbens prevents stereotyped
behavior, whereas destruction of the nucleus caudatus putamen has no effect. Others, however, have published opposite results (Fog, Randrup, and
Pakkenberg, 1970; Naylor and Olley, 1972). If one accepts McKenzie's
findings and extrapolates back to man, amphetamine psychoses may be
caused by increased dopamine-receptor stimulation in the limbic system.
Consequently, its reversal by neuroleptics might be mediated via their action
in the same area.

(3) The fact that antipsychotic drugs have an effect on the dopamine
system in the CNS is well established. It is argued that the antipsychotic
action of neuroleptics must be mediated through their effect on some part
of this system. The nigrostriatal dopamine system appears to be mainly involved in somatic motor mechanisms (Nauta and Mehler, 1966; DeLong,
1971). The tuberoinfundibular dopamine system is mainly concerned with
hormonal control (Martin, 1973). It may, of course, influence behavior indirectly through hormonal mechanisms. The mesolimbic dopamine system,
however, seems a far more likely candidate for the antipsychotic action of
neuroleptics in terms of what little is known about the areas it innervates:
nucleus accumbens, olfactory tubercles, and bed nucleus of the stria termi-
nalis.

Wilson (1972) has demonstrated that these structures are truly part of
the limbic system receiving afferents from the hippocampus, piriform cortex,
and amygdala. Various parts of the limbic system have been shown to be
involved in the production or control of sexual and aggressive behavior,
and implicated in the mediation of punishment and reward. The limbic

areas innervated by the dopamine system therefore make a tempting site of action for at least some of the antipsychotic properties of neuroleptics.

Recently, high levels of dopamine have been reported in the rat cortex which appear to be independent of known norepinephrine innervation of the area (Thierry, Stinus, Blanc, and Glowinski, 1973). Through the use of fluorescence histochemical techniques, dopamine terminals have also been demonstrated in the limbic and frontal cortex (Hökfelt, Ljungdahl, Fuxe, and Johansson, 1974; Lidbrink, Jonsson, and Fuxe, 1974). The location of the dopamine-containing cell bodies which innervate these areas is still unknown. It is highly possible that some of the antipsychotic effects of neuroleptics are mediated through an effect on this system. However, the subcortical limbic dopamine system may still be important here as there are demonstrated connections between this area and the limbic cortex.

Thus we feel that there is substantial evidence linking the site of action of the antipsychotic drugs to the dopamine system — extrapyramidal side effects to the nigrostriatal system and antipsychotic properties perhaps to the mesolimbic dopamine system. In addition, we have been provided with a detailed map of its anatomic location. For these reasons we choose the dopamine system for our model. However, rather than use a biochemical or behavioral approach for the development of our model, we directly measure the effect of drugs on the activity of dopaminergic neurons. The technique we use is extracellular single-unit recording. Briefly, this technique consists of stereotactically lowering microelectrodes into the brain of an anesthetized or paralyzed albino rat. Electrical activity of single dopamine-containing cells is picked up by the electrode and transferred to an oscilloscope and speaker through the use of various amplifiers and filters so that it can be monitored both visually and aurally. At the same time the amplified signal is passed through a rate meter and sent to a recorder where the activity of the cell is recorded in the form of a histogram, each line of which represents the integrated rate of firing expressed as spikes per second.

EXPERIMENTAL EVIDENCE SUPPORTING CHOICE OF DOPAMINE SYSTEM FOR MODEL

Using this technique, we have recently confirmed part of Carlsson's hypothesis. We have found that the systemic administration of many of the antipsychotic compounds including chlorpromazine and haloperidol does indeed cause an increase in the firing rate of dopamine-containing cells in both the ZC and VT areas (Bunney, Walters, Roth, and Aghajanian, 1973) (Fig. 2).

Another drug whose mechanism of action has been attributed to its effect on the dopamine system is *d*-amphetamine. A great deal of biochemical evidence has demonstrated that *d*-amphetamine affects both the dopamine and the norepinephrine system of the brain. *d*-Amphetamine is thought to

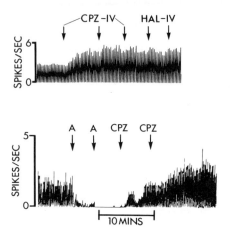

FIG. 2. **Upper:** Effect of chlorpromazine (CPZ) on the firing rate of a ZC dopaminergic cell. Intravenous administration of CPZ in a series of small doses (0.5, 0.5, and 1.0 mg/kg) maximally increases firing rate to double its baseline rate. Once a maximal rate of firing is obtained with CPZ, haloperidol (HAL; 0.1 and 0.5 mg/kg) has no further effect, suggesting that these antipsychotic agents act on the same dopamine receptors. (From Aghajanian and Bunney, 1973.) **Lower:** Antagonism by CPZ of d-amphetamine (A) induced depression of ZC dopaminergic cell activity. d-Amphetamine given intravenously in a total dose of 0.75 mg/kg stopped the cell completely. After CPZ (0.25 and 0.50 mg/kg) was administered intravenously cell firing resumed and increased to above baseline levels. (From Bunney et al., 1973.)

stimulate dopamine receptors indirectly through increasing the release of newly synthesized dopamine from nerve terminals and through blocking its reuptake (Carlsson, Fuxe, Hamberger, and Lindqvist, 1966; Besson, Cheramy, Fletz, and Glowinski, 1971a; Besson, Cheramy, and Glowinski, 1971b; Azzaro, Ziance, and Rutledge, 1974). Thus, through these two actions, d-amphetamine indirectly causes a stimulation of dopamine receptors by making more dopamine available in the synaptic cleft. In 1967, based on biochemical evidence, Corrodi, Fuxe, and Hökfelt hypothesized that increased dopamine-receptor stimulation would cause a decrease in dopamine cell-firing rate mediated through the same type of postsynaptic neuronal feedback pathway suggested by Carlsson in explaining the biochemical effects of antipsychotic drugs. Clinically, amphetamine has gained prominence both as a drug of abuse and as a research tool. Amphetamine, when administered in high doses in both amphetamine addicts and in normal experimental subjects, produces a paranoid psychosis that many feel is indistinguishable from acute paranoid schizophrenia in most cases (Snyder, 1972). Antipsychotic agents useful in the treatment of schizophrenia rapidly reverse the paranoid psychosis induced by amphetamine (Snyder, 1972).

For these reasons it was of interest to determine the effect of amphetamine on the activity of dopaminergic neurons. We found that, in small doses

(0.2 to 1.6 mg/kg, i.v.), amphetamine markedly inhibited both ZC and VT cells for prolonged periods of time, thus confirming Corrodi's hypothesis (Fig. 3). In addition, dopamine-receptor blockers, such as the antipsychotic drugs chlorpromazine and haloperidol, reverse the *d*-amphetamine-induced depression of dopamine cell activity (Fig. 2) (Bunney, Walters, Roth, and Aghajanian, 1973), thus providing a direct parallel with the interaction of these two drugs clinically in man.

In terms of building a predictive model, the above findings are of little significance unless we can show that the ability of chlorpromazine to increase dopamine cell-firing rate and to reverse amphetamine-induced depression of these cells is associated with the clinical properties of this drug. It was possible that a phenothiazine such as promethazine, which lacks antipsychotic properties and extrapyramidal side effects (Klein and Davis, 1969), might have the same effect on dopamine cell-firing rate.

Paralleling previous biochemical studies in which promethazine had no effect on dopamine metabolism (Carlsson and Lindqvist, 1964; Andén, Roos, and Werdinius, 1964*b;* Nybäck et al., 1968), promethazine was found to have no effect on baseline cell activity and did not reverse *d*-amphetamine-induced depression of dopamine cell activity in either the ZC or VT areas (Fig. 4). These findings suggested that the antipsychotic properties and/or extrapyramidal side effects of the phenothiazines are correlated with these drugs' ability to modify dopamine cell activity. However, from the data provided so far, it is impossible to distinguish between these possibilities.

To evaluate further the relationship between clinical effects and effects on firing rate we need to test in our model a phenothiazine which has one clinical property but not the other (e.g., no antipsychotic efficacy but one that can produce extrapyramidal side effects). Mepazine may be such a drug.

If we accept some of the hypotheses and assumptions mentioned earlier regarding the site of action of the antipsychotic properties and extrapyramidal side effects of phenothiazines, we should be able to make predictions about the effect mepazine will have on the activity of dopaminergic neurons in the ZC and VT areas. Since mepazine causes extrapyramidal symptoms and these symptoms are thought to be mediated through an action on the

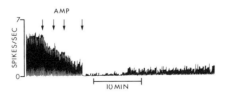

FIG. 3. Typical effect of *d*-amphetamine (AMP) on the activity of dopaminergic cells in the ZC and VT areas. Serial injections of *d*-amphetamine (totaling 2.0 mg/kg, i.v.) progressively depressed cell activity until firing ceased. Recovery was slow—approximately 25% in 30 min. (From Bunney and Aghajanian, 1973.)

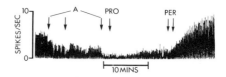

FIG. 4. Effect of promethazine (PRO) on dopamine cell activity subsequent to d-amphetamine (A) depression. d-Amphetamine (1.25 mg/kg, i.v., total dose) depressed unit activity. Promethazine (10 mg/kg, i.p.), a phenothiazine lacking antipsychotic efficacy or extrapyramidal side effects, failed to elicit the usual increase in firing rate induced by antipsychotic phenothiazines. The moderate increase in firing rate seen following promethazine administration is no greater than the spontaneous recovery from amphetamine seen with these cells. However, perphenazine (PER: 0.2 mg/kg, total dose), a clinically active phenothiazine, produced a rapid increase in rate to above baseline levels. (From Bunney et al., 1973.)

nigrostriatal dopaminergic system, we would predict that mepazine would reverse d-amphetamine-induced depression of ZC cell-firing rate. But if, as hypothesized, changes in the firing rate of VT cells are correlated more with the antipsychotic properties of the phenothiazines, mepazine should have no effect on d-amphetamine-induced depression of this cell group. As predicted, when tested for its effect on firing rate, mepazine was found to reverse d-amphetamine-induced depression of dopamine cells in the ZC group but not in the VT area (Bunney and Aghajanian, 1974a). These findings suggest that we may have a model which can be used to differentiate phenothiazines with antipsychotic properties from those lacking clinical efficacy by testing their ability to reverse amphetamine-induced depression of VT dopaminergic neurons.

Since antipsychotic efficacy in a given drug is often accompanied by a moderate to high incidence of extrapyramidal side effects, it would be useful if our model could distinguish between neuroleptics with a high versus low incidence of these side effects. To test the ability of our model system to distinguish between these two groups of drugs, we determined the effect on ZC dopamine cell activity of representatives from each of these two groups. We chose the nigrostriatal dopamine system because it is the one most implicated in the pathogenesis of these symptoms.

Antipsychotic drugs with a moderate to high incidence of extrapyramidal side effects such as chlorpromazine, perphenazine, trifluoperazine, and haloperidol (Klein and Davis, 1969) were found to increase the activity of ZC cells 50 to 100% above baseline rate. In addition they reversed d-amphetamine-induced depression of these cells to above baseline levels (Fig. 2). However, when neuroleptics with a low incidence of extrapyramidal side effects (e.g., thioridazine and clozapine) were tested, they never increased the firing rate of ZC dopamine cells to above baseline even when given in doses 10 times that needed to reverse d-amphetamine depression (Fig. 5). In addition, although they did reverse amphetamine-induced de-

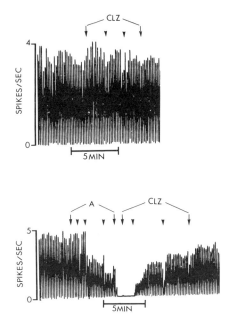

FIG. 5. Effects of clozapine (CLZ) on the firing rate of dopaminergic neurons in the substantia nigra VT (ZC cell group). **Upper:** Clozapine administered intravenously in a total dose of 8 mg/kg had no effect on baseline firing rate. Doses as high as 30 mg/kg, i.v. have been tested on other dopamine cells without effect. These results are in marked contrast to those with chlorpromazine where the average dose needed to increase baseline firing rate 50 to 100% is approximately 2.0 mg/kg. **Lower:** d-Amphetamine (A) (1.6 mg/kg, i.v.) stopped the firing of this dopamine cell. Clozapine given intravenously in a sequence of doses (1.0, 1.0, 2.0) increased unit activity to 50% of baseline rate. However, an additional 6 mg/kg still did not return activity to baseline levels. Chlorpromazine administered after a comparable dose of d-amphetamine would have markedly increased firing rate above baseline in a dose range of 1.5 to 2.0 mg/kg. (From Bunney and Aghajanian, 1974a.)

pression of these cells, they did so only back to baseline and never above. Thus antipsychotic drugs with a moderate to high incidence of extrapyramidal side effects increase ZC cell firing rate above baseline whether given alone or after d-amphetamine. Conversely, antipsychotic drugs with a low incidence of these side effects do not increase ZC cell activity. Therefore, there is a significant difference between drugs with a high versus low incidence of extrapyramidal side effects in terms of their effect on the firing rate of ZC cells. It is important to note, however, that there is no difference between these two groups of drugs in terms of their antipsychotic efficacy or effect on the firing rate of VT dopamine-containing cells.

How does one explain the fact that drugs equally effective as antipsychotic agents can differ markedly in the incidence of extrapyramidal side effects associated with them if both clinical actions are mediated through the DA system of the brain? One possible explanation suggested by the above data is that there may be important pharmacologic differences between dopamine receptors associated with different dopamine pathways (e.g., nigrostriatal versus mesolimbic). However, another possible explanation has recently been suggested. Anticholinergic drugs have been used for many years to treat the extrapyramidal side effects of neuroleptics. Based on "muscarinic receptor" binding studies (Miller and Hiley, 1974; Snyder, Banerjee, Yamamura, and Greenberg, 1974) and dopamine turnover studies (Andén and Stock, 1973), it has been hypothesized that clozapine and thioridazine may have a low incidence of extrapyramidal side effects due to central anticholinergic properties. We have recently shown that neurons in the zona reticulata of the substantia nigra are excited by acetylcholine applied micro-iontophoretically (Aghajanian and Bunney, 1973). This excitatory effect of acetylcholine is readily blocked by low systemic doses of the antimuscarinic drug scopolamine (0.5 to 1.0 mg/kg, i.v.). This block is highly specific in that excitatory responses to glutamate are unchanged by scopolamine. Because zona reticulata neurons show a uniform and marked sensitivity to acetylcholine it was possible to test for the proposed anticholinergic properties of clozapine at this site. Change in glutamate excitation was used as a control for nonspecific effects.

In doses effective in reversing d-amphetamine-induced depression of ZC dopamine neurons (1.0 mg/kg, i.v.) (Bunney and Aghajanian, 1974a), clozapine had little effect on the response of zona reticulata neurons to microiontophoretic actylcholine. However, at higher doses clozapine produced a selective and significant attenuation of acetylcholine excitation (Fig. 6). Glutamate excitation was unaffected by clozapine. Although 50% inhibition of acetylcholine-induced excitation could be achieved with doses of clozapine up to 10 mg/kg (i.v.), total inhibition was difficult to achieve even with much higher doses. On the other hand, scopolamine produced a total as well as selective block of acetylcholine in a dose of 1.0 mg/kg, i.v. Contrastingly, the acetylcholine response was unaffected by haloperidol (an antipsychotic drug with a high incidence of extrapyramidal side effects) even in relatively high doses (1.0 mg/kg, i.v.). Thus clozapine appears to have a weak cholinergic action at this site (Aghajanian and Bunney, 1974). Although lending support to Snyder and Miller's hypothesis, it is as yet unclear whether this weak anticholinergic action of clozapine would be sufficient to account for its low incidence of extrapyramidal side effects.

Whatever the mechanism involved, the difference in response of the ZC dopaminergic neurons to antipsychotic drugs with differing incidence of extrapyramidal side effects suggests that this model system may provide a means for predicting the incidence of extrapyramidal side effects of putative neuroleptics prior to clinical trials in man.

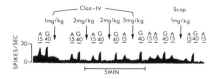

FIG. 6. Effects of intravenous clozapine (Cloz–i.v.) and scopolamine (Scop–i.v.) on the response of a zona reticulata cell to microiontophoretically applied acetylcholine (A) and glutamate (G). Initial responses to A and G are about equal. After a 10 mg/kg cumulative dose of clozapine there is approximately a 50% reduction in the response to A whereas the response to G is undiminished. Scopolamine (1 mg/kg, i.v.) abolishes the response to A. (From Aghajanian and Bunney, 1974.)

PREDICTIONS ON A CLINICALLY UNTRIED PUTATIVE
NEUROLEPTIC

The true test of this predictive system comes when we test a drug as yet untried in man, make predictions as to its antipsychotic efficacy and incidence of extrapyramidal side effects, and then test the drug clinically. We have recently had an opportunity to put our predictive model to this test. For years clinicians have noted that some schizophrenics respond to antipsychotic medication whereas others do not. One of the hypotheses proffered to explain this difference is that there are variations in the way individual patients metabolize antipsychotic drugs. During the last several years evidence has accumulated which suggests that several of the naturally oc-

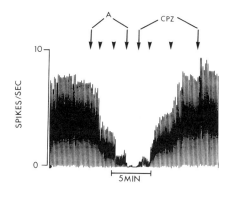

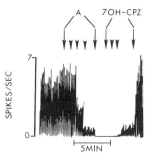

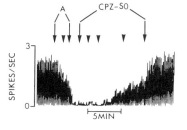

FIG. 7. **Upper:** Antagonism by chlorpromazine (CPZ) of *d*-amphetamine (A) induced slowing of VT dopaminergic neurons. *d*-Amphetamine in a total dose of 1.6 mg/kg (0.2, 0.2, 0.4, 0.8) temporarily stopped this cell. Chlorpromazine in a dose of 0.8 mg/kg (0.2, 0.2, 0.4) returned firing rate to baseline. An additional 0.8 mg/kg had little further effect. **Middle:** Antagonism by 7-hydroxychlorpromazine (7 OH-CPZ) of *d*-amphetamine (A) induced slowing of a VT dopaminergic neuron. *d*-Amphetamine (0.2, 0.2, 0.4, 0.8 mg/kg) stopped this cell. 7-Hydroxychlorpromazine reversed the *d*-amphetamine-induced depression back to baseline at a total dose of 0.8 mg/kg (0.1, 0.1, 0.2, 0.4). **Lower:** Effect of chlorpromazine sulfoxide (CPZ-SO) on VT dopaminergic neurons subsequent to *d*-amphetamine (A) depression. *d*-Amphetamine (0.2, 0.2, 0.4 mg/kg) markedly depressed this cell. Chlorpromazine sulfoxide in a total dose of 64 mg/kg (1.0, 1.0, 2.0, 4.0, 8.0, 16.0, 32.0) returned neuronal activity back to baseline.

All drugs in the three experiments were administered intravenously. (From Bunney and Aghajanian, 1974*b*.)

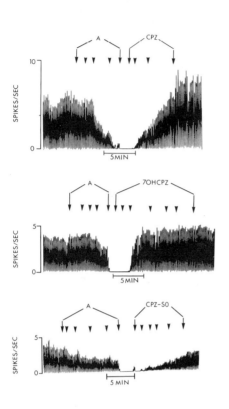

FIG. 8. **Upper:** Antagonism by chlorpromazine (CPZ) of *d*-amphetamine (A) induced slowing of a substantia nigra ZC dopaminergic neuron. *d*-Amphetamine in a total dose of 3.2 mg/kg (0.2, 0.2, 0.4, 0.8, 1.6) temporarily stopped this cell. Chlorpromazine in a total dose of 1.6 mg/kg (0.2, 0.2, 0.4, 0.8) increased firing rate to above baseline level. **Middle:** Reversal of *d*-amphetamine (A) induced depression of a ZC dopaminergic cell by 7-hydroxychlorpromazine (7 OH-CPZ). *d*-Amphetamine in a total dose of 1.6 mg/kg (0.1, 0.1, 0.2, 0.4, 0.8) caused this cell to stop firing. 7-Hydroxychlorpromazine in a total dose of 0.4 mg/kg (0.1, 0.1, 0.2) reversed the *d*-amphetamine-induced depression back to baseline levels. An additional 6.0 mg/kg of 7-hydroxychlorpromazine had no further effect on firing rate. **Lower:** Effect of chlorpromazine sulfoxide (CPZ-SO) on a ZC dopaminergic neuron subsequent to *d*-amphetamine (A) depression. *d*-Amphetamine in a total dose of 3.2 mg/kg (0.1, 0.1, 0.2, 0.4, 0.8, 1.6) stopped this cell temporarily. Chlorpromazine sulfoxide in a total dose of 64 mg/kg (2.0, 2.0, 4.0, 8.0, 16.0, 32.0) failed to return neuronal activity to baseline level. All drugs in the above three experiments were administered intravenously. (From Bunney and Aghajanian, 1974*b*.)

curring metabolites of chlorpromazine are pharmacologically active while others are not. Two metabolites of chlorpromazine (7-hydroxychlorpromazine and chlorpromazine sulfoxide) have been extensively studied in a variety of animal biochemical and behavioral tests. 7-Hydroxychlorpromazine was found to have almost as much activity as its parent compound whereas chlorpromazine sulfoxide was found to be relatively inactive (Manian, Efron, and Goldberg, 1965; Nybäck and Sedvall, 1972; Buckley, Steenburg, Barry, and Manian, 1973; Lal and Sourkes, 1972; Barry, Steenberg, Manian, and Buckley, 1974).

Clinical support for these findings has recently been reported by Sakalis, Chan, Gershon, and Park (1973). They found that four schizophrenics who improved on chlorpromazine therapy had high plasma levels of chlorpromazine and 7-hydroxychlorpromazine whereas four patients who did not respond had high plasma levels of chlorpromazine sulfoxide. Because of the animal and clinical evidence that 7-hydroxychlorpromazine might have antipsychotic properties and that chlorpromazine sulfoxide should not, we decided to test these two chlorpromazine metabolites in our model system and compare their effects with those previously determined for chlorpromazine

(Bunney and Aghajanian, 1974*b*). Small equivalent doses of chlorpromazine and 7-hydroxychlorpromazine were found to reverse readily amphetamine-induced depression of VT dopaminergic neurons (Fig. 7). Chlorpromazine sulfoxide was found to be 50 to 100 times less potent. In contrast to its effect on VT cells, the effect of 7-hydroxychlorpromazine on ZC neurons depressed by *d*-amphetamine was significantly different from that of chlorpromazine. The dose range of 7-hydroxychlorpromazine necessary to reverse completely amphetamine-induced depression was comparable to that of chlorpromazine. However, the final maximal firing rate obtained differed markedly. Thus, the dose of chlorpromazine required to reverse amphetamine-induced depression completely also increased cell activity above baseline (Fig. 8). 7-Hydroxychlorpromazine in doses up to 15 times that necessary to reverse completely amphetamine-induced depression of firing rate did not increase dopamine cell activity above baseline levels (Fig. 8).

From these findings we would predict that 7-hydroxychlorpromazine would have antipsychotic properties and a low incidence of extrapyramidal side effects. Chlorpromazine sulfoxide according to its effect on this model system should be virtually lacking in antipsychotic efficacy. Of course, clinical trials of 7-hydroxychlorpromazine in man will be the final test of our predictions.

SUMMARY

(1) Preliminary evidence suggests that the dopamine systems of the brain may provide a model which can predict antipsychotic efficacy and incidence of extrapyramidal side effects of putative neuroleptics. Specific changes in the firing rate of dopaminergic neurons appear to correlate with the clinical actions of known neuroleptics. These correlations are:

   (a) Antipsychotic drugs reverse the amphetamine-induced depression of dopamine-containing neurons in the midbrain VT area. Drugs lacking antipsychotic effects are inactive in this regard.

   (b) Drugs possessing a high to moderate incidence of extrapyramidal side effects increase the activity of substantia nigra ZC dopaminergic neurons above baseline and reverse amphetamine-induced depression of these cells to above baseline levels. Drugs with a low incidence of extrapyramidal side effects do not increase the firing rate of these cells even in high doses and do not reverse amphetamine-induced depression above baseline.

(2) Based on the above criteria we would predict that one metabolite of chlorpromazine (7-hydroxychlorpromazine) tested in this system would have antipsychotic effects and a low incidence of extrapyramidal side effects whereas another chlorpromazine metabolite (chlorpromazine sulfoxide) would be a poor antipsychotic agent.

(3) Antipsychotic drugs differ markedly in their propensity to cause extrapyramidal side effects. The reason for this is unclear. Preliminary results using microiontophoretic techniques support the suggestion that clozapine may lack these side effects because it has an anticholinergic action.

ACKNOWLEDGMENTS

This research was supported by NIMH Grants MH–17871 and MH–14459, a Scottish Rite Schizophrenia Research Grant, and the State of Connecticut.

REFERENCES

Aghajanian, G. K., and Bunney, B. S. (1973): Central Dopaminergic Neurons: Neurophysiological Identification and Responses to Drugs. In: *Frontiers in Catecholamine Research,* edited by S. H. Snyder and E. Usdin, pp. 643–648. Pergamon Press, Elmsford, N.Y.

Aghajanian, G. K., and Bunney, B. S. (1974): Dopaminergic and Nondopaminergic Neurons of the Substantia Nigra: Differential Responses to Putative Transmitters. In: *Proceed. 9th Internat. Congress of the Collegium Internationale Neuro Psychopharmacologicum,* Excerpta Medica Foundation (*in press*).

Andén, N. E., Carlsson, A., Dahlström, A., Fuxe, K., Hillarp, N. A., and Larsson, N. (1964a): Demonstration and mapping out of nigro-neostriatal dopamine neurons. *Life Sci.,* 3:523–530.

Andén, N. E., Corrodi, H., and Fuxe, K. (1972): Effect of neuroleptic drugs on central catecholamine turnover assessed using tyrosine and dopamine-β-hydroxylase inhibitors. *J. Pharm. Pharmacol.,* 24:177–182.

Andén, N. E., Corrodi, H., Fuxe, K., and Ungerstedt, U. (1971): Importance of nervous impulse flow for the neuroleptic induced increase in amine turnover in central dopamine neurons. *Eur. J. Pharmacol.,* 15:193–199.

Andén, N. E., Roos, B. E., and Werdinius, B. (1964b): Effects of chlorpromazine, haloperidol and reserpine on the levels of phenolic acids in rabbit corpus striatum. *Life Sci.,* 3:149–158.

Andén, N. E., Rubenson, A., Fuxe, K., and Hökfelt, T. (1967): Evidence for dopamine receptor stimulation by apomorphine. *J. Pharm. Pharmacol.,* 19:627–629.

Andén, N. E., and Stock, G. (1973): Effect of clozapine on the turnover of dopamine in the corpus striatum and in the limbic system. *J. Pharm. Pharmacol.,* 25:346–348.

Azzaro, A. I., Ziance, R. J., and Rutledge, C. O. (1974): The importance of neuronal uptake of amines for amphetamine-induced release of ^{3}H-norepinephrine from isolated brain tissue. *J. Pharmacol. Exp. Ther.,* 189:110–118.

Barry, H., III, Steenberg, M. L., Manian, A. A., and Buckley, J. P. (1974): Effects of chlorpromazine and three metabolites on behavioral responses in rats. *Psychopharmacologia,* 34: 351–360.

Besson, M., Cheramy, A., Fletz, P., and Glowinski, J. (1971a): Dopamine: Spontaneous and drug-induced release from the caudate nucleus in the cat. *Brain Res.,* 32:407–424.

Besson, M., Cheramy, A., and Glowinski, J. (1971b): Effects of some psychotropic drugs on dopamine synthesis in the rat striatum. *J. Pharmacol. Exp. Ther.,* 177:196–205.

Buckley, J. P., Steenburg, M. L., Barry, H., III, and Manian, A. A. (1973): Pharmacology of mono- and disubstituted chlorpromazine metabolites. *J. Pharm. Sci.,* 62:715–722.

Bunney, B. S., and Aghajanian, G. K. (1974a): Central Dopaminergic Neurons: A Model for Predicting the Efficacy of Putative Antipsychotic Drugs? In: *Use of Model Systems in Biological Psychiatry,* edited by D. Ingle, MIT Press, Cambridge.

Bunney, B. S., and Aghajanian, G. K. (1974b): A comparison of the effects of chlorpromazine, 7-hydroxychlorpromazine and chlorpromazine sulfoxide on the activity of central dopaminergic neurons. *Life Sci.,* 15:309–318.

Bunney, B. S., and Aghajanian, G. K. (1973): Electrophysiological Effects of Amphetamine on Dopaminergic Neurons. In: *Frontiers in Catecholamine Research,* edited by S. Snyder and E. Usdin, pp. 957–962. Pergamon Press, New York.

Bunney, B. S., Walters, J. R., Roth, R. H., and Aghajanian, G. K. (1973): Dopaminergic neurons: Effect of antipsychotic drugs and amphetamine on single cell activity. *J. Pharmacol. Exp. Ther.*, 155:560–571.

Butcher, L. L., and Engel, J. (1969): Behavioral and biochemical effects of L-DOPA after peripheral decarboxylase inhibition. *Brain Res.*, 15:233–242.

Caldwell, A. E. (1970): History of Psychopharmacology. In: *Principles of Psychopharmacology*, edited by W. G. Clark and G. delGuidise, pp. 9–30. Academic Press.

Carlsson, A., Fuxe, K., Hamberger, B., and Lindqvist, M. (1966): Biochemical and histochemical studies on the effects of imipramine-like drugs and (±)-amphetamine on central and peripheral catecholamine neurons. *Acta Physiol. Scand.*, 67:481–497.

Carlsson, A., and Lindqvist, M. (1963): Effect of chlorpromazine and haloperidol on formation of 3-methoxytryamine and normetanephrine in mouse brain. *Acta Pharmacol. Toxicol.*, 20:140–144.

Corrodi, H., Fuxe, K., and Hökfelt, T. (1967): The effect of some psychoactive drugs on central monoamine neurons. *Eur. J. Pharmacol.*, 1:363–368.

Dahlström, A., and Fuxe, K. (1964): Evidence for the existence of monoamine-containing neurons in the central nervous system. *Acta Physiol. Scand. (Suppl. 62)*, 232:1.

DeLong, M. R. (1971): Activity of pallidal neurons during movement. *J. Neurophysiol.*, 34: 414–427.

Ellinwood, E. H., Jr. (1967): Amphetamine psychosis: I. Description of the individuals and process. *J. Nerv. Ment. Dis.*, 144:273–283.

Ernst, A. M. (1967): Mode of action of apomorphine and dexamphetamine on gnawing compulsion in rats. *Psychopharmacologia*, 10:316–323.

Fog, R. L., Randrup, A., and Pakkenberg, H. (1970): Lesions in corpus striatum and cortex of rat brains and the effect on pharmacologically induced stereotyped, aggressive and cataleptic behavior. *Psychopharmacologia (Berl.)*, 18:346–356.

Glowinski, J., Axelrod, J., and Iversen, L. I. (1966): Regional studies of catecholamines in the rat brain. IV. Effects of drugs on the disposition and metabolism of H³-dopamine. *J. Pharmacol. Exp. Ther.*, 153:30–41.

Hassler, R. (1953): Extrapyramidalmotorische Syndrome and Erkrankungen. In: *Hb. Inn. Med. Vol. 5*, edited by G. V. Bergmann, W. Frey, H. Schwiegk, and R. Jung. Springer-Verlag, Berlin.

Hökfelt, T., Ljungdahl, A., Fuxe, K., and Johansson, O. (1974): Dopamine nerve terminals in the rat limbic cortex: Aspects of the dopamine hypothesis of schizophrenia. *Science*, 184: 177–179.

Horn, A. S., and Snyder, S. H. (1971): Chlorpromazine and dopamine: Conformational similarities that correlate with the antischizophrenic activity of phenothiazine drugs. *Proc. Nat. Acad. Sci. USA.*, 68:2325–2328.

Hornykiewicz, O. (1963): Die topische lokalisation und das Verhalten von Noradrenalin und dopamin-(3-hydroxytryamin) in der substantia nigra des normalin und Parkinsonkraken. *Menschen. Wien. Klin. Wschr.*, 75:309–312.

Klein, D. E., and Davis, J. M. (1969): *Diagnosis and Drug Treatment of Psychiatric Disorders.* Williams and Wilkins, Baltimore.

Lal, S., and Sourkes, T. L. (1972): Effects of various chlorpromazine metabolites on amphetamine induced stereotyped behavior in the rat. *Europ. J. Pharmacol.*, 17:283–286.

Lidbrink, P., Jonsson, G., and Fuxe, K. (1974): Selective reserpine-resistant accumulation of catecholamines in central dopamine neurons after DOPA administration. *Brain Res.*, 67: 439–456.

Manian, A. A., Efron, D. H., and Goldberg, M. E. (1965): A comparative pharmacological study of a series of monohydroxylated and methoxylated chlorpromazine derivatives. *Life Sci.*, 4:2425–2438.

Martin, J. B. (1973): Neural regulation of growth hormone secretion. *N. Engl. J. Med.*, 288: 1384–1393.

Matthysse, S. (1973): Antipsychotic drug actions: a clue to the neuropathology of schizophrenia? *Fed. Proc.*, 32:200–205.

McKenzie, G. M. (1972): Role of the tuberculum olfactorium in stereotyped behavior induced by apomorphine in the rat. *Psychopharmacologia*, 23:212–219.

Miller, R. J., and Hiley, C. R. (1974): Anti-muscarinic properties of neuroleptics and drug induced Parkinsonism. *Nature*, 248:596–597.

Nauta, W. J. H., and Mehler, W. R. (1966): Projections of the lentiform nucleus in the monkey. *Brain Res.*, 1:3–42.

Naylor, R. J., and Olley, J. E. (1972): Modification of the behavioral changes induced by amphetamine in the rat by lesions in the caudate nucleus, the caudate-putamen and globus pallidus. *Neuropharmacology*, 11:91–99.

Nobin, A., and Björklund, A. (1973): Topography of the monoamine neuron systems in the human brain as revealed in fetuses. *Acta Physiol. Scand. (Suppl.)*, 388:1–40.

Nybäck, H., Borzecki, A., and Sedvall, G. (1968): Accumulation and disappearance of catecholamines formed from tyrosine-14C in mouse brain: Effect of some psychiatric drugs. *Eur. J. Pharmacol.*, 4:395–403.

Nybäck, H., and Sedvall, G. (1971): Effect of nigral lesion of chlorpromazine-induced acceleration of dopamine synthesis from 14C tyrosine. *J. Pharm. Pharmacol.*, 23:322–326.

Nybäck, H., and Sedvall, G. (1972): Effect of chlorpromazine and some of its metabolites on synthesis and turnover of catecholamines formed from 14C-tyrosine in mouse brain. *Psychopharmacologia*, 26:155–160.

Olson, L., Nystrom, B., and Seiger, A. (1963): Monoamine fluorescence histochemistry of human post mortem brain. *Brain Res.*, 63:231–247.

Randrup, A., and Munkvad, I. (1972): Influence of amphetamines on animal behavior: Stereotypy, functional impairment and possible animal–human correlations. *Psychiatr. Neurol. Neurochem. (Amsterdam)*, 75:193–202.

Sakalis, G., Chan, T. L., Gershon, S., and Park, S. (1973): The possible role of metabolites in therapeutic response to chlorpromazine treatment. *Psychopharmacologia*, 32:279–284.

Snyder, S. H. (1972): Catecholamines in the brain as mediators of amphetamine psychosis. *Arch. Gen. Psychiatry*, 27:343–351.

Snyder, S. H., Banerjee, S. P., Yamamura, H. I., and Greenberg, D. (1974): Drugs, neurotransmitters and schizophrenia. *Science*, 184:1243–1253.

Stevens, J. R. (1973): An anatomy of schizophrenia? *Arch. Gen. Psychiatry*, 29:177–189.

Thierry, A. M., Stinus, L., Blanc, G., and Glowinski, J. (1973): Some evidence for the existence of dopaminergic neurons in the rat cortex. *Brain Res.*, 50:230–234.

Ungerstedt, U. (1971): Stereotaxic mapping of the monamine pathways in the rat brain. *Acta Physiol. Scand. (Suppl.)*, 367:1–48.

Wilson, R. D. (1972): *The Neural Associations of Nucleus Accumbens Septi in the Albino Rat.* Thesis. Massachusetts Institute of Technology.

DISCUSSION

Gershon: I think we've not only returned to the specific issue of prediction, but we've got more than a promise of a potential way out of the little closed-in black box.

Goldberg: Have you looked at any adrenergic-blocking agents in this system that might be expected to antagonize some of the effects of amphetamine and perhaps agents that might be peripherally active?

Bunney: We have not yet.

Weinryb: It appears that this system does not allow you to distinguish between a dopamine-receptor agonist and a compound that might release dopamine. Dr. Greengard at Yale, using a dopamine-receptor preparation to link with adenylate cyclase, has shown that amphetamine does not act at the dopamine receptor.

Bunney: You mean distinguish between drugs like amphetamine and apomorphine? I think we can, if you agree that *d*-amphetamine preferentially releases newly synthesized dopamine. We have found that pretreatment with the tyrosine hydroxylase inhibitor, alpha methyl paratyrosine, totally abolishes *d*-amphetamine induced depression of dopaminergic cell activity, whereas apomorphine induced depression is unaffected. If the drug's action is dependent upon ongoing dopamine synthesis, then one may be able to distinguish between those two categories.

Weinryb: As a point of interest, have you tried ET-495 (trivastal)?

Bunney: Yes, Dr. Judith Walters and I have tried trivastal and it looks quite similar to apomorphine. Apomorphine and trivastal probably have presynaptic as well as postsynaptic effects, and that is a complicating issue.

Weinryb: There are several of us using the Greengard adenylate cyclase type of preparation and we have not been able to show that trivastal acts at the receptor, but I do see recurring reports in the literature using behavioral models that suggest and conclude that trivastal is acting as a dopaminergic agonist. Your data appear to reinforce that conclusion.

Bunney: Yes. One of the things that is interesting about both apomorphine and trivastal is that a tachyphylaxis develops very rapidly. Thus, the first administration depresses the cell and it comes back after a time. However, if you give it again, you get much less of an effect, and after several doses you get no effect.

Gale: You mentioned the effects of thioridazine and clozapine on nigral cells, but I don't believe you mentioned the effects in comparison to these on the ventrotegmental cells.

Bunney: They both reverse *d*-amphetamine induced depression of both types of cells.

Gale: Do you get the overshoot phenomenon in ventrotegmental cells?

Bunney: I haven't said anything about overshoot in the ventrotegmental cells because the effects of a given drug are variable, and don't seem to correlate with anything. It's only with the zona compacta (ZC) cells that there seems to be a correlation between overshoot and drugs with a high and low incidence of extrapyramidal side effects.

Gale: Do you see an increase in the spontaneous firing rate in the ventrotegmental cells when you give thioridazine or clozapine?

Bunney: There is some, but it is variable.

Gale: Then the comparison between the two systems is not very secure yet?

Bunney: I'm not sure what you mean. We use one system for one thing and one for the other. ZC dopamine-containing cells are useful in our model for predicting incidence of extrapyramidal side effects, whereas ventral tegmental cells are useful for predicting antipsychotic efficacy.

Gershon: Is Dr. Gale saying that trivastal in the cat does not produce stereotypy? Wouldn't that relate to the fact that it does not have a behavioral endpoint that might tend to relate to its dopamine-agonist activity?

Gale: ET-495 is very poor in producing stereotypy in rats. You have to go up to very high doses and it doesn't look like apomorphine behavior at all.

Knill: Have you done any dose-response studies to see whether those agents associated with extrapyramidal side effects are correlated with a return to baseline without the overshoots?

Bunney: Yes, we have. Starting with very low doses and increasing sequentially, there is just no difference. When you finally hit the dose that is effective, it goes over.

Klerman: Can you separate those compounds which have either adrenergic or dopaminergic effects, for example, pimozide, which is thought to be almost exclusively dopaminergic?

Bunney: You can separate them, but one must use a different system. We record from the locus coeruleus and look at the effect of the drugs on the firing rate of those cells and then compare the difference between the locus coeruleus cells and the dopamine cells. In Dr. Roth's lab at Yale, Dr. Walters has done some work along this line. Interestingly enough, what she found was that all of the antipsychotic drugs she tested have very little effect on the activity of the locus coeruleus cells, and although *d*-amphetamine has an equal ability to depress locus cells and dopamine cells (approximately the same dose range), antipsychotic drugs are not very effective in reversing *d*-amphetamine induced depression of these cells.

Klerman: All this is presumed to be due to postsynaptic drug effects. What about looking at drugs with presynaptic effects, like the tricyclic antidepressants as opposed to the tricyclic antipsychotics?

Bunney: They have no effect on the dopamine system, in terms of firing rate. They do not change firing rate. Henrick Nybäck, who is now working in Bob Roth's lab with us, is doing the tricyclic antidepressant studies on the locus at this time and he has found that they are highly effective there.

Klerman: What about compounds like the thioxanthenes which have a modified tricyclic structure and mixed reports as to having both antipsychotic and antidepressant activity?

Bunney: We haven't tried them yet. Someone asked before about differences between *d*- and *l*-amphetamine, in terms of their effect on firing rate. Obviously, an interesting study is to see what the effects of *d*- and *l*-amphetamine are on the ZC dopamine-containing cells versus the noradrenergic locus coeruleus cells. Our data are a little different from Dr. Snyder's. We find that *d*- and *l*-amphetamine are equally potent in depressing dopamine-containing cells, the exact opposite of what one would predict from Dr. Snyder's biochemical studies. So, if you want to put together a hypothesis for schizophrenia, you might have to reverse it and make it the norepinephrine hypothesis, rather than the dopamine.

Domino: This is obviously a very elegant work and Dr. Bunney should be congratulated. My concern is that you're recording from the cell bodies and presumably the action of these drugs is way up there at the nerve endings and presumably far away where the nerve endings are, there are feedback systems that then affect the cell bodies. I know that Dr. Aghajanian got into difficulty with this sort of problem when it came to the LSD story and the raphe neurons, because LSD then started acting on the cell body, whereas it should have acted way up there. My question is, if you remove the business end of these drugs which is supposed to be, for example, in the caudate or in the striatum, will these agents still affect the cell bodies in the same way? In other words, one might record from a dopaminergic neuron in various sites and then remove the terminal end of that system, for example, by lesioning the striatum, the hippocampus, or other areas.

Bunney: I think you are asking if you can determine whether drugs are having a presynaptic effect, as well as a postsynaptic one. There would be a couple of ways of getting at that. One way would be to cut the brain in such a way that any possible neuronal feedback mechanism is eliminated. We've done that to help us study the action of amphetamine and found that severing neuronal feedback pathways blocked very nicely its ability to depress the firing rate of these cells. Another way to get at it is to iontophoretically apply the drug directly to the cell body and see whether it has an effect or not. We've done that with amphetamine. It has no effect. However, apomorphine, when applied directly to dopamine cell bodies in the ZC, continues to inhibit them after all possible neuronal feedback pathways have been cut. That's why we're saying there is evidence for presynaptic effects. When you get to the antipsychotic drugs, microiontophoresis doesn't work too well, because many are quite insoluble, so that is a problem. We have been able to use chlorpromazine to some extent. Chlorpromazine by itself, when so applied to the cell, doesn't do very much. But I don't think that necessarily rules out a *presynaptic* action of these drugs. Of course, there is also a direct way to determine the *postsynaptic* effects of these drugs. One can go to postsynaptic cells (such as the caudate nucleus or accumbens nucleus) where we know there is a good dopamine input and, while recording from them, determine the effect of antipsychotic drugs on their activity. These experiments are currently in progress.

Domino: What about LSD affecting the dopaminergic neuron, etc.? Have you done that?

Bunney: Yes, that was one of our controls – no effect. However, 5HT does seem to have some kind of a modulating effect on the activity of dopamine-containing neurons.

Domino: Will you identify that a little further, since that's going to be a topic of my discussion?

Bunney: Yes. As you know, there's a serotonergic input to the substantia nigra and the question is whether it forms synapses with reticulata cells or with ZC cells. The ZC cells send dendrites way down in the reticulata, so it's especially hard to tell how things are hooked up. If you apply 5HT iontophoretically onto reticulata cells and onto ZC cells, you find that some reticulata cells are somewhat depressed, but there is a mixed response. When you apply 5HT directly to dopamine cells, you get a partial depression of firing rate, but they do not stop completely. You can eject more and more 5HT and you don't get any further effect. This is quite different from other postsynaptic areas in which one iontophoreses 5HT and sees a very nice depression of activity that is dose dependent. ZC cells are exquisitely sensitive to glutamate when you apply it locally. All you have to do is to turn off the retaining current and they speed up tremendously. If you give 5HT and glutamate at the same time, you find that glutamate no longer has much effect on these cells, suggesting that 5HT may actually have a modulating role, although it isn't quite classical in terms of other postsynaptic areas. If that's true, then one would think that LSD ought to have an effect on the activity of these cells. At the doses in which LSD acts presynaptically (in which it turns off the raphe neuron), it doesn't seem to affect dopaminergic cell activity and it does not act as a 5HT agonist. We have not yet been able to reconcile these two findings. Perhaps an effect of 5HT (and LSD) on these cells can be seen only when they are excessively activated.

Wade: You mention that chlorpromazine produces a high percentage increase in firing rate.

Bunney: Yes, 25 to 100%.

Wade: Does that represent a maximum firing rate of the cell?

Bunney: In some cases, but not always.

Wade: Does the firing rate in an undrugged animal remain stable?

Bunney: Yes, quite stable. The interesting thing about dopamine cells is that they speed up with some anesthetics. They go faster with chloral hydrate, so you have to say which preparation you are using. There is no difference, however, in the effect of the drug whether they are paralyzed or whether they are anesthetized, except that in anesthetized animals the cells are going a little faster to begin with, so the amount of increase that you see when you administer a neuroleptic like chlorpromazine or haloperidol to an anesthetized animal won't be quite as great. That's why

I said 25 to 100% increase. In a paralyzed animal we see a 100% increase in rate. In anesthetized animals the cells are already going faster and you usually see only a 25 to 50% increase. There seems to be a ceiling on these cells. They actually go into depolarization block when they get going fast.

Wade: Would this firing rate then possibly represent a definition of psychosis?

Bunney: That is an interesting idea, but I really doubt it.

Ayd: There are several things that happen clinically that I would like you to speculate on, on the basis of your work. I would also like you to tell me if you have given chlorpromazine and then given an antiparkinsonian drug in your test. Ed Domino and I were wondering whether giving the antiparkinsonian drugs blocks some of the phenothiazine effects (even its therapeutic effects).

Bunney: Of course, that's another very interesting question—how do the anticholinergics interact with this whole system? Interestingly enough, a drug like scopolamine used alone doesn't seem to have much effect. It doesn't block the increase in firing rate induced by haloperidol. A drug like benztropine does, but the problem is that benztropine has several effects. It's not only a good anticholinergic, but also probably blocks the uptake of dopamine, so what it may be doing is actually getting more dopamine into the synaptic cleft.

Ayd: Take the patient and give him a particular dose, say 5 mg of haloperidol, and you may get very severe extrapyramidal reactions. You give this same patient 50 mg of haloperidol and you get no extrapyramidal reactions at all. How would you explain this?

Bunney: I find it hard to explain this effect of an increase in dose unless you are starting to affect some other system. I mean, does haloperidol have enough anticholinergic properties, for instance, so that when you push the dose high enough you put the balance back into the system? That would be a possible explanation.

Klerman: That's in part what Steve Matthysse has tried to do and that's probably why thioridazine may not produce so much extrapyramidal effect. Beside the anticholinergic components found in clozapine or thioridazine, can a given compound, as the dose gets higher, produce anticholinergic effects so that the drug is treating its own produced extrapyramidal effects?

Bunney: That is Sol Snyder's work. He has measured, *in vitro*, the antimuscarinic properties of many neuroleptics and suggests that thioridazine and clozapine may not have as many extrapyramidal side effects because they are good anticholinergics. Again, we are very interested in whether or not that's true because, in a sense, what we have been suggesting is a difference between the dopamine receptor in the nigrostriatal system versus the mesolimbic system. But Dr. Snyder's work suggests another alternative—it may be it's just an anticholinergic effect. One way to further investigate this possibility is to record from zona reticulata cells which are quite sensitive to iontophoretic acetylcholine (almost as sensitive as the hippocampal cells, but not quite), and although there has never been a good anatomical demonstration of where the acetylcholine comes from in the reticulata, there do seem to be receptors for it, because they are activated by acetylcholine applied directly. This is a specific effect as the acetylcholine excitation is selectively blocked by intravenous or iontophoretically applied scopolamine. If you record from a zona reticulata cell and you give acetylcholine, you get a marked increase in firing rate. And if you iontophorese glutamate onto the cell, you get a marked increase in firing rate. Now, what happens if you give clozapine i.v. and then try to excite the cell with acetylcholine and glutamate? If clozapine is an anticholinergic, one would expect that the response to acetylcholine would be diminished, but there would be no effect on the glutamate excitation. Glutamate excitation is thus a control for whether it's a specific or non-specific effect. What you find is that if you give clozapine i.v. at about 10 mg/kg, you get a 50% depression of the response. But even 75 mg/kg i.v. has little further effect. Scopolamine, however, totally blocks acetylcholine excitation at 0.5 to 1.0 mg/kg. That doesn't necessarily discount Snyder's theory because you wouldn't want clozapine to have the same effect as scopolamine or it would be toxic at the high doses used clinically. It might be that it just takes enough of the edge off at a low dose. It's going to take a lot more study, I think, before we can really say whether or not its weak anticholinergic properties can account for its low incidence of extrapyramidal side effects.

Goldberg: I would like you to speculate on whether you would expect gamma hydroxybutyrate (GHB) to behave like the phenothiazine in this model.

Bunney: GHB has been studied extensively in this system by Judith Walters working with Dr. Roth in our laboratory complex. What GHB does is to depress these cells. It takes a fair amount of it to do it, but it does depress them. It's not a specific effect as the GHB will depress some other cells – not just dopamine cells. What these findings mean in terms of possible GABAergic inputs to these neurons is not clear.

Gale: On the basis of what you just said and what you said before about the lack of action of scopolamine on the haloperidol effect on the nigral cells, do you want to speculate about this proposed feedback system and what it might be mediated by?

Bunney: I can review the evidence for it. It most likely leads back from the caudate into the substantia nigra and is probably GABAergic. McGeer and others have provided substantial evidence for this. The fact that we get the excitatory responses to acetylcholine that I described certainly says there are probably acetylcholine receptors there also. Whether or not there is a cholinergic interneuron there, or some other cholinergic input from someplace else, we don't know. We have tried, in preliminary experiments, pretreating rats with bicuculline and seeing if it would block the amphetamine induced depression of ZC neurons. In a couple of experiments that we've done that's worked. The trouble is that bicuculline and even picrotoxin are sort of "dirty" drugs. They are not really specific for blocking GABA, so we're planning to try picrotoxin and see if that works also and then maybe we can say more about it.

Predictability in Psychopharmacology: Preclinical and Clinical Correlations, edited by A. Sudilovsky, S. Gershon, and B. Beer. Raven Press, New York © 1975.

The Indole Hallucinogen Model: Is It Worth Pursuing?

Edward F. Domino

Department of Pharmacology, University of Michigan, Ann Arbor, Michigan 48104 and Lafayette Clinic, Detroit, Michigan 48207

In this chapter, I would like to systematically offer evidence that the indole hallucinogen model is worth pursuing in order to find new drugs of possible value in treating schizophrenic patients. Our current antipsychotic drugs are useful during the first year or two of medication, but if they are still of value three, five, or 10 years after being given in the long-term management of schizophrenia is a debatable issue. We desperately need long-term follow-up studies on this point. Nevertheless, it is generally agreed that several classes of neuroleptics including the substituted phenothiazines, thioxanthenes, and butyrophenones are effective antipsychotics. Central dopamine antagonists seem to be especially effective. Most of these compounds have been screened in animals using the amphetamine model of psychosis. This model has provided us with many new drug treatments which vary markedly in potency, duration, and side effects. It is generally recognized that approximately one-third of our schizophrenic patients do not respond favorably to phenothiazine medication. Part of this may be explained on the basis of differences in metabolism between phenothiazine-sensitive and resistant patients as noted by Bunney (*this volume*) in reference to some of the research of Gershon and his associates. However, it may also be that some schizophrenic patients simply do not have a disturbance of dopamine metabolism but instead have a different disease. In fact, Bleuler's characterization of the schizophrenias as a group of diseases should be emphasized. For example, the childhood schizophrenic who becomes an adult is, in many respects, quite a different schizophrenic than the schizophrenic of young adulthood. In line with this is the hypothesis that we are dealing with a variety of different diseases in which neuroleptic-resistant patients represent one type and neuroleptic responders, another. I would like to take the position that some of these patients have a different disease involving a different amine than dopamine. Perhaps instead of a quantitative disturbance in amines (as there might be in depression), there may indeed be a qualitative disturbance in amines in at least some schizophrenic patients.

Current Biologic Theories of Schizophrenia

Some of the current biologic theories of schizophrenia are listed in Table 1. Most will agree that genetic factors are very important. Perhaps the most controversial hypothesis is that involving excess transmethylation. This can lead to a large variety of abnormal phenethylamines like dimethoxy-phenethylamine (DMPEA) or various methylated indoles such as di-methyltryptamine (DMT) and 5-methoxy DMT (5-MODMT). This list could be extended considerably. For example, we now know that the "pink" spot is not just one phenethylamine, but actually eight to 10 different compounds with this particular color and Rf value.

There are two major hypotheses regarding blood protein abnormalities in schizophrenia. Both hypotheses have been severely criticized and, to this day, controversy abounds as to their significance. However, at the Lafayette Clinic, Frohman and Gottlieb have continued to attempt to develop a potential treatment based upon the presence of an abnormal helical conformation of an S protein (S for schizophrenia or stress). The key issue is not if such a protein exists, but rather if it is merely a hemolysin which acts to alter artifactually amine metabolism, particularly of indoles. The treatment approach of these researchers is to isolate, identify, and obtain in large amounts through synthesis an anti-S small polypeptide.

The other blood protein hypothesis is that of Heath and co-workers (1967a,b) regarding a γ-globulin (taraxein) as an autoimmune disease in which the body produces antibodies to brain antigen. Other hypotheses of schizophrenia suggest a disturbance in histamine, zinc and copper metabolism, Mauve factor (kryptopyrole), gluten intolerance, etc. Although additional hypotheses could be added to this list, I'd venture to say that if we were to select a young biochemist who knows absolutely nothing about schizophrenia and say, "We give you six months to go to the medical

TABLE 1. *Current biological theories of schizophrenia*

Genetic
  Recessive
Transmethylation excess
  Abnormal amines
    DMPEA
    DMT
    5-MODMT
Blood Protein Abnormalities
  $\alpha2$ Globulin — S Factor
  γ Globulin — Autoimmune
Histamine Abnormality
Zn/Cu Imbalance
Mauve factor — Kryptopyrole
Gluten intolerance

---

library and read everything you can regarding the biochemistry of schizo-phrenia and then pick the most fruitful area to work in," he might easily come to the conclusion that it's hopeless. Then again he might conclude, "It's all a dopamine abnormality." If we then said, "You can't work on dopamine, it must be something else," I'd predict that our young biochemist would probably work with the indole alkylamines. Why? Because it turns out that of the many substances that are hallucinogenic, the only ones that can apparently be made endogenously are the methylated indole alkyla-mines. This is a basic fact that implies that this area may give rise to po-tential, fruitful research. However, it is first important to ask how well our current drug models of schizophrenia apply to the natural disease.

Models of Schizophrenia

As listed in Fig. 1, patients with the natural mental disorder of schizo-phrenia show a number of primary as well as secondary mental symptoms. The primary symptoms include the four As: autism, ambivalence, dis-turbance of association, and affect. The secondary symptoms include hallucinations and motor and autonomic disturbances. There is a difference if the symptoms of either acute or chronic schizophrenic patients are being discussed. Chronic schizophrenics show especially the primary symptoms, whereas acute schizophrenics have a mixture of both primary and secondary. Acute patients may have especially prominent hallucinations, particularly auditory.

Most psychotomimetic drugs readily mimic the secondary symptoms of schizophrenia. There is no doubt that the best drug model of paranoid schizophrenia is chronic amphetamine.

Primary symptoms of schizophrenia are mimicked rather infrequently in various experimental models of this disease except for sensory and sleep deprivation, and phencyclidine. We've been very interested in the phen-cyclidine model because of its current widespread abuse in the state of Michigan (Domino and Luby, 1973). It should be studied further, particu-

SCHIZOPHRENIA
natural disorder

SCHIZOPHRENIA
model disorder

PRIMARY SYMPTOMS
  Autism
  Ambivalence
  Association
  Affect

SECONDARY SYMPTOMS
  Hallucinations
  Motor
  Autonomic

Amphetamine
Deprivation:
  sleep
  sensory
Phencyclidine

LSD-25
Psilocybin
Mescaline
DMT
Hashish

FIG. 1. Relation of various models of schizophrenia to the natural disorder. The primary symptoms of schizophrenia are best mimicked by chronic amphet-amine, sleep and sensory deprivation, and phencyclidine. The secondary symp-toms of schizophrenia are best mimicked by the hallucinogens.

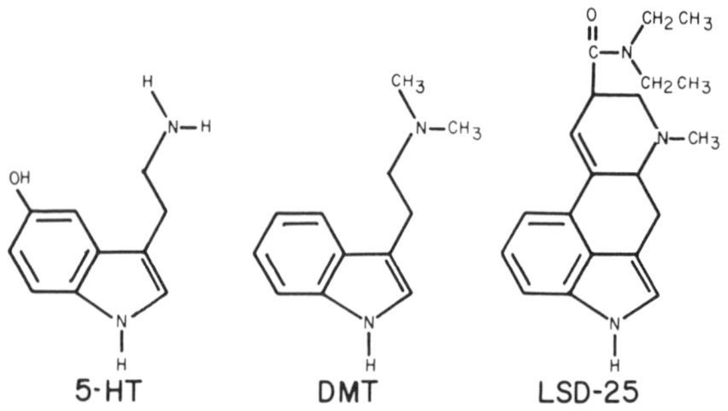

FIG. 2. Structural relations between 5-HT, DMT and LSD-25. Note the similarity of the basic indole ethylamine structure in all three agents.

larly regarding mechanisms and potential antagonists. A large number of well-known hallucinogens mimic the secondary symptoms of schizophrenia. However, as far as I know, only the indole hallucinogens such as DMT and 5-MODMT can be made endogenously in the body. Although LDS-25 cannot be made in the human organism, it is of interest to note the marked structural similarities between serotonin (5-HT), DMT, and LSD-25 (see Fig. 2). One can see in LSD-25 the phenethylamine structure of methamphetamine in the molecule. Hence, I was very interested in Bunney's remarks (*this volume*) that LSD-25 did not act on dopaminergic neurons like amphetamine but acted instead on serotonergic neurons.

Biosynthetic Pathways for Formation of Indole Hallucinogens

As illustrated in Fig. 3, the enzyme systems for making hallucinogenic indoles are present in all of us. Why? Why did nature endow us with the ability to make hallucinogens? Snyder (Snyder, Banarjee, Yamamura, and Greenberg, 1974) reviewed the relationship of neurotransmitters to schizophrenia. In his section dealing with the endogenous formation of hallucinogenic indoles, he suggests that rather than worrying about these compounds in relationship to schizophrenia, we ought to worry about why the synthetic mechanisms are present in us. He feels that perhaps some of the mental changes during stress, instantaneous or religious conversion, isolation in mountains, woods, or on the sea may, in fact, be related to the production of some of these uniquely different kinds of indole alkylamines.

The major source of all indoles is tryptophan (TP). TP is an essential amino acid necessary for proper growth and development. An individual's diet is the major source of TP, although it can be made biosynthetically via chorismate and several intermediates to indole-3-glycerolphosphate and thence to TP. The metabolism of TP is complex. Most of the TP is utilized by cells to form essential proteins. Approximately 1% of the TP is hydroxyl-

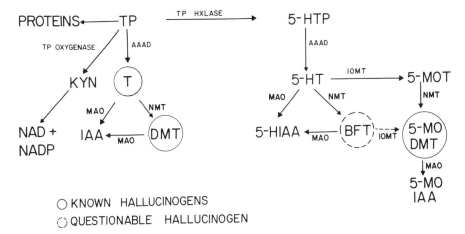

FIG. 3. Formation of hallucinogenic amines from tryptophan metabolism. See text for description and symbols. Most of the TP forms proteins. Only a small percentage is converted to T and 5-HT. Negligible amounts to none of the hallucinogenic substances can be identified although the enzymatic pathways are known.

ated to form 5-hydroxytryptophan (5-HTP). Another portion is converted in the liver by tryptophan oxygenase (L-TP: oxygen oxidoreductase, TP pyrrolase) to form kynurenine (KYN), quinolate and thence nicotinate, the essential vitamin B_3 necessary to form the cofactors nicotinamide adenine dinucleotide (NAD) and nicotinamide adenine dinucleotide phosphate (NADP). A very small portion of TP is decarboxylated by aromatic amino acid decarboxylase (AAAD) to tryptamine (T). The same enzyme also decarboxylates 5-HTP to 5-hydroxytryptamine (5-HT). 5-HT is thought to be an important putative neurotransmitter involved in many bodily functions. In fact, the vast majority of 5-HT is in the GI tract and is necessary for proper GI function. Only a small amount of it is important in brain function. The major 5-HT containing neurons in the brain are in the raphe system of the brainstem. Lesions of the raphe nuclei and surrounding area in animals produce a state of relative insomnia, at least in the cat. There are species differences in this regard, and the relationship of 5-HT to sleep, analgesia, and a variety of other behavioral states is an active area of research. In any event, 5-HT can then be converted to the corresponding aldehyde by type A MAO, and then by aldehyde dehydrogenase to 5-HIAA. This can be removed from the brain by an acid transport system into the circulation, and ultimately via the kidneys through an acid transport system excreted into the urine. A parallel system exists for the synthesis of T, the immediate decarboxylation product of TP. AAAD is not as efficient to form T as it is to form 5-HT from 5-HTP. Nevertheless, there is T in a large variety of species but in lower concentration in the brain than 5-HT itself.

There is evidence that T (Martin and Sloan, 1970), BFT (Fabing, 1956;

Hawkins and Fabing, 1956; Fisher, 1968), and DMT (Szara, 1956, 1957) are hallucinogenic in man. These same substances are constituents of various snuffs taken by certain South American Indian tribes. The evidence, pro and con, that some of these compounds are hallucinogenic as well as proof that they are constituents of various snuffs has been elegantly summarized by Holmstedt and Lindgren (1967). These substances have significant autonomic and motor effects. There is some question as to whether BFT is hallucinogenic (Isbell, 1967). Studies in animals indicate that 5-methoxy DMT (5-MODMT) is more behaviorally toxic than DMT (Gessner and Page, 1962; Benington, Morin, and Clark, 1965; Vasko, Lutz, and Domino, 1974). Hence, 5-MODMT is of special significance. Shulgin (*personal communication*) has data that 5-MODMT is a potent hallucinogen in man. The intoxication produced is qualitatively like DMT but 5-MODMT is more potent. The effective dose is 10 mg, and usually less. The onset of action is within 1 min and is shorter in duration than DMT. Both hallucinogens are ineffective orally and must be given parenterally. The inhalation route is usually employed. The N-homologues (N,N-diethyl and N,N-diisopropyl-5-methoxytryptamine) are less potent as is true of their counterparts without the 5-methoxy group. Again, all of these agents must be given parenterally to be effective.

It is a paradox that nature should provide us with the biosynthetic pathways for making hallucinogenic indoles. Axelrod (1962) first reported the presence of a nonspecific N-methyltransferase (NMT) in rabbit lung capable of forming N-methyltryptamine (NMET) from T and S-adenosylmethionine (SAM), and DMT from NMET and SAM. Both Mandel (1975) and we have shown, by TLC separations, that T is converted primarily to NMET. When NMET is used, it is readily converted to DMT by the rabbit lung enzyme. Amazingly, Axelrod's important observation was not pursued for approximately seven years. Then other investigators observed a similar enzyme as well as a more specific indole amine-N-methyltransferase (INMT) in many tissues of both animals (Morgan and Mandell, 1969; Mandel, Rosenzweig, and Kuehl, 1971; Saavedra and Axelrod, 1972*a*; Thithapandha, 1972; Walker, Ahn, Mandel, and Vanden Heuvel, 1972; Ahn, Walker, Vanden Heuvel, Rosegay, and Mandel, 1973; Hsu and Mandell, 1973; Saavedra, Coyle, and Axelrod, 1973) and man (Heller, 1971; Mandell and Morgan, 1971; Mandel, Ahn, Vanden Heuvel, and Walker, 1972; Narasimhachari, Plaut, and Himwich, 1972; Domino, Krause, and Bowers, 1973; Wyatt, Saavedra, and Axelrod, 1973*c*).

In addition to SAM, 5-methyltetrahydrofolic acid (MTHF) has been reported to be an alternative methyl donor for forming DMT (Banarjee and Snyder, 1973; Hsu and Mandell, 1973). However, Mandel (1975) has been unable to show that it acts as a methyl donor for NMT. Instead, he has shown MTHF methylates 5-HT to 5-methoxytryptamine (5-MOT) and more importantly forms norharmaline analogues. 5-HT could be converted to 5-MOT, and IOMT enzyme could then N-methylate this amine to form 5-MODMT. Mandel and Walker (1974) have demonstrated the synthesis of 5-MODMT through such a mechanism *in vitro* using 5-MOT, SAM, and rabbit or human lung IOMT.

Mandel et al. (1971) reported that INMT from rabbit lung had a K_m for T of 3.3×10^{-4} M and for NMET of 5×10^{-5} M. Mandel et al. (1972) reported that with the purified human lung enzyme NMET had the lowest K_m of several indole amine substrates (2.8×10^{-4} M) and that the products of the reaction, BFT and DMT, were inhibitory. Saavedra et al. (1973) reported that for rat brain NMT the K_m for both T and NMET is 2.8 and 3.7×10^{-5} M and for SAM 5.1×10^{-5} M. Research in our laboratories at the Lafayette Clinic has indicated that K_m for the rabbit lung NMT for T is approximately 7.7×10^{04} M and for NMET 1.5×10^{-4} M. It should be noted that Hsu and Mandell have pointed out that in the presence of MTHF rat brain NMT has a high K_m and hence low enzyme affinity indicating that enzymatic N-methylation only occurs with high amine concentrations. High tissue concentrations of T in the rabbit, at least, are made into DMT *in vivo!* T given intracisternally to rats is converted to NMET as well as to DMT (Saavedra and Axelrod, 1972*a*). Furthermore, Ahn et al. (1973) have shown that the rabbit can make DMT from NMET *in vivo.* It is especially important to note that most researchers agree that in human tissues the enzymatic activity of either the nonspecific NMT or the more specific INMT enzyme is very low. Our own studies using brain tissue obtained from autopsy of deceased chronic schizophrenic, organic brain syndrome, or mentally normal patients who died of various physical causes have been very sobering. We have been able to find only extremely low levels of NMT activity in human brain. Furthermore, we have been unable to find a difference in regional NMT activity among those three groups of patients (Domino et al., 1973). Narasimhachari et al. (1972) reported enhanced NMT activity in the serum of most acute and some chronic schizophrenic patients. Wyatt et al. (1973*c*) have also reported enhanced NMT activity in the platelets of schizophrenic patients compared to mentally normal controls. When the enzyme from both the normal controls and the schizophrenic patients was dialyzed, it showed similar activity, suggesting that the schizophrenic platelets lacked a small dialyzable inhibitor. Demethylated SAM, better known as S-adenosylhomocysteine (SAH), immediately comes to mind as a possibility inasmuch as this agent is a potent NMT inhibitor as discussed below.

It is well known that the amine substrates for the methylated indoles exist in various tissues of animals and man. These include 5-HT (Lewis, 1958; Garattini and Valzelli, 1965) and T (Martin, Sloan, Christian, and Clements, 1972; Saavedra and Axelrod, 1972*b*; Sloan, Martin, Clements, Bridges, and Buchwald, 1974). In addition, living organisms contain adequate levels of the N-methyl donors SAM (Baldessarini and Kopin, 1966;

Gaitonde, 1970) and MTHF (Korevaar, Geyer, Knapp, Hsu, and Mandell, 1973). After the MAO inhibitor isocarboxazid, dog brain and spinal cord T is increased two- to threefold (Martin et al., 1972). Both isocarboxazid and pargyline increase dog blood T as well, but isocarboxazid does not elevate cat brain T levels (Sloan et al., 1974). As described above, Frohman (1973) and Gottlieb and Frohman (1974) have suggested that these bio-synthetic pathways for forming hallucinogenic indoles are excessively utilized in schizophrenic patients with a plasma alpha helical S protein. According to their view this protein facilitates the uptake of TP into cells and hence makes TP more available for all of the synthetic pathways shown in Fig. 3.

The MAO enzymes play a key role in regulating the levels of the various amines. There are two basic families of MAO, the A and B types (Yang and Neff, 1974). The A type MAO oxidizes 5-HT and NE, whereas the B type MAO oxidizes phenethylamine and benzylamine. Amines such as T are oxidized by both types of MAO. Utena, Kanamura, Suda, Nakamura, Machiyama, and Takahashi (1968) determined the regional MAO activity from the brains of five deceased chronic schizophrenic and five cancer patients. They used 5-HT as the substrate; hence they were measuring type A MAO. In the 24 regional brain areas studied they were unable to find any difference between the two groups. However, when the areas were combined into functional brain systems MAO activity from the schizo-phrenic patients was lower in all areas except in the cerebral cortex. Vogel, Orfei, and Century (1969) used T as the substrate to measure both A and B type MAO activity in the brains of two deceased schizophrenic and three other psychiatric patients. These investigators found no differences in MAO activity in the neocortex of all of the patients, but the schizophrenic patients had low MAO activity in the hypothalamus and caudate. The lowered MAO observed in the caudate of the two schizophrenics is partly consistent with an older study of Birkhäuser (1941) who observed that pallidal MAO activity using tyramine as the substrate was enhanced in schizophrenic patients over 60 years old. However, in six patients below 60 years at the time of death, pallidal MAO activity was decreased below normal ($p < 0.052$). In our preliminary studies (Domino et al., 1973) in which T was used as substrate there were no differences in MAO activity in 15 regional brain areas of four deceased mentally normal versus six chronic schizophrenic patients. Similarly, Schwartz, Aikens, Neff, and Wyatt, (1974a) reported that there was no difference in MAO activity during T as substrate in 14 different brain regions of nine schizophrenic and nine men-tally normal individuals. Wise and Stein (1973, 1975) also found normal MAO activity in the brains of deceased schizophrenic patients, but dopa-mine-beta-hydroxylase activity was markedly reduced in all brain areas studied. In addition to the numerous variables associated with studying brain tissue of cadavers there is also an age variable for MAO activity which has been reported to be positively correlated with age (Birkhäuser, 1941; Robinson, Davis, Nies, Colburn, Davis, Bourne, Bunney, Shaw, and Coppen, 1972). Nevertheless, it is reasonable to conclude that there seems to be no significant alteration in schizophrenic brain MAO activity, although more detailed studies using selective type A or B substrates and inhibitors are indicated. Recently, Schwartz, Aikens, and Wyatt (1974*b*) extended their initial studies and characterized human platelet MAO activity as primarily type B. In their studies of autopsied material they showed that both types A and B MAO were found distributed throughout the brain. There were no significant differences in MAO A and B activity between the brains of eight chronic schizophrenics and nine mentally normal individuals. Wyatt et al. (1975) recently reported that in a preliminary study they were unable to confirm the decrease in dopamine-beta-hydroxylase as specific for schizophrenic brains. He suggested that the decrease observed by Wise and Stein was related to time after death for this enzyme is much less stable than MAO.

These predominantly negative results for brain MAO are in marked contrast to the findings that chronic schizophrenic patients as a group have a marked reduction in type B MAO activity in platelets compared to mentally normal controls (Murphy and Wyatt, 1972; Wyatt et al., 1973*b*). The mechanism by which platelet MAO activity is reduced in schizophrenic patients is unclear. It should be noted that normal mono- and dizygotic twins have a high inheritability for platelet MAO activity (Nies et al., 1973). Similarly platelet type B MAO activity in 13 monozygotic twin pairs discordant for schizophrenia have a high correlation of type B MAO activity between twins (Wyatt et al., 1973*b*). Low platelet MAO activity in the schizophrenic twins was mirrored by similarly low activity in their phenotypically normal co-twins. These investigators interpreted their findings that platelet type B MAO activity is associated with a diathesis toward schizophrenia and not secondary in some way to this condition. It seems most crucial to study the MAO activity of other tissues of schizophrenic patients to determine the generality of this deficit in peripheral type B MAO activity. It is not known whether type A or B MAO oxidizes DMT. This has obvious implications for treatments which can facilitate MAO activity and hence may be beneficial for schizophrenic patients.

Are Schizophrenic Patients Walking Hallucinogen Factories?

If the biosynthetic pathways for making hallucinogenic indoles are present in humans, do schizophrenics have such compounds in their body fluids or tissue? Not long ago the answer to this question would have been a qualified "yes" (Franzen and Gross, 1965; Gross and Franzen, 1965; Fisher, 1968; Rosengarten, Szemis, Piotrowski, Romaszewska, Matsumato, Stencka, and Jus, 1970; Narasimhachari, Heller, Spaide, Haskovec, Fujimori, Tabushi, and Himwich, 1971a; Narasimhachari, Heller, Spaide, Haskovec, Meltzer, Strahilevitz, and Himwich, 1971b; Greenberg, 1973; Himwich, Narasimhachari, Heller, Spaide, Haskovec, Fujimori, and Tabushi, 1973; Juntunen, Struck, Warner, Frohman, and Gottlieb, 1974). Now the answer seems a qualified "no" — at least for the majority of schizophrenics because of the recent publications of Mandel (1975) and his associates who used a GC-MS isotope dilution assay specific for DMT (Walker, Ahn, Albers-Schonberg, Mandel, and Vanden Heuvel, 1973; Wyatt, Mandel, Ahn, Walker, and Vanden Heuvel, 1973a; Bidder, Mandel, Ahn, Walker, and Vanden Heuvel, 1974; Lipinski, Mandel, Ahn, Vanden Heuvel, and Walker, 1974; Wyatt, Mandel, Ahn, Walker, and Vanden Heuvel, 1974). Their studies indicate that a large percentage of acute and chronic schizophrenic patients have no significant plasma levels of DMT to the minimum detection level of their assay, which was 0.5 to 1.8 ng/ml of plasma. However, there is a very sobering observation made by these researchers who gave DMT in hallucinogenic doses to mentally normal volunteers (Kaplan, Mandel, Walker, Vanden Heuvel, Stillman, Gillin, and Wyatt, 1974). They were only able to measure very low plasma levels of DMT for a very short time using the same GC-MS assay method, indicating that this hallucinogen disappears from the plasma very rapidly. This finding in man is in agreement with data in rats using a less specific fluorometric method (Cohen and Vogel, 1972). Narasimhachari et al. (1974) reported positive identification of both BFT and DMT in the urine of six drug-free chronic schizophrenic patients placed on a diet low in foods containing preformed indoleamines. The patients showed exacerbations of their symptoms during the drug-free period of 13 weeks in which urines were assayed after the fourth week of their drug holiday. BFT was identified for all six patients using a TLC separation and confirmed by gas chromatography–mass spectrometry. Very low urinary levels of DMT were also found using TLC separation and identification by gas chromatography and mass spectrometry. The base peak at m/e 58 was used primarily for quantification. However, the mass spectra of the DMT standard and a DMT peak urine sample were identical. The fact that a small percentage of schizophrenic patients have detectable plasma or urine levels of DMT indicates that they probably produce endogenously very large amounts of this substance. Investigators who have used chromatographic assays have consistently reported enhanced blood or urine levels of DMT and related indoles (Narasimhachari et al., 1971a,b; Greenberg, 1973; Himwich et al., 1973). It would appear that these latter investigators may be measuring not only DMT but also other amines with similar retention times. The issue of whether schizophrenic patients have enhanced hallucinogen levels is still wide open. It is especially important to measure T, BFT, DMT, and 5-MODMT simultaneously before and during TP, and methionine loading with and without an MAO inhibitor in both normals and schizophrenic patients of all types before this question can be answered definitively.

Perhaps one reason that DMT and related hallucinogenic agents are not readily found in the body fluids and tissue may be related to product feedback inhibition. Both SAH (Lin, Narasimhachari, and Himwich, 1974) and DMT (Krause and Domino, *unpublished observations*) are feedback inhibitors of the NMT enzyme that forms DMT from SAM. It may be very significant that Saavedra et al. (1973) reported that the NMT activity of platelets from schizophrenic patients is greater than those from mentally normal subjects due to the absence of a dialyzable NMT inhibitor. SAH immediately comes to mind as such a possible candidate. We are planning to examine SAH levels in the platelets of schizophrenics and mentally normal controls.

Possible New Therapeutic Approaches

The advantage of the indole hallucinogen model is that it suggests a number of novel treatment approaches for those schizophrenic patients who produce hallucinogenic indoles. These are summarized in Table 2. Inasmuch as TP is an essential amino acid that humans cannot biosynthesize in sufficient quantity, one approach could be to reduce TP intake in selected patients. One of the major problems is to reduce the TP content of the diet to a sufficient degree that would still be palatable and sufficiently nutritious to maintain life. Himwich (1971) has used this approach in the treatment of a few schizophrenic patients. Unfortunately, his low TP diet did not improve the patients. However, no blood TP measurements were done in order to determine how effective the diet was. In addition, one would have to select schizophrenic patients on the basis that they produced hallucinogenic indoles, otherwise a low TP diet would be of little value. The low TP diet seems an especially rational approach in view of its analogy to the low

TABLE 2. *Possible therapeutic measures to treat schizophrenic patients producing an excess of indole hallucinogens*

1. Low TP diet + Nicotinamide
2. Selective competitors with TP for AAAD
3. Enhance TP oxygenase activity
4. Selective inhibitors of NMT and INMT
5. Compounds which trap methyl groups from SAM and MTHF, penetrate BBB, and are pharmacologically inactive
6. Enhance breakdown of indole hallucinogens
   a. MAO
   b. Demethylation
   c. *N*-oxide formation
   d. Hydroxylation (?)
7. Develop a T, DMT, and 5-MODMT antagonist

phenylalanine diet in the treatment of children with phenylketonuria. Of course, nicotinic acid supplements would have to be given to patients on a low TP diet to prevent pellagra. It is of interest that many schizophrenic patients eat very poorly during an exacerbation of their illness. Whether this makes the mental disturbance worse or is beneficial to the patient is not known. It is a fact that acute schizophrenics have plasma TP levels significantly below normal (Gilmour, Manowitz, Frosch, and Shopsin, 1973; Manowitz, Gilmour, and Racevskis, 1973; Domino and Krause, 1974). As the acute patients recover in the hospital, plasma TP levels gradually return toward normal. Manowitz et al. (1973) pointed out that acute schizophrenic patients had normal plasma phenylalanine and tyrosine levels at a time when plasma TP was reduced. They concluded that the selective decrease in TP could not be due to starvation but they did not do a food deprivation control to rule this out. It is well known that during periods of starvation and stress (e.g., prisoners held in concentration camps or patients undergoing severe weight reducing diets) there is an increased incidence of psychoses. Mentally normal people with severe dietary restrictions and great stress would presumably have low plasma TP levels in addition to low levels of many other important nutrients as well. Our present knowledge does not allow us to decide conclusively if selective low TP intake in schizophrenic patients would be beneficial therapy. Obviously, such a therapeutic approach would be relatively simple and could surely be justified on grounds of its potential merit. However, one must be certain that the patient is an indole hallucinogen producer and that blood TP measurements be taken to insure a proper low TP intake.

As previously discussed, four major enzymes are involved in the biosynthesis of hallucinogenic indoles. AAAD is responsible for the decarboxylation of TP to T. Normally very low levels of brain T are present but after a MAO inhibitor the levels of T increase two- to threefold but there are marked species differences as mentioned earlier (Martin, 1972; Sloan et al., 1974). AAAD is also involved in the decarboxylation of 5-HTP to 5-HT. There are much higher levels of 5-HT than T in the brain, so, apparently, 5-HTP is a much more effective substrate than TP for AAAD. The use of synthetic TP derivatives such as alpha-methyltryptophan would be an interesting approach to reduce brain levels of T and 5-HT. The rationale would be analogous to that of alpha-methyl DOPA as a competing substrate for L-DOPA. Alpha-methyltryptophan has been shown to cause a prolonged decrease in brain 5-HT (Sourkes, 1971). A similar reduction in brain T would be expected. This agent also induces TP oxygenase activity in the liver which would further shunt TP away from the synthesis of hallucinogenic indoles. Selective 5-HTP supplements might be necessary to maintain brain 5-HT at reasonable levels. One of the disadvantages of alpha-methyltryptophan is that probably alpha-methyltryptamine would accumulate as a false neurotransmitter. Inasmuch as alpha-methyltryptamine is psychotoxic in both man (Murphree, Dippy, Jenney, and Pfeiffer, 1961) and animals (Vasko et al., 1974), the limiting factor to this therapeutic approach would be its accumulation in the brain.

Since T and 5-HT are substrates of both a nonspecific NMT and a more specific INMT, another approach would be to find selective inhibitors of these enzymes. An important clue is the fact that SAH and DMT are product inhibitors of the NMT from rabbit lung (Krause and Domino, *unpublished observation*). As shown in Fig. 4, SAH is an especially potent inhibitor of the rabbit lung enzyme as was first shown by a medical student, Ms. Bonnie Smith, and a premedical student, Mr. Laurence Domino, working in my laboratory at the University of Michigan in the summer of 1972. Since then, Lin, Narasimhachari, and Himwich (1973) have described further kinetics of SAH inhibition. It is known that SAH also inhibits a wide variety of methyltransferase reactions including phenethanolamine *N*-methyltransferase (PNMT) which catalyzes the methylation of norepinephrine to epinephrine (Deguchi and Barchas, 1972), catechol-*O*-methyltransferase (COMT) which methylates norepinephrine to normetanephrine (Coward, D'Urso-Scott, and Sweet, 1972; Deguchi and Barchas, 1972), acetylserotonin *O*-methyltransferase (IOMT) which forms melatonin (Deguchi and Barchas, 1972), nicotinamide *N*-methyltransferase which forms *N*-methylnicotinamide (Swiatek, Simon, and Chao, 1973), SAM-homocysteine-*S*-methyltransferase which forms methionine (Shapiro, Almenas, and Thomson, 1965), glycine methyltransferase which forms sarcosine (Kerr, 1972), histamine *N*-methyltransferase which forms *N*-methylhistamine (Zappia, Zydek-Cwick, and Schlenk, 1969), and tRNA methyltransferase which forms methylated polynucleotides (Kerr, 1972). Methylation of DNA which involves SAM as the methyl donor has been suggested as playing a role in switching off genes when their need in development is over (Adams, 1973). SAH should be studied as an inhibitor of this methylation reaction.

In view of the lack of specificity of SAH as a methyltransferase inhibitor *in vitro* it probably is fairly toxic *in vivo*. However, I do not know of any data on the pharmacology and toxicology of SAH. There would be no great

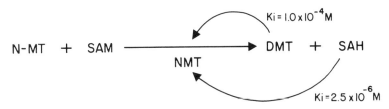

FIG. 4. Dimethyltryptamine and especially *S*-adenosylhomocysteine are product inhibitors of *N*-methyltransferase. Using rabbit lung enzyme, the Kis of both DMT and SAH were determined. Note that SAH is an especially potent feedback inhibitor.

harm to the patient if PNMT and COMT were inhibited. Inhibition of IOMT would reduce melatonin levels which would not be too crucial for man and would be beneficial because 5-MODMT would not be formed. Since methionine is already in the diet, its formation *in vivo* from homocysteine does not seem important nor does the *N*-methylation of histamine. The only systems which might be adversely affected by inhibition are the methylation of tRNA and DNA, but we need data to support this assumption. Even if SAH were active *in vivo* and not toxic, one would still be concerned about its stability (for it is enzymatically broken down) (Deguchi and Barchas, 1972) as well as its absorption and penetration through cell membranes and the blood-brain barrier. Furthermore, SAH is extremely expensive. It is therefore unlikely that it can be tested in animals for toxicity and specificity of inhibition of methylations *in vivo* in the near future. It is important to find more specific derivatives of SAH and related compounds that are effective NMT inhibitors. Lin et al. (1974) reported that the brains of several animal species, human brain and blood, and bovine pineal gland contain two substances which appear to be small peptides with molecular weights of 600 (I, minor) and 500 (II, major). It is especially important to pursue these findings for they indicate that other endogenous inhibitors beside SAH are present which inhibit NMT. Should INMT be selectively inhibited these substances would indeed be a major breakthrough toward new treatment approaches. It is intriguing that Bigelow (1974) has used pineal extracts in the successful treatment of some schizophrenics. Could it be they contain NMT inhibitors? Synthetic cogeners of such peptides as well as SAH and DMT would be of considerable interest to test as potential selective NMT inhibitors and, if nontoxic, as therapeutic agents. We are actively pursuing this approach in our laboratory at the Lafayette Clinic.

   The use of nicotinic acid and nicotinamide in large doses as treatments for schizophrenia was based on their ability to be *N*-methylated and hence to trap excess methyl groups (Hoffer, Osmond, Callbeck, and Kahan, 1957). Baldessarini (1967) has been unable to show that nicotinamide lowers SAM levels in the rat brain. This would be expected for nicotinamide should not readily penetrate the blood-brain barrier because of its charged form at pH 7.4. The megavitamin approach using this substance unfortunately has not proved effective in the treatment of schizophrenia as reported by the American Psychiatric Association task force on megavitamins (Lipton, Ban, Kane, Mosher, and Wittenborn, 1973) and by Lehman, Ban, and Ananth (1973) in Canada. Nevertheless, the approach of using alternate substrates for trapping methyl groups is still valid. Some agents which lower tissue SAM levels (e.g., chlorpromazine) are antipsychotic whereas others (e.g., L-DOPA, imipramine, and pargyline) apparently make schizophrenic patients worse. No simple correlation exists. Nevertheless this approach is most intriguing. Schatz, Diez Altares, and Sellinger (1973) and Schatz, Ashcraft, and Sellinger (1974) have shown that L-methionine sulfoximine depresses rat brain SAM levels. Perhaps this may explain the curious finding of Heath, Nesselhof, and Timmons (1966) that D,L-methionine-*d,l*-sulfoximine in doses which produce psychotic symptoms and EEG changes in control subjects cause a significant diminution of psychotic symptoms and no EEG changes in chronic schizophrenics. However, because a compound reduces brain SAM levels does not mean it will be of value in schizophrenics; a reduction in SAM levels can be due to many different mechanisms. For example, SAM synthesis may be reduced, or SAM utilization enhanced. Furthermore, toxic methylated metabolites may be formed. Although L-methionine sulfoximine depresses brain SAM, it apparently does not do this by decreased SAM synthesis. Instead brain histamine methyltransferase and COMT activity are enhanced. Schatz et al. (1974) suggested that the convulsant actions of methionine sulfoximine may be related to the formation of seizure-inducing methylated products.

Another approach for more effective treatments of schizophrenia would be to enhance the breakdown of hallucinogenic indoles. Most of the hallucinogenic indoles are tertiary amines. Only T is a primary amine. The MAO enzymes are involved in their breakdown. Hence MAO inhibitors should enhance DMT effects. However, Sai-Halász (1963) showed that subjects given 100 mg of iproniazid/day for four days followed by a two-day drug-free period had remarkably few hallucinations and an attenuation of the DMT effect when given DMT on the seventh day. The volunteers did have an odd feeling of a changed personality following DMT which resembled the schizophrenic *wahnstimmung* which precedes the outbreak of a psychosis. In addition, Sai-Halász (1962*a,b*) showed that *l*-methyl-D-lysergic acid butanolamide (Deseril®), a 5-HT antagonist, accentuated the experimental psychosis induced by DMT. This investigator felt that by elevating 5-HT brain levels one would protect against DMT hallucinations whereas blocking 5-HT would enhance the effects of DMT. It is of interest that Wyatt, Vaughan, Galanter, Kaplan, and Green (1972) reported that the administration of 5-HTP to some schizophrenic patients had a beneficial effect. Unfortunately, this was not consistent or reproducible in all schizophrenic patients indicating a heterogeneity of disease types. There is an obvious discrepancy between the human studies of Sai-Halász and the findings from our own laboratory using animal models of DMT effects. For example, DMT-induced depression of rat shuttle box acquisition is potentiated by iproniazid (Domino and Lutz, *unpublished observation*). This is shown by a shift to the left in the dose-effect curve of DMT in suppressing one-way acquisition. Similarly, in rats trained for a FR_4 milk reward, single doses of iproniazid potentiate the suppression of DMT-induced bar pressing (Kovacic and Domino, 1973). Pretreatment with iproniazid enhances rat brain and liver levels of DMT (Fig. 5; Lu, Wilson, Moore, and Domino, 1974). In addition, DMT-induced hyperthermia and pupillary dilatation in the rabbit is also prolonged by iproniazid (Moore, Demetriou, and

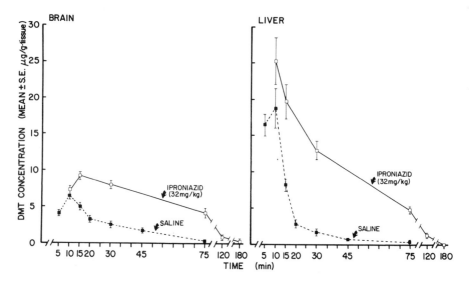

FIG. 5. Pretreatment with iproniazid elevates and prolongs rat brain and liver DMT concentrations. In groups of six to eight rats given 10 mg/kg of DMT i.p., a dose of 32 mg/kg i.p. of iproniazid given the day before markedly enhances and prolongs the tissue concentration of DMT compared to 0.9% NaCl (saline). (From Lu et al., 1974.)

Domino, *unpublished observation*). From these animal findings it would appear that one pathway for the biodegradation of DMT is through MAO. *In vitro* DMT is a very poor substrate for MAO compared to T (Domino and Krause, *unpublished observation*). However, iproniazid *in vivo* appears to be far better in prolonging rat brain and liver levels of DMT than would be expected from *in vitro* studies.

These results do not rule out a prior demethylation of DMT to T before oxidation by MAO. This possibility is being pursued in our laboratory using demethylase inhibitors. If MAO is important for biotransforming DMT in man, it becomes most intriguing that platelet MAO activity is reduced in schizophrenic patients as discussed above.

There are several other theoretical pathways by which DMT and related indole hallucinogens can be biotransformed. These include demethylation, N-oxide formation, and hydroxylation. In view of the essential role of the liver microsomal enzymes in these metabolic reactions, it would be of considerable interest to study the effects of inhibitors of drug metabolism such as SKF-525A, or liver microsomal enzyme inducers such as phenobarbital on the behavioral effects of DMT as well as on tissue levels of this substance. Perhaps by selectively enhancing the breakdown of DMT and related indoles one might be able to develop a novel treatment.

Another approach is to find better DMT antagonists. Although there is evidence that LSD-25 and DMT do not involve identical mechanisms, it is pertinent to ask what are clinically effective LSD and DMT antagonists. Years ago, Marrazzi and Hart (1957) showed that chlorpromazine antagonized the effects of LSD-25 on the transcallosal pathway of the cat. I could never quite understand why, in an emergency situation, chlorpromazine is not a very good antagonist of LSD-25. You talk a patient down instead of giving an antagonist! To a pharmacologist, it is fundamentally repulsive to talk down a patient instead of giving a drug antagonist. I would like to argue that chlorpromazine and related phenothiazines are not good antagonists of LSD. The issue these days is did a patient even take LSD-25 or something else such as DOM? I've been impressed by a statement that Aghajanian made to me years ago that chlorpromazine was not a good antagonist of LSD-25 either in man or in his raphe neuron rat preparation. Although chlorpromazine antagonizes the hyperthermia, pupillary dilatation, and behavioral excitation of DMT in the rabbit, other neuroleptic agents with more selective anti-5-HT actions such as methiothepin (Monachon, Burkard, Jalfre, and Haefely, 1972) are more effective (Moore et al., *unpublished observations*). DeFrance, Kitai, McCrea, and Yosihara (1975) also found methiothepin to antagonize the effects of DMT on the cat hippocampal-septal circuit. It is important to study other more selective antagonists of indole hallucinogens. Such studies are currently proceeding in our laboratory.

To my knowledge the only potent agent that antagonizes DMT blockade of the lateral geniculate is methiothepin. Furthermore, it antagonizes rabbit hyperthermia induced by DMT. It seems as though methiothepin is something new among neuroleptic agents. Although it is a dopamine and norepinephrine antagonist, there is evidence that it is a 5-HT antagonist as well (Lloyd and Bartholini, 1974).

I would like to suggest that various drug companies ought to determine the best DMT models in animals to find potential DMT antagonists. The real problem is that the rat, cat, and rabbit might be completely different from man. In our own laboratories we observed that a wide variety of MAO inhibitors potentiate various endpoints of DMT effect in animals and yet Sai-Halász (1963) notes that iproniazid antagonizes DMT in man.

One can again ask the same question as when we started. Is the indole hallucinogen model worth pursuing? Are you a gambler? If you are, and I think the drug companies have to be, instead of getting another "me too" dopamine antagonist, how about a selective DMT antagonist instead?

REFERENCES

Adams, R. L. P. (1973): Delayed methylation of DNA in developing sea urchin embryos. *Nature (New Biol.)*, 244:131, 27–29.
Ahn, H. A., Walker, R. W., Vanden Heuvel, W. J. A., Rosegay, A., and Mandel, L. R. (1973): Studies on the *in vivo* biosynthesis of N,N-dimethyltryptamine (DMT) in the rabbit and rat. *Fed. Proc.*, 32:511.

Axelrod, J. (1962): The enzymatic N-methylation of serotonin and other amines. *J. Pharmacol. Exp. Ther.*, 138:28–33.

Baldessarini, R. J. (1967): Factors influencing S-adenosyl methionine levels in mammalian tissue. In: *Amines and Schizophrenia*, edited by H. E. Himwich, S. S. Kety, and J. R. Smythies, pp. 199–207. Pergamon Press, New York.

Baldessarini, R. J., and Kopin, I. J. (1966): S-Adenosylmethionine in brain and other tissues. *J. Neurochem.*, 13:769–777.

Banarjee, S. P., and Snyder, S. H.: Methyltetrahydrofolic acid mediates N- and O-methylation of biogenic amines. *Science*, 182:74–75.

Benington, F., Morin, R. D., and Clark, L. C. (1965): 5-Methoxy N,N-dimethyltryptamine, a possible endogenous psychotoxin. *Ala. J. Med. Sci.*, 2:397–403.

Bidder, T. G., Mandel, L. R., Ahn, H. S., Vanden Heuvel, W. J. A., and Walker, R. W. (1974): Blood and urinary dimethyltryptamine in acute psychotic disorders. *Lancet*, 1:165.

Bigelow, L. B. (1974): Effects of acqueous pineal extract in chronic schizophrenia. *Biol. Psychiatry*, 8:1.

Birkhäuser, H. (1941): Cholinesterase und maono-aminoxydase im zentralen nervensystem. *Schweiz. Med. Wochenschr.*, 71:750–752.

Cohen, I., and Vogel, W. H. (1972): Determination and physiological disposition of dimethyltryptamine and diethyltryptamine in rat brain, liver and plasma. *Biochem. Pharmacol.*, 21:1214–1218.

Coward, J. K., D'Urso-Scott, M., and Sweet, W. D. (1972): Inhibition of catechol-O-methyltransferase by S-adenosylhomocysteine and S-adenosylhomocysteine sulfoxide, a potential transition-state analog. *Biochem. Pharmacol.*, 21:1200–1203.

DeFrance, J. F., Kitai, S. T., McCrea, R. A., and Yosihara, H. (1975): Effects of N,N-dimethyltryptamine (DMT) on the hippocampal-septal circuit and antagonism by methiothepin (*in preparation*).

Deguchi, T., and Barchas, J. (1972): Inhibitions of transmethylations of biogenic amines by S-adenosylhomocysteine. *J. Biol. Chem.*, 246:3175–3181.

Domino, E. F., Krause, R. R., and Bowers, J. (1973): Various enzymes involved with putative neurotransmitters—regional distribution in the brain of deceased mentally normal, chronic schizophrenics or organic brain syndrome patients. *Arch. Gen. Psychiatry*, 29:195–201.

Domino, E. F., and Krause, R. R. (1974): Plasma tryptophan tolerance curves in drug free normal controls, schizophrenic patients and prisoner volunteers. *J. Psychiatr. Res.*, 10: 247–261.

Domino, E. F., and Luby, E. D. (1973): Abnormal mental states induced by phencyclidine as a model of schizophrenia. In: *Psychopathology and Psychopharmacology*, edited by J. O. Cole, A. Friedhoff, and A. M. Friedman, Chapter 3, pp. 35–50. Proc. 62 Meeting of Amer. Psychopath. Assoc., Johns Hopkins Press, Baltimore.

Fabing, H. D. (1956): On going berserk: A neurochemical inquiry. *Am. J. Psychiatry*, 113: 409–415.

Fisher, R. (1968): Chemistry of the brain. *Nature (Lond.)*, 220:411.

Franzen, Fr. and Gross, H. (1965): Tryptamine, N,N-dimethyltryptamine, N,N-dimethyl-5-hydroxytryptamine and 5-methoxytryptamine in human blood and urine. *Nature (Lond.)*, 206:1052.

Frohman, C. E. (1973): Plasma proteins and schizophrenia. In: *Biological Psychiatry*, edited by J. Mendels, pp. 131–148. John Wiley and Sons, New York.

Gaitonde, M. K. (1970): Sulfur amino acids. In: *Handbook of Neurochemistry*, edited by A. Lajtha, Vol. 3, Chapter 8, pp. 225–285. Plenum Press, New York.

Garattini, S., and Valzelli, L. (1965): *Serotonin*, pp. 392. Elsevier Publishing Co., Amsterdam.

Gessner, P. K., and Page, I. H. (1962): Behavioral effects of 5-methoxy N,N-dimethyltryptamine, other tryptamines and LSD. *Am. J. Physiol.*, 203:167–172.

Gilmour, D. G., Manowitz, P., Frosch, W. A., and Shopsin, B. (1973): Association of plasma tryptophan levels with clinical change in female schizophrenic patients. *Biol. Psychiatry*, 6:119–128.

Gottlieb, J. S., and Frohman, C. E. (1974): Towards a biologic mechanism in schizophrenia. In: *Biological Mechanisms of Schizophrenia and Schizophrenia-like Psychoses*, edited by H. Mitsuda and T. Fukuda, pp. 154–166. Igaku Shoin Ltd., Tokyo.

Greenberg, R. (1973): N,N-Dimethylated and N,N-diethylated indoleamines in schizophrenia. In: *Chemical Modulation of Brain Function—A Tribute to J. E. P. Toman*, edited by H. C. Sabelli, pp. 277–296. Raven Press, New York.

Gross, V. H., and Franzen, F. (1965): Zur bestimmung korpereigener amine in biologischen substraten. *Z. Klin. Chem.,* 3:99–102.

Hawkins, R., and Fabing, H. D. (1965): Intravenous bufotenine injection in human beings. *Science,* 123:886–887.

Heath, R. G., and Krupp, I. M. (1967a): Schizophrenia as an immunologic disorder. I. Demonstration of antibrain globulins by fluorescent antibody techniques. *Arch. Gen. Psychiatry,* 16:1.

Heath, R. G., Krupp, I. M., Byers, L. W., and Liljekvist, J. I. (1967b): Schizophrenia as an immunologic disorder. II. Effects of serum protein fractions on brain function. *Arch. Gen. Psychiatry,* 16:10.

Heath, R. G., Nesselhof, W., Jr., Bishop, N. P., and Byers, L. W. (1965): Behavioral and metabolic changes associated with administration of tetraethylthiuram disulfide. *Dis. Nerv. Syst.,* 26:99–106.

Heath, R. G., Nesselhof, W., Jr., and Timmons, E. (1966): D,L-Methionine-d,1-sulfoximine effects in schizophrenic patients. *Arch. Gen. Psychiatry,* 14:213–217.

Heller, B. (1971): N-Methylating enzyme in blood of schizophrenics. *Psychosomatics,* 12:273–274.

Himwich, H. E. (Ed.) (1971): *Biochemistry, Schizophrenias and Affective Illnesses,* pp. 500. Williams and Wilkins Co., Baltimore.

Himwich, H. E., Narasimhachari, N., Heller, B., Spaide, J., Haskovec, L., Fujimori, M., and Tabushi, K. (1973): Biochemical approaches to the study of schizophrenia. In: *Chemical Modulations of Brain Function—A Tribute to J. E. P. Toman,* edited by H. E. Sabelli, pp. 297–311. Raven Press, New York.

Hoffer, A., Osmond, H., Callbeck, M. J., and Kahan, I. L. (1957): Treatment of schizophrenia with nicotinic acid and nicotinamide. *J. Clin. Exp. Psychopathol.,* 18:131–158.

Holmstedt, B., and Lindgren, J. B. (1967): Chemical constituents and pharmacology of South American snuffs. In: *Ethnopharmacologic Search for Psychoactive Drugs,* edited by D. H. Efron, pp. 339–382. Publication No. 1645, Public Health Service, Washington, D.C.

Hsu, L. L., and Mandell, A. J. (1973): Multiple N-methyltransferases for aromatic alkylamines in brain. *Live Sci.,* 13:847–858.

Isbell, H. (1967): Quoted In: *Ethnopharmacologic Search for Psychoactive Drugs,* edited by D. H. Efron, p. 369. Publication No. 1645, Public Health Service, Washington, D.C.

Kaplan, J., Mandel, L. R., Walker, R. W., Vanden Heuvel, W. J. A., Stillman, R., Gillin, J. C., and Wyatt, R. J. (1974): Blood and urine levels of N,N-dimethyltryptamine following administration of psychoactive dosages to human subjects. *Psychopharmacologia (Berl.),* 38:239–245.

Kerr, S. J. (1972): Competing methyltransferase systems. *J. Biol. Chem.,* 247:4248–4252.

Korevaar, W. C., Geyer, M. A., Knapp, S., Hsu, L. L., and Mandell, A. J. (1973): Regional distribution of 5-methyltetrahydrofolic acid in brain. *Nature (New Biol.),* 245:244–245.

Kovacic, B., and Domino, E. F. (1973): Effects of various drugs on DMT-induced disruption of rat bar pressing behavior. *The Pharmacologist,* 15:218.

Lehman, H. E., Ban, T. A., and Ananth, J. V. (1973): Nicotinic acid and the transmethylation hypothesis of schizophrenia. In: *Psychopathology and Psychopharmacology,* edited by J. O. Cole, A. Friedhoff, and A. M. Friedman, Chapter 14, pp. 219–230. Proc. 62 Meeting of Amer. Psychopath. Assoc., Johns Hopkins Press, Baltimore.

Lewis, G. P. (Ed.) (1958): *5-Hydroxytryptamine,* pp. 253. Pergamon Press, London.

Lin, R. L., Narasimhachari, N., and Himwich, H. E. (1973): Inhibition of indolethylamine-N-methyltransferase by S-adenosylhomocysteine. *Biochem. Biophys. Res. Commun.,* 54:751–759.

Lin, R., Narasimhachari, N., and Himwich, H. E. (1971): Specific endogenous inhibitors for indolethylamine-N-methyltransferase. *Trans. Am. Soc. Neurochem.,* 5:156.

Lipinski, J., Mandel, L. R., Ahn, H. S., Vanden Heuvel, W. J. A., and Walker, R. W. (1974): Blood dimethyltryptamine concentrations in psychotic disorders. *Biol. Psychiatry,* 9:1,89–91.

Lipton, M. A., Ban, T. A., Kane, Levine, J., Mosher, L. R., and Wittenborn, R. (1973): Megavitamin and orthomolecular therapy in psychiatry. A report of the APA Task Force on vitamin therapy in psychiatry. Task Force Report 7, July American Psychiatric Association, Washington, D.C.

Lloyd, K. G., and Bartholini, G. (1974): The effect of methiothepin on cerebral monoamine neurons. In: *Advances in Biochemical Pharmacology, Vol. 10, Serotonin—New Vistas—*

Histochemistry and Pharmacology, edited by E. Costa, G. L. Gessa, and M. Sandler. Raven Press, New York.

Lu, L. J., Wilson, A. E., Moore, R. H., and Domino, E. F. (1974): Correlation between brain N,N-dimethyltryptamine (DMT) levels and bar pressing behavior in rats: Effect of MAO inhibition. *The Pharmacologist,* 16:237.

Mandel, L. R. (1975): Dimethyltryptamine: Its biosynthesis and possible role in mental disease. In: *Neurotransmitter Balances Regulating Behavior,* edited and published by E. F. Domino and J. Davis. Ann Arbor.

Mandel, L. R., and Walker, R. W. (1974): The biosynthesis of 5-methoxy-N,N-dimethyltryptamine *in vitro. Life Sci.,* 15:1457–1463.

Mandel, L. R., Ahn, H. S., Vanden Heuvel, W. J. A., and Walker, R. W. (1972): Indoleamine-N-methyltransferase in human lung. *Biochem. Pharmacol.,* 21:1197–1200.

Mandel, L. R., Rosenzweig, S., and Kuehl, F. A., Jr. (1971): Purification and properties of indoleamine-N-methyltransferase. *Biochem. Pharmacol.,* 20:712–716.

Mandell, A. J., and Morgan, M. (1971): Indole(ethyl)amine N-methyltransferase in human brain. *Nature (Lond.),* 230:85–87.

Manowitz, P., Gilmour, D. G., and Racevskis, J. (1973): Low plasma tryptophan levels in recently hospitalized schizophrenics. *Biol. Psychiatry,* 6:109–118.

Marrazzi, A. S., and Hart, E. R. (1957): An electrophysiological analysis of drugs useful in psychotic states. In: *Tranquilizing Drugs,* edited by H. E. Himwich, p. 9. A.A.A.S., Washington, D.C.

Martin, W. R., and Sloan, J. W. (1970): Effects of infused tryptamine in man. *Psychopharmacologia (Berl.),* 18:231–237.

Martin, W. R., Sloan, J. W., Christian, S. T., and Clements, R. H. (1972): Brain levels of tryptamine. *Psychopharmacologia (Berl.),* 24:331–346.

Monachon, M. A., Burkard, W. P., Jalfre, M., and Haefely, W. (1972): Blockage of central 5-hydroxytryptamine receptors by methiothepin. *Naunyn Schmiedebergs Arch. Pharmacol.,* 274:192–197.

Morgan, N., and Mandell, A. J. (1969): Indole (ethyl) amine N-methyltransferase in the brain. *Science,* 165:492–493.

Murphree, H. B., Dippy, R. H., Jenney, E. H., and Pfeiffer, C. C. (1961): Effects in normal man of α-methyltryptamine and α-ethyltryptamine. *Clin. Pharmacol. Ther.,* 2:722–726.

Murphy, D. L., and Wyatt, R. J. (1972): Reduced monoamine oxidase activity in blood platelets from schizophrenic patients. *Nature (Lond.),* 238:225–226.

Narasimhachari, N., Baumann, P., Pak, H. S., Carpenter, W. T., Locchi, A. F., Hokanson, L., Fujimori, M., and Himwich, H. E. (1974): Gas chromatographic–mass spectrometric identification of urinary bufotenin and dimethyltryptamine in drug-free chronic schizophrenic patients. *Biol. Psychiatry,* 8:293–305.

Narasimhachari, N., Heller, B., Spaide, J., Haskovec, L., Fujimori, M., Tabushi, K., and Himwich, H. E. (1971a): Urinary studies of schizophrenics and controls. *Biol. Psychiatry,* 3: 9–20.

Narasimhachari, N., Heller, B., Spaide, J., Haskovec, L., Meltzer, H., Strahilevitz, M., and Himwich, H. E. (1971b): N,N-Dimethylated indoleamines in blood. *Biol. Psychiatry,* 3: 21–23.

Narasimhachari, N., Plaut, J. M., and Himwich, H. E. (1972): Indole ethylamine-N-methyltransferase in serum samples of schizophrenics and normal controls. *Life Sci.,* 11:221–227.

Nies, A., Robinson, D. S., Lamborn, K. R., and Lampert, R. P. (1973): Genetic control of platelet and plasma monoamine oxidase activity. *Arch. Gen. Psychiatry,* 28:834–838.

Robinson, D. S., Davis, J. M., Nies, A., Colburn, R. W., Davis, J. N., Bourne, H. R., Bunney, W. E., Shaw, D. M., and Coppen, A. J. (1972): Ageing, monoamines and monoamine-oxidase levels. *Lancet,* 1:290–291.

Rosengarten, H., Szemis, A., Piotrowski, A., Romaszewska, K., Matsumato, H., Stencka, K., and Jus, A. (1970): N,N-Dimethyltryptamine and bufotenin in the urine of patients with chronic and acute schizophrenic psychoses. *Psychiatr. Pol.,* 4:519–521.

Saavedra, J. M., and Axelrod, J. (1972a): Psychotomimetic N-methylated tryptamines: Formation in brain *in vivo* and *in vitro. Science,* 172:1365–1366.

Saavedra, J. M., and Axelrod, J. (1972b): A specific and sensitive enzymatic assay for tryptamine in tissues. *J. Pharmacol. Exp. Ther.,* 182:363–369.

Saavedra, J., Coyle, J. R., and Axelrod, J. (1973): The distribution and properties of the non-specific N-methyltransferase in brain. *J. Neurochem.,* 20:743–752.

Sai-Halász, A. (1962*a*): The effect of antiserotonin on the experimental psychosis induced by dimethyltryptamine. *Experientia (Basel),* 18:137–138.

Sai-Halász, A. (1962*b*): The role of serotonin antagonism in the model-psychoses. *Iddeggyog-Szle (Hung.),* 15:301–305.

Sai-Halász, A. (1963): The effect of MAO inhibition on the experimental psychosis induced by dimethyltryptamine. *Psychopharmacologia (Berl.),* 4:385–388.

Schatz, R., Ashcraft, E. A., and Sellinger, O. Z. (1974): The elevation by methionine sulfoximine of rat brain histamine methyltransferase and catechol-O-methyltransferase activity. *Trans. Am. Soc. Neurochem.,* 5:184.

Schatz, R., Diez Altares, M. C., and Sellinger, O. Z. (1973): Effect of methionine (MET) and methionine sulfoximine (MSO) on rat brain S-adenosyl methionine (SAM). *Trans. Am. Soc. Neurochem.,* 4:74.

Schwartz, M. A., Aikens, A. M., Neff, N. H., and Wyatt, R. J. (1974*a*): MAO activity in brains from schizophrenics and others. New Research Abstracts, p. 26, May. American Psychiatric Association Annual Meeting, Detroit.

Schwartz, M. A., Aikens, A. M., and Wyatt, R. J. (1974*b*): Monoamine oxidase activity in brains from schizophrenic and mentally normal individuals. *Psychopharmacologia,* 38: 319–328.

Shapiro, S. K., Almenas, A., and Thomson, J. F. (1965): Kinetics and mechanism of reaction of S-adenosylmethionine: Homocysteine methyltransferase. *J. Biol. Chem.,* 240:2512–2518.

Sloan, J. W., Martin, W. R., Clements, T. C., Bridges, S. R., and Buchwald, W. F. (1974): Brain levels of tryptamine (T) in the cat, dog, guinea pig and rat. *Fed. Proc.,* 33:468.

Snyder, S. H., Banarjee, S. P., Yamamura, H. I., and Greenberg, D. (1974): Drugs, neurotransmitters, and schizophrenia. *Science,* 184:4143,1243–1253.

Sourkes, T. L. (1971): *Alpha*-methyltryptophan and its actions on tryptophan metabolism. *Fed. Proc.,* 30:897–903.

Swiatek, K. R., Simon, L. N., and Chao, K. -L. (1973): Nicotinamide methyltransferase and S-adenosylmethionine: 5¹-methylthioadenosine hydrolase. Control of transfer ribonucleic acid methylation. *Biochemistry,* 12:4670–4674.

Szara, S. (1956): Dimethyltryptamine: Its metabolism in man, the relation of its psychotic effect to serotonin metabolism. *Experientia (Basel),* 12:441–442.

Szara, S. (1957): The comparison of the psychotic effect of tryptamine derivatives with the effects of mescaline and LSD-25 in self-experiments. In: *Psychotropic Drugs,* edited by S. Garattini and V. Ghetti, pp. 460–467. Elsevier Publishing Co., Amsterdam.

Thithapandha, A. (1972): Substrate specificity and heterogeneity of N-methyltransferase. *Biochem. Biophys. Res. Commun.,* 47:301–308.

Utena, H., Kanamura, H., Suda, S., Nakamura, R., Machiyama, Y., and Takahashi, R. (1968): Studies on the regional distribution of monoamine oxidase activity in the brains of schizophrenic patients. *Proc. Jap. Acad.,* 44:1078–1083.

Vasko, M., Lutz, M. P., and Domino, E. F. (1974): Structure activity relations of some indole-alkylamines in comparison to phenethylamines on motor activity and acquisition of avoidance behavior. *Psychopharmacologia (Berl.),* 36:49–58.

Vogel, W. H., Orfei, V., and Century, V. (1969): Activities of enzymes involved in the formation and destruction of biogenic amines in various areas of human brains. *J. Pharmacol. Exp. Ther.,* 165:195–203.

Walker, R. W., Ahn, H. W., Mandel, L. R., and Vanden Heuvel, W. J. A. (1972): Identification of N,N-dimethyltryptamine as the product of an *in vitro* enzymatic methylation. *Anal. Biochem.,* 47:228–234.

Walker, R. W., Ahn, H. S., Albers-Schonberg, G., Mandel, L. R., and Vanden Heuvel, W. J. A. (1973): Gas chromatographic–mass spectrometric isotope dilution assay for N,N-dimethyltryptamine in human plasma. *Biochem. Med.,* 8:105–113.

Wise, C. D., and Stein, L. (1973): Dopamine-β-hydroxylase deficits in the brains of schizophrenic patients. *Science,* 181:344–347.

Wise, C. D., and Stein, L. (1975): Evidence of a central noradrenergic deficit in schizophrenia. In: *Neurotransmitter Balances Regulating Behavior,* edited and published by E. F. Domino and J. Davis. Ann Arbor.

Wyatt, R. J., Vaughan, T., Galanter, M., Kaplan, J., and Green, R. (1972): Behavioral changes of chronic schizophrenic patients given L 5-hydroxytryptophan. *Science,* 177:1124–1126.
Wyatt, R. J., Mandel, L. R., Ahn, H. S., Walker, R. W., and Vanden Heuvel, W. J. A. (1973a): Gas chromatographic–mass spectrometric isotope dilution determination of N,N-dimethyl-tryptamine concentrations in normals and psychiatric patients. *Psychopharmacologia (Berl.),* 31:265–270.
Wyatt, R. J., Mandel, L. R., Ahn, H. S., Walker, R. W., and Vanden Heuvel, W. J. A. (1974): DMT – a possible relationship to schizophrenia. Proc. 1st Int. Serotonin Conference. *Adv. Biochem. Pharmacol.,* 11:299–313.
Wyatt, R. J., Murphy, D. L., Belmaker, R., Donnely, D., Cohen, S., and Pollin, W. (1973b): Reduced monoamine oxidase activity in platelets: a possible genetic marker for vulnerability to schizophrenia. *Science,* 179:916–918.
Wyatt, R. J., Saavedra, J. M., and Axelrod, J. (1973c): A dimethyltryptamine (DMT) forming enzyme in human blood. *Am. J. Psychiatry,* 130:754–760.
Yang, H. Y. T., and Neff, N. H. (1974): The monoamine oxidases of brain: Selective inhibition with drugs and the consequences of the metabolism of the biogenic amines. *J. Pharmacol. Exp. Ther.,* 189:733–740.
Zappia, V., Zydek-Cwick, C. R., and Schlenk, F. (1969): The specificity of S-adenosylmethionine derivatives in methyl transfer reactions. *J. Biol. Chem.,* 244:4499–4509.

DISCUSSION

Fink: All the substances on the last slide supposedly block DMT. One of them, an MAO inhibitor, can activate schizophrenic symptoms. We gave MAO inhibitors and produced a flagrant increase in their psychosis. Maybe we don't know what the biochemistry was, but, if anything, the clinical experience of MAO inhibition in schizophrenics who are passive, withdrawn, and apathetic produces a florid, delusional, hallucinatory, excited kind of patient.

Domino: I am well aware of that observation. It fits with our thinking. Every MAO inhibitor that we tried in animals potentiated and prolonged the behavioral toxicity of DMT, including various physiologic endpoints like hypertension. What doesn't fit (and that is really the message that I wanted to convey) is the finding of Sai-Halász that iproniazid for four days, and three days later DMT, antagonized DMT hallucinations in man. This does not fit our animal model and needs to be repeated. If it is true, it means that the endogenous hallucinogen is not DMT. From every other point of view, the clinical observation that MAO inhibitors enhance the symptoms of schizophrenia fits beautifully with the indole hallucinogen model.

Fink: In laboratory studies of excitement produced in schizophrenic patients by administration of LSD, intravenous administration of chlorpromazine would block the LSD excitement state in a matter of 4 to 8 min.

Domino: Some time ago, I asked Dr. Aghajanian if he had ever found an agent that antagonizes LSD inhibition of raphe, specifically chlorpromazine. His answer was negative. It doesn't work in the rat. Furthermore, only very large doses of chlorpromazine antagonize DMT depression in the lateral geniculate.

Fink: I don't know about the raphe. I know about the patients.

Domino: The sympathomimetic effects of LSD are antagonized in patients by chlorpromazine. The issue is that not all of the effects of LSD are antagonized by our present neuroleptics which are more effective as dopamine antagonists.

Predictability in Psychopharmacology: Preclinical and Clinical Correlations, edited by A. Sudilovsky, S. Gershon, and B. Beer. Raven Press, New York © 1975.

Biochemically Identified Receptors in the Design of New Psychotropic Drugs*

Solomon H. Snyder

Departments of Pharmacology and Experimental Therapeutics and Psychiatry and the Behavioral Sciences, Johns Hopkins University School of Medicine, Baltimore, Maryland 21205

For many years new drugs have been developed by the rather loosely coordinated activities of chemists and pharmacologists. The chemists synthesized vast numbers of potential drugs based more or less on structures known to possess therapeutic activity. However, there is no detailed structure-activity analysis in the synthesis of series of agents, primarily because of limitations in methods employed for pharmacologic evaluation of the drugs. Specifically, drugs are generally screened in whole animal systems after administration usually by the oral route. Screening tests employed are those which have empirically been shown to correlate with pharmacologic potency in man. There may or may not exist a demonstrated relationship between biochemical or physiologic mechanisms affected by the drugs in the animals and the clinical effects of the drug in man.

One of the strongest rationales for using the approach described above is the general experience in the drug industry over the years that seemingly more sophisticated and painstaking approaches are no more, and probably less, effective. The most dramatic pharmacologic actions of drugs often involve systems for which the drug was not designed initially; it seems as if most therapeutic breakthroughs are unplanned accidents. If this is the case, the most intelligent approach to drug development should certainly involve a systematic plan to take advantage of happenstances, a programmed serendipity.

The prevalence of systematic serendipity in new drug development as opposed to more purely rational approaches can be attributed primarily to our general ignorance of the precise molecular mechanisms of drug action. Biochemical effects which correlate with drug activity usually do not seem to involve the precise focus of drug activity but simply some secondary effect which "correlates" and represents a biochemical screen as opposed to an *in vivo* pharmacologic screen. In a few cases where biochemical mechanisms are apparent, they have provided extremely efficient means for pre-

---

* Paper presented by K. Taylor.

cise development of more potent agents. For instance, the understanding that the monoamine oxidase-inhibiting antidepressants might exert their therapeutic effects by inhibiting monoamine oxidase enabled scientists to perform a straightforward enzyme assay evaluation of potential drugs. Similarly, the fact that tricyclic antidepressants inhibit biogenic amine uptake has provided a straightforward system to evaluate new agents. However, for a vast number of important psychotropic drugs, such approaches have not been feasible.

In the last few years, it has been possible to identify biochemically the receptor sites for several neurotransmitters and for opiates in the brain. A direct *in vitro* analysis of the influence of many drugs on these receptors has provided new insight into certain mechanisms of drug activity. A direct evaluation of the effects of drugs on the molecular receptor whereupon the therapeutic actions of the drug are exerted affords a means for developing new psychotropic drugs logically and rationally. In the short as well as the long run, this approach probably has much greater commercial potential than the traditional approach to drug evaluation. First, to screen a drug one need not synthesize large quantities. Less than 1 milligram would suffice for screening a new chemical's effects on 10 or 20 different brain receptors. Instead of synthesizing vast numbers of compounds based solely on simplicity of synthesis, the chemist might coordinate his activities more closely with the biochemist and systematically develop drugs according to apparent optimal "fit" to the receptor. When drugs are screened by *in vivo* tests, this approach is not possible, because differential metabolism and variable penetration to the receptor site obfuscate the variations in drug potency which are determined strictly by receptor affinity. With the molecular approach, if a particular agent is active at the receptor, it should be far simpler to systematically develop other compounds with vastly increased potency than when *in vivo* screens are the pharmacologic endpoint.

As an example of how receptor research can be applied profitably to new drug development, research related to the opiate receptor, the glycine receptor, and the muscarinic cholinergic receptor will be described. The differential actions of opiate agonists and antagonists on the opiate receptor provide a valuable screen for agonist-antagonist analgesics which have less addictive potential than conventional analgesics. Interactions of benzodiazepines with the glycine receptor appear to predict the therapeutic actions of these agents. The relative affinities of phenothiazines for the muscarinic cholinergic receptor in the brain predict the incidence of extrapyramidal side effects of phenothiazines.

THE OPIATE RECEPTOR

Because of the common properties of a large number of opiates, it has generally been assumed that opiates exert their therapeutic effects by interacting with selective receptor sites in the brain. Numerous investigators have attempted to identify opiate receptors by measuring the binding of radioactive opiates to brain tissue. However, in most cases the nonspecific binding was so great that no selective interactions could be demonstrated. Based on the suggestion of Goldstein, Lowney, and Pal (1971) that a simple preliminary criterion for specific opiate receptor binding is stereospecificity, we identified binding of ^{3}H-naloxone to brain tissue which represents an interaction with the pharmacologically relevant opiate receptor (Pert and Snyder, 1973a,b). These findings were confirmed independently (Simon, Hiller, and Edelman, 1973; Terenius, 1973) and subsequently (Hitzemann and Loh, 1973; Klee and Streaty, 1974). The stereospecific criterion is important because the analgesic effects of opiates are highly stereospecific, elicited by (−) but not by (+) isomers. However, because stereospecific binding can occur to biologic and nonbiologic substances unrelated to the opiate receptor (in our laboratory we have observed stereospecific binding to glass filters), it was important to show that a wide range of opiates bind to the receptor with affinities paralleling their pharmacologic activity and that nonopiates have negligible affinity for the receptor (Table 1).

The opiate receptor assay is simple, sensitive, and specific and has enabled us to answer many important questions about how opiates act. For instance, we showed that there are marked regional differences in opiate receptor binding in the monkey and man (Kuhar, Pert, and Snyder, 1973) as confirmed in man by Hillman, Pearson, and Simon (1973). The distribution of the opiate receptor through the brain parallels the medially located paleospinothalamic and spinoreticular pathways which are thought to regulate affective components of pain responses. These are also the areas in which morphine implantation most effectively induces analgesia. Such areas include the periaqueductal grey, the medial nuclei of the thalamus, the hypothalamus, and other areas of the limbic system. Clearly detailed analysis of regional variations in opiate receptor binding may greatly elucidate the physiology of pain.

Subcellular localization studies enabled us to demonstrate that the opiate receptor is most enriched in synaptosomal, nerve ending fractions of brain homogenates. After hypotonic lysis of synaptosomes, the opiate receptor binding is recovered primarily in synaptic membrane fractions. This is consistent with speculations that opiate effects occur at synapses (Pert, Snowman, and Snyder, 1974).

Detailed studies of chemical features of the opiate receptor may pave the way for its purification and isolation. The opiate receptor is exquisitely sensitive to protcolytic enzymes and to certain phospholipases (Pasternak and Snyder, 1974).

Of greatest importance for the thesis of this chapter is the fact that the opiate receptor assay is highly reproducible and that the affinity of opiates for the receptor correlates closely with their pharmacologic activity. How-

TABLE 1. *Effects of sodium on inhibition by opiate agonists and antagonists of stereo-specific ^{3}H-naloxone binding to rat brain homogenates*

| Nonradioactive opiates | ED$_{50}$ of stereospecific ^{3}H-naloxone binding (nM) | | ED$_{50}$ ratio +NaCl/−NaCl |
	No NaCl	100 mM NaCl	
GPA 2163	100	20	0.2
Naloxone	1.5	1.5	1.0
Naltrexone	0.5	0.5	1.0
Diprenorphine	0.5	0.5	1.0
Cyclazocine	0.9	1.5	1.7
Levallorphan	1.0	2.0	2.0
Nalorphine	1.5	4.0	2.7
Etonitazene	1.0	3.0	3.0
Pentazocine	15	50	3.3
Etorphine	0.5	6.0	12
Phenazocine	0.6	8.0	13
Meperidine	3,000	50,000	17
Levorphanol	1.0	15	15
Methadone	7.0	200	28
Oxymorphone	1.0	30	30
Morphine	3.0	110	37
Dihydromorphine	3.0	140	47
Normorphine	15	700	47
(±)-Propoxyphene	200	12,000	60

Inhibition of stereospecific ^{3}H-naloxone binding was determined in the presence and absence of 100 mM NaCl for 14 nonradioactive opiates, employing 100 nM (+)- and (−)-3-hydroxy-N-allylmorphinan to assess specificity. Rat brain with cerebellum removed was homogenized (Polytron PT-10, 3000 rev/min) in 100 volumes of 0.05 M Tris buffer and centrifuged at 40,000 g for 10 min. After the supernatant fluid (which contains no specific binding) was discarded, the pellet was reconstituted in the original volume of Tris buffer. Seven to 10 concentrations of each drug were incubated with 1.5 nM ^{3}H-naloxone in the presence and absence of 100 mM NaCl. The concentration of drug that produced 50% inhibition of control stereospecific binding (ED$_{50}$) was determined by log probit analysis. Control ^{3}H-naloxone binding values in the absence and presence of 100 mM NaCl (0.05 M Tris-HCl buffer, pH 7.4 at 37°C) were 1,163 ± 104 and 2,806 ± 198 counts/min, respectively, at 44% counting efficiency.

ever, to simply predict the potency of opiates themselves is not especially crucial. There are more than enough available opiates. The aim in development of new drugs is to obtain relatively nonaddicting analgesics. The closest approximation to such drugs involves agents combining opiate agonist and antagonist activities.

The existence of opiate antagonists is one of the most dramatic aspects of opiate pharmacology. Antagonists are usually obtained by small chemical modifications, specifically the conversion of the *N*-methyl substituent of opiates to *N*-allyl, *N*-cyclopropylmethyl, or similar groups. Because of their chemical similarity, one might expect opiate antagonists to compete molecule-for-molecule with the opiates. However, the antagonists are much more potent than opiate agonists themselves. Small doses of antagonists can reverse the effects of 10 to 100 times greater doses of opiates.

Some opiate antagonists, such as naloxone and naltrexone, are "pure" antagonists, which possess no agonist activity, eliciting neither analgesia nor euphoria. Other opiate antagonists are "mixed." For instance, the first clinically utilized opiate antagonist nalorphine (Nalline®) antagonizes the actions of morphine but can itself elicit analgesia. Nalorphine has never been employed widely to treat pain because, like any other mixed agonist-antagonists, it elicits anxiety and psychotomimetic effects at doses not much greater than those required to produce analgesia. However, some agonist-antagonist opiates can relieve pain without psychotomimetic side effects at clinically utilized doses. The best example is the benzomorphan pentazocine (Talwin®). Pentazocine and other agonist-antagonist drugs are less capable of inducing physical dependence than pure opiate agonists and therefore offer genuine promise as relatively nonaddicting analgesics. Traditional pharmacologic screens have been ineffective in identifying such drugs. Agents such as pentazocine do not behave as analgesics in screening tests such as the hot plate test and are only detected in other analgesic tests. Moreover, their antagonist properties are difficult to demonstrate rigorously *in vivo* in animals. The opiate receptor assay affords probably the most reliable and rigorous means of identifying agonist-antagonists. In addition, their relative agonist and antagonist properties can be quantified, providing us with a numerical "index" which seems to predict drugs which will have the appropriate combination of agonist and antagonist activity which is associated with nonaddicting analgesia with minimal side effects.

In initial studies, our receptor assay did not distinguish between opiate agonists and antagonists. Agonists had essentially the same affinity for the receptor as their corresponding antagonists. These early assays were conducted in the absence of sodium. When physiologic concentrations of sodium are employed, we find a dramatic difference between the binding of opiate agonist and antagonists (Table 1). Sodium increases the binding of opiate antagonists and markedly decreases the binding of agonists. Interestingly, sodium-induced enhancement of binding is greatest for the pure antagonist naloxone and less for the antagonists which are contaminated with some agonist activity, such as nalorphine and levallorphan. The "sodium effect" explains the greater clinical potency of antagonists than of agonists. At normal body concentrations of sodium, the antagonists will bind to the opiate receptor much more efficiently than the agonists and therefore exert pharmacologic effects at lower doses (Pert, Pasternak, and Snyder, 1973; Pert and Snyder, 1974).

In this screening test, we measure the effect of sodium on the concentration of the drug necessary to displace ^{3}H-naloxone binding 50% (ED$_{50}$). The opiate antagonists show a decrease of inhibitory potency in the presence of sodium by a factor of 12 to 60. Antagonists with some agonist properties, such as cyclazocine, levallorphan, and nalorphine are slightly affected by sodium with inhibitory potency decreased by a factor of 1.7 to 2.7 in the presence of sodium. The most interesting results are obtained with pentazocine (Talwin®) whose inhibitory potency falls by a factor of 3.3, a value intermediate between predominantly agonist and antagonist opiates. For several other mixed agonist-antagonists which offer clinical potential as relatively nonaddicting analgesics, we have obtained ratios between 3.3 and 6.

Thus, the degree to which a drug's interaction with the opiate receptor is altered by sodium enables one to rate the drug along the agonist-antagonist dimension. Of a large number of agonist-antagonist agents which we have screened and which have shown the greatest therapeutic potential in terms of relieving pain without causing addiction, opiate receptor binding has impressively predicted their pharmacologic actions *in vivo*.

BENZODIAZEPINES AND THE GLYCINE RECEPTOR

During the last decade a large body of evidence from neurochemical and neurophysiologic sources has revealed that glycine is a major inhibitory transmitter of interneurons in the spinal cord and brainstem. In these areas, glycine appears to be the neurotransmitter at 25% of all synapses. The synaptic effects of glycine are potently antagonized by strychnine, which is a potent antagonist of natural synaptic inhibition in these locations in the central nervous system (CNS). We have identified a specific binding of ^{3}H-strychnine to the glycine receptor in synaptic membranes of the spinal cord and brainstem of mammals (Young and Snyder, 1973, 1974). Proof that the strychnine binding represents an interaction with the glycine receptor derives from several types of experiments. The regional distribution of strychnine binding correlates closely with regional variations in endogenous glycine, high affinity synaptosomal uptake, unique glycine accumulating synaptosomes, and the synaptic neurophysiologic actions of glycine. Strychnine binding cannot take place to the glycine uptake site, because strychnine has negligible affinity for this uptake system. In addition, the ability of a variety of amino acids to mimic glycine neurophysiologically closely parallels their affinity for strychnine binding sites.

The glycine receptor assay using ^{3}H-strychnine binding to synaptic membranes is simple, sensitive, and specific, much like the opiate receptor assay. Accordingly, we were able to screen a large number of psychotropic drugs for their ability to inhibit ^{3}H-strychnine binding (Young, Zukin, and Snyder, 1974b). A large number of drugs have negligible effects on strychnine binding (Table 2). However, the benzodiazepines, such as diazepam (Valium®), are as potent in inhibiting ^{3}H-strychnine binding as glycine itself. Diazepam inhibits strychnine binding 50% at a concentration of approximately 2 μM, similar to blood and brain levels of diazepam at pharmacologic doses. To determine whether benzodiazepine effects on the glycine receptor are related to clinical effects of the drug, we examined a series of 21 benzodiazepines whose pharmacologic activities have been evaluated extensively in

TABLE 2. Benzodiazepines: Correlation of behavioral effects with displacement of ^{3}H-strychnine binding

Behavioral test	No. of drugs tested	Statistical significance (p)	Spearman correlation coefficient
Human bioassay	20	< 0.001	0.74
Fighting mouse test	21	< 0.001	0.71
Antipentylenetetrazol test, mice	20	< 0.004	0.63
Continuous avoidance, shock rate increase, rat	20	< 0.004	0.63
Cat muscle relaxation	19	< 0.005	0.67
Monkey taming	19	< 0.005	0.65
Mouse muscle relaxation	20	< 0.005	0.61
Antimaximal electroshock, mice	19	< 0.05	0.46
Discrete trials "trace" avoidance, noise response failure, rat	14	< 0.10	0.51
Antiminimal electroshock, mice	19	< 0.20	0.33
Continuous avoidance, escape failure, rat	19	< 0.45	0.20

Central muscle relaxants which had no effect on ^{3}H-strychnine binding at 10^{-2} M: carisoprodol, chloroxazone, meprobamate, methocarbamol, mephenesin, methaqualone, tybamate.

Drugs having no effect on ^{3}H-strychnine binding at 10^{-4} M: tetracycline, aminosalicylic acid, nicotinamide, pyridoxal HCl, Dilantin, naphthylthiourea, urea, acetazolamide, ethoxyzolamide, methyldopa, ergocristine, methylsergide, hippuric acid, melatonin, tolbutamide, alloxan, ketamine, lithium carbonate, ethanol, reserpine, benactyzine, haloperidol, hydroxyzine, diethylcarbamazine, lidocaine HCl, dichlorphenamide, chlorphenesin, ethosuximide, phenacemide, carbamazepine, acetophenetidine.

Data adapted from Young et al., 1974b.

animal tests and in humans. (Table 2). There is a 50-fold variation in the potency of these drugs in inhibiting ^{3}H-strychnine binding with half-maximal inhibition ranging from 19 μM to more than 1,000 μM. We compared the clinical potency of the drugs in pharmacologic tests in animals and man with their potency to displace ^{3}H-strychnine binding. Their ability to displace bound ^{3}H-strychnine correlates very closely with their potencies in "human bioassay." Similar close correlations occur with several behavioral tests in animals which are effective predictors of drug potency in man. Considerably lower correlations are obtained with tests such as discrete trial conditioning, the effect of the drugs on escape failure from electric shock, and convulsions elicited by minimal and maximal electroshock, tests which are also less effective predictors of benzodiazepine actions in humans (Zbinden and Randall, 1967).

The close correlation between pharmacologic activity of benzodiazepines and their displacement of strychnine binding strongly suggests that the drugs exert their pharmacologic actions via the glycine receptor. However, it is still conceivable that the varying pharmacologic potencies relate simply to the ability of the drugs to reach brain receptors because of factors such as lipid solubility which might also determine the access of the drugs to strychnine binding sites in our synaptic membrane preparations. If this were the case, these same factors should govern interactions of benzodiazepines with other brain receptors in synaptic preparations. Accordingly, we measured the ability of benzodiazepines to interact with opiate and muscarinic cholinergic brain receptors (Young et al., 1974b). At concentrations 10 to 50 times higher than those needed for displacement of strychnine, benzodiazepines did displace opiate receptor and muscarinic cholinergic receptor binding. However, inhibition of opiate and muscarinic receptor binding by benzodiazepines does not correlate with any of the pharmacologic tests. It is therefore highly unlikely that the correlation of pharmacologic activity of benzodiazepines with their ability to displace strychnine binding can result from nonspecific membrane effects.

Drugs other than the benzodiazepines, most notably propanediols such as meprobamate (Miltown® and Equanil®), also exert some muscle relaxant effects. These agents fail to displace ^{3}H-strychnine binding in concentrations as high as 10 mM (Table 2). However, the bearing of these data on the mechanism of action of these drugs must be viewed with caution, since these agents are pharmacologically quite weak compared to the benzodiazepines. For instance, meprobamate is less than 1% as potent as diazepam in clinical practice.

The major clinical actions of the benzodiazepines are relief of anxiety and muscle relaxation. Since these effects are closely correlated with each other, muscle relaxation may be responsible for amelioration of anxiety. Alternatively, the two effects might be exerted at different parts of the CNS but utilize a common mechanism. Glycine neurons and receptors exist in the spinal cord, brainstem, and diencephalic structures. We propose that benzodiazepines produce their antianxiety, muscle relaxant, and probably anticonvulsant effects by mimicking glycine receptors in the CNS. One would expect the synaptic effects of glycine, inhibiting the firing of motor neurons in the spinal cord, to be associated with muscle relaxation. Indeed, the glycine antagonist strychnine causes muscle tenseness followed by convulsions. Conceivably, muscle relaxant actions involve an enhancement of glycine-mediated inhibition in the spinal cord, whereas antianxiety effects result from enhanced synaptic inhibition in the brainstem or higher centers. Effects of benzodiazepines on seizure activity, both cortically and subcortically induced, may result from potentiating inhibitory pathways from the brainstem reticular activating system.

An understanding of the molecular mechanism of therapeutic action of benzodiazepines clearly affords a new avenue for designing antianxiety drugs. One need not restrict oneself to benzodiazepines. The glycine receptor assay affords one major advantage over most in vivo screens. Since barbiturates display cross-tolerance for their sedative actions with the benzodiazepines, it is likely that sedative effects of both classes of drugs occur via the same mechanism. The sedative actions of the benzodiazepines probably do not involve the glycine receptor, because barbiturates have no effect on glycine receptor binding. It might therefore be possible to design a drug which mimics glycine at very low doses but which is devoid of sedative properties. The resultant agent might be a nonsedating antianxiety drug. Most *in vivo* screens of benzodiazepine action, especially in man, rely to a greater or lesser extent on the sedative actions of the benzodiazepines. Obviously, sedative action is a property of the drugs one would ideally like to avoid.

PHENOTHIAZINES AND THE MUSCARINIC CHOLINERGIC RECEPTOR

It appears quite likely that antischizophrenic phenothiazines and butyrophenones exert their antipsychotic effects and elicit extrapyramidal side effects by blocking dopamine receptors in the brain. There are numerous dopamine pathways in the brain. The extrapyramidal side effects presumably arise from dopamine receptor blockade in the corpus striatum, mimicking endogenous Parkinson's disease to a certain extent. It is unclear which dopamine pathway is associated with relief of schizophrenic symptoms. The best candidates include pathways with dopamine terminals in the nucleus accumbens, the olfactory tubercle, and the dopamine projections to the cingulate gyrus of the cerebral cortex. Dopamine receptor blockade by phenothiazines occurs to the same extent and at the same concentrations of the drugs at all the dopamine receptor sites in the brain. Phenothiazine drugs are, with just a few exceptions, equally effective in alleviating schizophrenic symptoms. Clinicians generally titrate the dose until optimal antischizophrenic effects are obtained. These therapeutic doses are probably associated with optimal dopamine receptor blockade at crucial areas of the brain. Because the drugs act similarly at all dopamine receptors, at therapeutic antischizophrenic doses all butyrophenones and phenothiazines should produce the same incidence of extrapyramidal side effects. Whereas all antischizophrenic drugs do produce extrapyramidal effects, the frequency varies considerably. The piperidine phenothiazine thioridazine produces these side effects less frequently than chlorpromazine, and the recently introduced antipsychotic agent clozapine elicits few if any of these untoward actions (Table 3). By contrast, the piperazine phenothiazines and butyrophenones evoke a much higher incidence of extrapyramidal actions.

These discrepancies seriously challenge the dopamine hypothesis of schizophrenia. More relevant to questions of drug design, standard pharmacologic screening tests actually select for the drugs with the highest incidence of extrapyramidal signs. These screening tests, such as antagonism of amphetamine stereotypy or blockade of apomorphine effects and probably even the conditioned avoidance test, all involve dopamine receptor block-

TABLE 3. *Relative affinities of phenothiazines and butyrophenones for muscarinic cholinergic receptor binding in brain correlates inversely with extrapyramidal side effects*

Drug class	ED_{50} concentration (M)[a]	Relative affinity for muscarinic receptor	Frequency of extrapyramidal side effects rank by class (1 = most side effects)
Dibenzodiazepine			
Clozapine	2.6×10^{-8}	385	5
Piperidine phenothiazine			
Thioridazine	1.5×10^{-7}	66.7	4
Alkylamino phenothiazine			
Promazine	6.5×10^{-7}	15.2	3
Chlorpromazine	1.0×10^{-6}	10.0	
Trifluopromazine	1.0×10^{-6}	10.0	
Piperazine phenothiazine			
Acetophenazine	1.0×10^{-5}	0.90	2
Perphenazine	1.1×10^{-5}	0.91	
Trifluoperazine	1.3×10^{-5}	0.78	
Fluphenazine	1.2×10^{-5}	0.83	
Butyrophenone			
Haloperidol	4.8×10^{-5}	0.21	1

[a] Affinity for the muscarinic receptor is defined as the reciprocal $\times 10^{-5}$ of the ED_{50} value, defined as the molar concentration of drug which displaced by 50% the specific binding of ^{3}H-QNB (1 nM) to whole rat brain homogenates. ED_{50} values were obtained by log probit plots of the effects of four concentrations of each drug assayed in triplicate. Each experiment was replicated twice.

ade, which will elicit extrapyramidal side effects. Because all presently available phenothiazines are equally antischizophrenic and quite effective in this regard, the major impetus for new drug development is to produce agents which might be devoid of extrapyramidal side effects. In this way, many traditional *in vivo* screens select out as effective the drugs which should be discarded.

Recent studies of the muscarinic acetylcholine receptor in the brain may help resolve some of these problems. For many years muscarinic antagonists such as atropine and its synthetic analogues have been used to treat Parkinson's disease. Phenothiazines themselves elicit anticholinergic effects, such as dry mouth and difficulty in urination. Clozapine, which has few extrapyramidal actions, is a fairly potent anticholinergic agent in smooth muscle experiments. We speculate that for all phenothiazines and butyrophenones, extrapyramidal effects vary inversely with anticholinergic potency (Snyder, Banerjee, Yamamura, and Greenberg, 1974a; Snyder, Greenberg, and Yamamura, 1974b). Certain phenothiazines may block muscarinic receptors in the corpus striatum, thereby attenuating the extrapyramidal side effects which they evoke via dopamine receptor blockade. The most potent anticholinergics should evoke the fewest extrapyramidal effects and, conversely, drugs with the highest incidence of side effects should be the weakest anticholinergics.

To evaluate this hypothesis, one must be able to quantify the affinity of drugs for muscarinic receptors in the brain. In our laboratory we measure the reversible binding of 3-quinuclidinyl benzilate (QNB), a potent muscarinic antagonist, to membrane preparations of the CNS. The binding of radioactive QNB represents an almost exclusive interaction with muscarinic receptors (Yamamura and Snyder, 1974a,b). Possessing a simple, sensitive, and specific assay for the muscarinic receptor, we evaluated the relative affinities of a variety of antischizophrenic drugs (Table 3). Their affinity for the muscarinic receptor in whole brain correlates inversely in an impressive fashion with their tendency to elicit extrapyramidal side effects. Clozapine, which is almost devoid of these side effects, has the greatest potency, similar to that of standard antiparkinsonian drugs. Thioridazine, which next to clozapine elicits the fewest extrapyramidal symptoms, is second most potent. The alkylamino phenothiazines, whose moderate incidence of extrapyramidal actions is greater than that of thioridazine, have correspondingly less affinity for the acetylcholine receptor. Piperazine phenothiazines and the butyrophenones, whose frequency of extrapyramidal effects is greatest, have the least affinity for the muscarinic receptor. According to this formulation, at antischizophrenic doses of phenothiazines and butyrophenones, brain levels of all the drugs produce comparable dopamine receptor blockade so that all have about the same tendency to elicit extrapyramidal side effects. Blockade of acetylcholine receptors by drugs such as clozapine and thioridazine combats these extrapyramidal effects whereas the piperazine phenothiazines and butyrophenones elicit many more extrapyramidal symptoms because of their negligible anticholinergic activity.

Pharmacologists have traditionally screened for muscarinic receptor activity of drugs by measuring the contractions of the guinea pig ileum. In general, we have found a good correlation between the affinity of drugs for the muscarinic receptor of the brain and for the guinea pig ileum receptor (Snyder et al., 1974a; Yamamura and Snyder, 1974b). However, there are some important exceptions. For instance, although several phenothiazines have the same affinity for the receptor of brain and intestine, clozapine is four times as potent in the brain as in the intestine. This may prove to be a valuable lead. One doesn't want to develop phenothiazines which are extremely potent peripheral anticholinergics. One would then trade in the extrapyramidal side effects for perhaps equally troublesome anticholinergic effects such as dry mouth, blurred vision, constipation, and difficulty in urinating. Thus screening for anticholinergic effects of phenothiazines on smooth muscle contraction is probably not ideal. Screening for central anticholinergic effects *in vivo* by antagonism of oxotremorine tremors is also questionable, since drugs can block oxotremorine by effects unrelated to the cholinergic nervous system. Like the other receptor assays, the muscarinic cholinergic receptor can be quantitated precisely, with great sensitivity and considerable ease. One can screen more drugs more rapidly and at considerably lesser expense on the muscarinic receptor of the brain *in vitro* than even on smooth muscle preparations.

CONCLUSIONS

In summary, it appears likely that in the future decade biochemical quantification of specific neurotransmitter and drug receptors in the brain may afford a valuable new means to developing psychotropic agents. The neurotransmitter receptors identified thus far are only a few of the receptors which probably exist in the brain. Glutamic acid is probably a major excitatory transmitter in the brain. It is certainly the neurotransmitter of the granule cells in the cerebellum, the most prevalent neuronal population within the cerebellum (Young, Oster-Granite, Herndon, and Snyder, 1974*a*). Drugs which would mimic glutamic acid at its receptors might be useful stimulants, whereas glutamic acid antagonists could conceivably provide valuable antiepileptic agents. The GABA receptor in mammalian brain has been identified biochemically only recently (Zukin, Young, and Snyder, 1974). Drugs which mimic GABA might be valuable sedatives. Several peptides such as substance P and angiotensin may well be prominent neurotransmitters. Substance P is almost certainly the major sensory neurotransmitter (Konishi and Otsuka, 1974).

In light of the new developments in neurotransmitter receptor identification, it might be wise to shift strategy in new drug identification. Heretofore we have been looking for drugs which will reproduce the property of drugs already available. There may, however, be important therapeutic actions which might be produced by drugs, which we have not yet conceptualized. Thus, in the early 1940s it would never have occurred to anyone to search for a selective antianxiety agent. Presently, although we have drugs available which are useful in the treatment of psychotic depression, agents for ameliorating the symptoms of neurotic depression do not exist. What I conceive of as neurotic depression is a constellation of lethargy and dejection, essentially the "blues" from which all of us suffer at one time or another. Such depression is as pervasive as is anxiety in our society. Perhaps, as neurotransmitter receptors are identified biochemically, one should endeavor to develop agents with great affinity for the receptors, both agonists and antagonists, and then proceed to find out their pharmacologic and possible therapeutic actions *in vivo*. We are confronted with receptors in search of drugs, which may be an exceedingly happy circumstance for the future of psychopharmacology and the treatment of mental illness.

ACKNOWLEDGMENTS

These studies were carried out in collaboration with Anne Young, Steven Zukin, Candace Pert, Gavril Pasternak, Henry Yamamura, and David Greenberg. Research was supported in part by USPHS grants DA-00266, MH-18501, and RSDA award MH-33128 to S.H.S.

REFERENCES

Goldstein, A., Lowney, L. I., and Pal, B. K. (1971): Stereospecific and nonspecific interactions of the morphine congener levorphanol in subcellular fractions of the mouse brain. *Proc. Nat. Acad. Sci. USA*, 68:1742–1747.

Hillman, J. M., Pearson, J., and Simon, E. J. (1973): Distribution of stereospecific binding of the potent narcotic analgesic etorphine in the human brain: Predominance in the limbic system. *Res. Commun. Chem. Pathol. Pharmacol.*, 6:1052–1061.

Hitzemann, R. J., and Loh, H. H. (1973): Characteristics of the binding of ^{3}H-naloxone in the mouse brain. *Proc. Soc. Neuroscience*, 3:350.

Klee, W. A., and Streaty, R. A. (1974): Narcotic receptor sites in morphine dependent rats. *Nature*, 248:61–63.

Konishi, S., and Otsuka, M. (1974): The effects of substance P and other peptides on spinal neurons of the frog. *Brain Res.*, 65:397–410.

Kuhar, M. J., Pert, C. B., and Snyder, S. H. (1973): Regional distribution of opiate receptor binding in monkey and human brain. *Nature*, 245:447–451.

Pasternak, G. W., and Snyder, S. H. (1974): Opiate receptor binding: Effects of enzymatic treatments. *Mol. Pharmacol.*, 10:183–193.

Pert, C. B., Pasternak, G., and Snyder, S. H. (1973): Opiate agonists and antagonists discriminated by receptor binding in brain. *Science*, 182:1359–1361.

Pert, C. B., Snowman, A. M., and Snyder, S. H. (1974): Localization opiate receptor binding in synaptic membranes of rat brain. *Brain Res.*, 70:184–188.

Pert, C. B., and Snyder, S. H. (1973a): Opiate receptor: demonstration in nervous tissue. *Science*, 179:1011–1014.

Pert, C. B., and Snyder, S. H. (1973b): Properties of opiate receptor binding in rat brain. *Proc. Nat. Acad. Sci. USA*, 70:2243–2247.

Pert, C. B., and Snyder, S. H. (1974): Opiate receptor binding of agonists and antagonists affected differentially by sodium. *Mol. Pharmacol.*, 10:868–879.

Simon, E. J., Hiller, J. M., and Edelman, I. (1973): Stereospecific binding of the potent narcotic analgesic ^{3}H-etorphine to rat brain homogenate. *Proc. Nat. Acad. Sci. USA*, 70:1947–1949.

Snyder, S. H., Banerjee, S. P., Yamamura, H. I., and Greenberg, D. (1974a): Drugs, neurotransmitters and schizophrenia. *Science*, 184:1243–1253.

Snyder, S. H., Greenberg, D., and Yamamura, H. I. (1974b): Antischizophrenic drugs and brain cholinergic receptors: affinity for muscarinic sites predicts extrapyramidal effects. *Arch. Gen. Psychiatry*, 31:58–61.

Terenius, L. (1973): Characteristics of the "receptor" for narcotic analgesics in synaptic plasma membrane fraction from rat brain. *Acta Pharmacol. Toxicol.*, 33:377–384.

Wong, D. T., and Horng, J. S. (1973): Stereospecific interaction of opiate narcotics in binding of ^{3}H-dihydromorphine to membranes of rat brain. *Life Sci.*, 13:1543–1556.

Yamamura, H. I., and Snyder, S. H. (1974a): Muscarinic cholinergic binding in rat brain. *Proc. Nat. Acad. Sci. USA*, 71:1725–1729.

Yamamura, H. I., and Snyder, S. H. (1974b): Muscarinic cholinergic receptor binding in the longitudinal muscle of the guinea pig ileum with ^{3}H-quinuclidinyl benzilate. *Mol. Pharmacol.*, 10:861–867.

Young, A. B., Oster-Granite, M. L., Herndon, R. M., and Snyder, S. H. (1974a): Glutamic acid: selective depletions by viral induced granule cell loss in hamster cerebellum. *Brain Res.*, 73:1–13.

Young, A. B., and Snyder, S. H. (1973): Strychnine binding associated with central nervous glycine receptors. *Proc. Nat. Acad. Sci. USA*, 70:2832–2836.

Young, A. B., and Snyder, S. H. (1974): Strychnine binding in rat spinal cord membranes associated with the synaptic glycine receptor: cooperativity of glycine interactions. *Mol. Pharmacol. (in press)*.

Young, A. B., Zukin, S. R., and Snyder, S. H. (1974b): Interaction of benzodiazepines with central nervous glycine receptors: possible mechanism of action. *Proc. Nat. Acad. Sci. USA (in press)*.

Zbinden, G., and Randall, L. O. (1967): Pharmacology of benzodiazepines: laboratory and clinical correlations. *Adv. Pharmacol.*, 5:213–291.

Zukin, S. R., Young, A. B., and Snyder, S. H. (1974): Gamma-aminobutyric acid binding to receptor sites in the rat central nervous system. *Proc. Nat. Acad. Sci. USA*, 71:4802–4807.

DISCUSSION

Horovitz: Do you know why glycine was picked as the receptor of strychnine?

Taylor: There is much neurophysiologic evidence indicating that glycine is the neurotransmitter involved in postsynaptic inhibitory neurons in the spinal cord and brainstem and that strychnine acts by blocking these nerves. The idea that diazepam might displace strychnine may have come from the fact that if glycine is a transmitter in the spinal cord, this might be the sight of action of muscle relaxant drugs.

Horovitz: Has metrazol been looked at? The correlations published in the 1960s show a much better correlation between antimetrazol effects than antistrychnine.

Taylor: Metrazol is not on the list of compounds that have been tested in the binding assay. In correlating the strychnine displacement data with results of the clinical efficacy of benzodiazepines, the Speakman correlation coefficient is 0.74. Between the antimetrazol induced convulsion assay in animals and the clinical efficacy, it is 0.63.

Bunney: Has anybody tried scopolamine in terms of relative affinity for the binding sites?

Haubrich: Atropine has been used (*Neuropharmacology*, 13:53, 1974), but I know of no data on scopolamine.

Bunney: And how does atropine stack up with this kind of a system compared with clozapine, for example?

Haubrich: I don't think it's been done with atropine. However, there is a paper in *Nature* (Vol. 248, p. 596, 1974) using ^{3}H-propylbenzylylcholine mustard to alkylate the muscarinic receptors. Using the agent to measure the antimuscarinic activity of antipsychotics, these investigators found an inverse correction between the ratio antimuscarinic/antidopaminergic activity and the reported incidence of extrapyramidal side effects for a series of compounds.

Blackwell: One of the really exciting possibilities for me that may sound a little ghoulish is that you have the possibility for the first time of getting around species differences and that you possibly could use human autopsy material.

Taylor: I haven't tried it and I know that with the binding of the opiate receptor they have used human brain material to map out the binding sites in the whole brain. The tissue is not as fragile as if you were making isolated nerve endings or some preparation like that. You can really mash it up and maybe there isn't such a thing as postmortem loss of receptor sites. I think that definitely is a possibility.

Domino: I need some help with regard to logic. With respect to the acetylcholine receptor, one is taking an antagonist and phenothiazines which are likewise cholin-

ergic antagonists and then studying relative displacement for binding of one antagonist against the other. In the case of glycine or strychnine there is physiologic
evidence that strychnine is, in fact, a glycine antagonist. But are the benzodiazepines agonists or antagonists? They obviously cannot be antagonists at the glycine
receptor site because then they would be convulsants. So in that situation, there is a
switch in logic and now one has to, of necessity, say they are agonists of glycine
rather than antagonists.

Taylor: There is no direct way of determining if the benzodiazepines act as agents
or antagonists at glycine receptor sites such as is possible with the opiate receptor
where there is a method for separating antagonists from agonists and that's the displacement in the presence of excess sodium. However, concentration of labeled
strychnine used in the binding experiment is about 1nM. The benzodiazepines
displace strychnine with ID_{50}s in the mM range. This, plus the fact that benzodiazepines have anticonvulsant activity rather than a convulsant action like strychnine,
suggests that they are agonists rather than antagonists at glycine receptor sites.
Maybe this suggests that glycine could have antianxiety effects.

Domino: But if it is, why is it down in the spinal cord? It ought to be higher up in
the limbic system, cortex . . .

Taylor: Yes. The localization of glycine suggests that any action of benzodiazepines at glycine receptor sites is more likely to be involved with the muscle relaxant
rather than the antianxiety effect of these compounds. However, these two pharmacological effects of the benzodiazepines may not be mutually exclusive. Unfortunately, with *in vitro* receptor binding studies, it is not possible to measure the consequences of the drug-receptor interaction.

Author and Subject Indexes

Author Index

A

B

C

J

Jalfre, M., 263
Jalland, B. F., 214
Janssen, P. A. J., 180, 182
Jenney, E. H., 259
Johansson, O., 229
Jones, H. S., 73
Jones, T., 75
Jonsson, G., 229
Jori, A., 166
Jus, A., 255

K

Kahan, I. L., 260
Kanamura, H., 254
Kane, L. J., 260
Kaplan, J., 144, 256, 261
Kaplan, R., 144
Kast, E. C., 189
Kelly, D. H. W., 126, 127, 128
Kerr, S. J. 259
Kimble, D. P., 145
King, H. E., 189
Kitai, S. T., 263
Klee, W. A., 271
Klein, D. E., 231, 232
Klerman, G. L., 159, 161, 163, 165
    166, 184
Kline, N. S., 165
Kluver, H., 145
Knapp, S., 254
Kochansky, G. E., 132
Koetschet, P., 180
Kolsky, M., 180
Konishi, S., 280
Kopin, I. J., 253
Korevaar, W. C., 254
Kovacic, B., 261
Kraepelin, E., 189
Kraupl-Taylor, F., 189
Krause, R. R., 258, 259
Kuehl, F. A., Jr., 252
Kugelmass, S., 144
Kuhar, M. J., 271

Kuhn, R., 165
Kuriansky, J. P., 1, 3

L

Lacey, J. I., 128
Lader, M. H., 125, 126, 127, 143, 144
Laffan, R. J., 215
Lal, H., 190
Lal, S., 236
Lang, P. J., 130, 131
Lapierre, Y. D., 144, 155
Larsson, N., 225
Lauener, H., 214
Lauter, J., 144
Lawlor, W. G., 144
Lawrence, J., 132
Lazarus, A. A., 144
Lazovick, A. D., 131
Leaf, R. C., 151, 184
Lehmann, H. E., 129, 260
Levine, J., 67
Lewinsohn, P. M., 172
Lewis, G. P., 253
Lidbrink, P., 229
Lin, R., 260
Lindgren, J. B., 252
Lindqvist, M., 227, 230, 231
Lindsley, O. R., 129
Linoff, J. M., 214
Lipinski, J., 256
Lipman, E., 130
Lipton, M. A., 260
Ljungdahl, A., 229
Lloyd, K. G., 263
Lobb, H., 144
Loh, H. H., 271
Longo, V. G., 190
Loomer, H. P., 165
Lowney, L. I. 271
Lu, L. J., 261, 262
Luby, E. D., 249
Lutz, M. P., 252

Subject Index

A

A-34, 519
  EEG, 76
Acetazolamide, glycine receptor, 275
Acetophenazine, muscarinic cholin-
    ergic receptor, 278
Acetophenetidin, glycine receptor,
    275
Adenyl cyclase, 240-241
Affective disorder diagnostic sheet
    (ADDS), 56-59, 62
Affective disorders
  biogenic amines, 166-167
  diagnosis, 51
AHR-1118, EEG, 75-76, 89
Alcohol
  EEG, 68-69
  separation model, 168
  stimulant-depressant continuum,
    164
Alcoholism, 2, 5
  RDC, 36-37
Alloxan, glycine receptor, 275
Aminosalicylic acid, glycine receptor,
    275
Amitriptyline
  antianxiety effects of, 155
  conflict procedure, 151
  depression, 163-165
  diagnostic criteria, 122
  EEG, 69, 75-77
  separation model, 170
Amobarbital
  EEG, 66, 68-69, 73-74, 89-90
  Geller conflict procedure, 151
Amphetamine
  conflict procedure, 151
  depression, 163-164
  dopamine, 229-236, 240-245
  EEG, 68-69
  geriatrics, 131
  GSR, 144
  pediatrics, 131

Amphetamine *(Contd.)*
  psychosis, 228, 230
  schizophrenia, 249
  stereotypy, 190, 214
  stimulant-depressant continuum,
    164
Analgesics, opiate receptor, 271-274
Anesthetics, stimulant-depressant con-
    tinuum, 164
Animal-environment relationship,
    BRIDGE, 193-194
Antianxiety agents
  antipunishment effects, 182-184
  approach-avoidance continuum, 123
  behavioral evaluation, 121-137
  behavioral measures, 131-137
  clinical evaluation, 105-119
  conflict avoidance, 129
  GSR, 143-145
  performance measures, 128-131
  physiologic measures, 125-128
Anticholinergic agents, extrapyramidal
    effects, 233
Antidepressive agents
  amygdala, 184
  animal model, 159-178
  digital vasoconstriction, 127-128
  EEG, 67-70
  GSR, 127-128
Antipsychotic agents, *see* Neuroleptics
Antisocial personality, 5
  RDC, 35-36
Anxiety
  forearm blood-flow measure, 126-
    128
  human test model, 124-125
  rating scales, 132
  stereotypy, 128
Anxiety, types
  behavioral, conditioned emotional
    stimulus, 150
  neurosis, 143

295